Veterinary Medicine: An Animal Health Perspective

Veterinary Medicine: An Animal Health Perspective

Editor: Ryan Jaxon

FOSTER ACADEMICS
www.fosteracademics.com

www.fosteracademics.com

Cataloging-in-Publication Data

Veterinary medicine : an animal health perspective / edited by Ryan Jaxon.
p. cm.
Includes bibliographical references and index.
ISBN 978-1-63242-860-8
1. Veterinary medicine. 2. Animal health. 3. Animals--Diseases. I. Jaxon, Ryan.
SF745 .V48 2019
636.089--dc23

Foster Academics,
118-35 Queens Blvd., Suite 400,
Forest Hills, NY 11375, USA

ISBN 978-1-63242-860-8 (Hardback)

Printed and bound in China.

Contents

Preface IX

Chapter 1 **Effect of a low dose of BCG-Phipps vaccine on the development of reactivity to tuberculin skin test in neonatal calves and adult cows** 1
Lizzet Corona-Gómez, Laura Jaramillo-Meza, Rafael Pérez-González, Fernando Diosdado-Vargas, Julio Santiago-Cruz, Clara I Espitia-Pinzón, Ricardo Lascurain and Fernando Díaz-Otero

Chapter 2 **Study on veterinary antibiotic drugs handling and utilization in and around Holeta** 10
Seblewongel Ayichew Megerrsa and Taddesa Bezu Ashine

Chapter 3 **Anthelmintic resistance in gastrointestinal nematodes of goats** 15
Alsácia Atanásio-Nhacumbe, Maria Consuêlo Carybé Ayres, Sabrina Mota Lambert and Bárbara Paraná Souza

Chapter 4 **Epidemiological investigation of Middle East respiratory syndrome corona virus (mers-cov) among dromedary camels** 22
Getnet Fekadu, Gelagay Ayelet and Fufa Abunna

Chapter 5 **Composition, prevalence and abundance of Ixodid cattle ticks at Ethio-Kenyan Border, Dillo district of Borana Zone, Southern Ethiopia** 30
Golo Dabasa, Wubishet Zewdei, Tadelle Shanko, Kula Jilo, Gete Gurmesa and Garu Lolo

Chapter 6 **Prevalence of bovine of schistosomosis in and around Nekemte, East Wollega zone, Western Ethiopia** 38
Abriham Kebede, Jiregna Dugassa, Geremew Haile and Berhanu Wakjira

Chapter 7 **Prevalence of bovine trypanosomiosis in Gamogoffa Zone, Ouba Debrestahay District, Southern Ethiopia** 43
Migbaru Keffale Bezabih and Mabure Shille Bisho

Chapter 8 **A study on the sero epidemiology of African horse sickness in three woredas of Sidama Zone, Hawassa, Ethiopia** 48
Getaw Yeshitila and Dejene Bekele

Chapter 9 **Gastrointestinal nematodes of donkeys and horses in Gondar town northwest, Ethiopia** 53
Anteneh Wondimu and Getachew Sharew

Chapter 10 **Bacterial pathogens of pigs with particular reference to *Escherichia coli*** 57
Rukayya Hussain Abubakar, Evelyn Madoroba, Olubukola Adenubi, Darshana Morar-Leather and Folorunso O. Fasina

Chapter 11 **Clinical survey on major ruminant diseases in Kola Tembein and Tanqua Abergelle Districts, Central Zone of Tigray, Northern Ethiopia** 84
Guash Abay, Mulalem Zenebe, Daniel Desta, Hailai Hagos, Minister Berhanie and Tsegay Teame

Chapter 12 **Public health risk and transmission route of Middle East respiratory syndrome (MERS): MERS coronavirus in dromedary camel** 91
Andualem Yimer and Sisay Fanta

Chapter 13 **Cross-sectional study on the prevalence and risk factors for major skin diseases of cattle** 99
Zekarias Fantaye and Berhanu Mekibib Melake

Chapter 14 **Serological prevalence of *Babesia caballi* and *Theileria equi* in camels and donkeys** 106
Jesca Nakayima, Mary L. Nanfuka, Daniel Aleper and Duke Okidi

Chapter 15 **Bursa body index as a visual indicator for the assessment of bursa of Fabricius** 112
A. A. Raji, B. Mohammed, S. B. Oladele, L. Saidu, A. H. Jibril and C. Cazaban

Chapter 16 **Tick resistance of two breeds of cattle in Wolaita Zone, Southern Ethiopia** 119
Desie Sheferaw

Chapter 17 **Tsetse density and bovine trypanosomosis in selected sites of Konta, Ethiopia** 126
Anteneh Wondimu, Endeshaw Reta and Asnake Fekadu

Chapter 18 **Health and welfare status of donkeys in and around Hawassa Town, Southern Ethiopia** 131
Agegnehu Ashinde, Abebaw Gashaw and Nejash Abdela

Chapter 19 **Prevalence and species of major gastrointestinal parasites of donkeys** 144
Temesgen Kassa Getahun and Tihune Zeleke Kassa

Chapter 20 **Eukaryotic expression and characterization of BHV-1 glycoprotein D (gD) as a potential diagnostic antigen** 153
M. Sylvestre, Ramneek Verma, Ravi Kant Agrawal and Dipak Deka

Chapter 21 **Incidence and the history of *Echinococcus granulosus* infection in dogs within the past few decades** 160
Mohamed, M. Ibrahem, Wafa, M. Ibrahem, Kawther, M. Ibrahem, Badereddin and B. Annajar

Chapter 22 **Prevalence of tick-borne haemoparasitic diseases (TBHDS) and haematological changes in sheep and goats in Maiduguri abattoir** 170
Egbe-Nwiyi T. N., Sherrif G. A. and Paul B. T

Chapter 23 **A cross-sectional study on bovine Schistosomiasis in and around Kemissie, Dawa Cheffa District** 176
Alemu Aylate, Mohammed Hussen, Alebachew Tilahun and Ashenafi Kiros

Chapter 24 **Aerobic and anaerobic bacterial isolates from the respiratory tract of sheep slaughtered at Addis Ababa Abattoirs Enterprises, Central Ethiopia** 181
Addisu Awukew Yegoraw, Addis Kassahun Gebremeskel, Tesfaye Sisay Tesema and Biruk Tesfaye Birhanu

Chapter 25 **Prevalence of endo-parasites in donkeys and camels in Karamoja sub-region, North-eastern Uganda** 187
Jesca Nakayima, William Kabasa, Daniel Aleper and Duke Okidi

Chapter 26 **A study on sero prevalence of foot and mouth diseases in West and South West Shoa zones of Oromia regional state, central Ethiopia** 192
Kebede Shanko Hordofa, Tesfaye Rufael Chibsa and Enquibaher Kasaye

Chapter 27 **Detection of *Mycobacterium avium* subspecies paratuberculosis excretion in bovine feces, using quantitative real time polymerase chain reaction (Q-PCR)** 199
Adriana Guadalupe Martínez-Covarrubias, Marco Antonio Santillán-Flores, Dionicio Córdova-López and Claudia Celic Guzmán-Ruíz

Chapter 28 **Microbiological quality of frozen raw and undercooked Nile tilapia (*Oreochromis niloticus*) fillets and food safety practices of fish handlers** 206
Wendwesen Teka, Dagmar Nölkes, Yitbarek Getachew and Matusala Mulachew

Permissions

List of Contributors

Index

Preface

This book has been an outcome of determined endeavour from a group of educationists in the field. The primary objective was to involve a broad spectrum of professionals from diverse cultural background involved in the field for developing new researches. The book not only targets students but also scholars pursuing higher research for further enhancement of the theoretical and practical applications of the subject.

The field of veterinary medicine deals with the treatment and prevention of animal diseases and injuries. A number of diseases occur in bovines, cats and dogs such as anthrax, buffalo pox, bovine mastitis, bladder stones, rabies, pyometra, brachycephalic airway obstructive syndrome, diabetes, obesity, etc. Animals are also prone to injuries such as bite wounds and wounds acquired from stepping on or running into objects. Depending on the injury, wounds may be cleaned and sutured, explored, lavaged and debrided, or left open and allowed to heal. Orthopedic surgeries such as hip replacement, leg amputation, bone fracture repair, etc. may be done to manage traumatic injuries. Zoonoses, such as Ebola, salmonellosis, bird and swine flu, early HIV infections, etc. are caused by bacteria, viruses, fungi and parasites. These may be transmitted to humans through bites and saliva, or through air. Humans can also infect animals with diseases such as influenza, pneumonia, measles, tuberculosis and leishmaniasis. This book is a valuable compilation of topics, ranging from the basic to the most complex advancements in the field of veterinary medicine. The objective of this book is to give a general view of the different areas of veterinary medicine and their applications. The extensive content of this book provides the readers with a thorough understanding of the subject.

It was an honour to edit such a profound book and also a challenging task to compile and examine all the relevant data for accuracy and originality. I wish to acknowledge the efforts of the contributors for submitting such brilliant and diverse chapters in the field and for endlessly working for the completion of the book. Last, but not the least; I thank my family for being a constant source of support in all my research endeavours.

Editor

1

Effect of a low dose of BCG-Phipps vaccine on the development of reactivity to tuberculin skin test in neonatal calves and adult cows

Lizzet Corona-Gómez[1], Laura Jaramillo-Meza[1], Rafael Pérez-González[2], Fernando Diosdado-Vargas[2], Julio Santiago-Cruz[3, 4], Clara I Espitia-Pinzón[5], Ricardo Lascurain[6] and Fernando Díaz-Otero[1*]

[1]Departamento de Inmunología, Centro Nacional de Investigación Disciplinaria en Microbiología Animal, INIFAP, Toluca, Mexico.

[2]Facultad de Estudios Superiores Cuautitlán, Universidad Nacional Autonoma de México, México City, Mexico.
[3]Departamento de Microbiología y Parasitología, Facultad de Medicina, Universidad Nacional Autonoma de México, México City, Mexico.

[4]Instituto Nacional de Enfermedades Respiratorias Ismael Cosío Villegas, Secretaria de Salud, Mexico.
[5]Instituto de Investigaciones Biomédicas, Universidad Nacional Autonoma de México, México City, Mexico.
[6]Departamento de Bioquímica, Facultad de Medicina, Universidad Nacional Autonoma de México, México City, Mexico.

Bovine tuberculosis (bTB) has a direct impact in the productive and reproductive efficiency of dairy cattle. Nowadays, disease control programs based on tuberculin testing and removal of infected cattle are unaffordable for the developing countries, since there is no program of financial compensation, especially in high bTB-prevalence herds. Thus, control strategies based on vaccination are considered the best alternative. The aim of this study was to evaluate whether a low dose of BCG-Phipps vaccine induces reactivity to tuberculin skin test and its duration in neonatal calves and adult cows. For the analysis of the former, 69 TB-free Holstein-Friesian calves less than one-month old were used; of which, 54 calves were subcutaneously inoculated with 10^4 CFU of the BCG-Phipps vaccine, while the rest remained without vaccination. Under similar conditions of immunization, 133 single intradermal comparative cervical (SICCT) reactors and 133 non-reactors Holstein-Friesian cows of different age were also analyzed. In calves, the SICCT-reactivity was evaluated periodically in the first 14 months post-vaccination (mpv) while, in adult cows, the effect of vaccination on the test was evaluated at six months post-vaccination. A comparative ELISA was used by measuring the antibody levels in the groups. In calves, reactivity frequencies of 7.4 and 3.7% at 3 and 5 mpv, respectively were recorded. This reactivity disappeared at six months. None calves in the control group were reactor during the study. There were no variations in the degree of reactivity in the group adult reactor cows. However, in the non-reactor group, a conversion of 12.8% at six mpv was recorded. In addition, the conversion percentage was higher in older cows than in younger cows ($p<0.05$). The specific antibody levels did not increase in the vaccinated groups. Data indicate that the low dose of BCG-Phipps vaccine used had a reduced effect on the development of a delayed type hypersensitivity to tuberculin in neonatal calves, and heifers lesser than one-year-old.

Key words: *Bacillus* Calmette-Guérin, bovine tuberculosis, *M. bovis*, single intradermal comparative tuberculin test.

INTRODUCTION

Bovine tuberculosis (bTB) is one of the main diseases causing economic losses to dairy industry, and its incidence has been increasing in recent years. The severity of disease is more in immunosuppressed animals or in concurrent infections (Gupta et al., 2009). Therefore, it is required to develop effective control strategies. Hence, the use of Bacillus Calmette-Guérin (BCG) *Mycobacterium bovis* vaccine could be one of the most viable tools for this purpose. In this regard, it has been pointed out that vaccination with BCG in cattle at an early age diminishes pathological scores, so it could be an approach to decrease bacterial loads and reduce the transmission risk both from bovine to bovine and bovine to human (Lienhardt et al., 2012; Waters et al., 2012; Kaufmann et al., 2014).

However, field trials investigating protection have reported variable efficacies; furthermore, revaccination did not improve protective effect. Potential explanations of the variable levels of field protection includes the use of different BCG strains, administration of very high doses of BCG, different routes of inoculation, and previous exposure to *M. bovis* in maternal milk from infected cows, circumstances that diminish the effective protective immunity (González et al., 2007; Hope et al., 2011; Thom et al., 2012).

With respect to the optimum age of vaccination against tuberculosis, it has been determined that vaccine efficacy is higher in very young calves, lesser than one month old, compared to calves between five and six months old (Buddle et al., 2003; Hope et al., 2005). Why calves lesser than one month old develop higher levels of protection, may be that they have been lesser exposed to environmental mycobacteria which interferes with development of a protective immune response against bTB, compared to older calves (Siddiqui et al., 2012). It is therefore incontrovertible that eventual future application of vaccines will be used to improve the control of bTB. Thus, it is relevant to improve the knowledge of factors determining the development of a delayed type hypersensitivity (DTH) response, if it really develops when vaccine is given under a number of different modalities and stages (Cockle et al., 2002; Logan et al., 2005). Few studies talk about the development of a DTH response or conversion of tuberculin skin test (TST); as a result of the vaccine application, one of this studies demonstrated that DTH reaction is developed in the first months and lost in 90% of the vaccinated animals at nine months post-vaccination (Whelan et al., 2011; Buddle et al., 2013).

However, the theoretical framework of the BCG vaccine application indicates that it primes the animals to respond to the tuberculin test, and it is an impediment to use the BCG as a vaccine since this test is the primary tool for epidemiological surveillance used in many countries as a main strategy of bTB control, in México (Mexican Official Norm NOM-031-ZOO-1995; Good and Duignan, 2011; OIE, 2012). Today, the rate of conversion induced by the BCG, the correlation of DTH with protective immunity, and the factors determining the development of protection are unknown. These observations could have useful implications at some point in the future, for a solid improvement of BCG vaccines designed for the bovine cattle. The objective of this study was to determine whether the BCG-Phipps vaccine at low dose (10^4 CFU) induces reactivity to tuberculin skin test and its duration in neonatal calves as well as evaluate its effect on reactors and non-reactors adult dairy cows.

MATERIALS AND METHODS

Ethics statement

Animals used in this study belong to a commercial farm and have been submitted only to the standard clinical practices specifically regulated by the Mexican legislation on tuberculosis control program (Mexican Official Norm NOM-031-ZOO-1995), which were vaccination and blood sampling.

Experimental design for neonatal calves

Sixty-nine female calves between 6 to 30 days of age obtained from herds with no history of bTB were used. All animals were tested and confirmed negative for *M. bovis* by antigen-induced IFN-gamma produced by peripheral blood mononuclear cells (PBMCs), ELISA for detection of specific antibodies to a culture filtrate protein extract (CFPE), and PCR on nasal swabs were used. Fifty-four of these calves were inoculated subcutaneously on the neck with a dose of 10^4 CFU of BCG-Phipps strain in PBS. To avoid prime calves to bovine Purified Protein Derivative (PPD) by repeated tuberculin tests, they were divided in two groups for alternative testing; half of the animals were tested at 0, 3, 7 and 11 months post-vaccination, the other half, at 0, 5, 9 and 14 months, and results were analyzed altogether. Fifteen control animals were inoculated with PBS. All animals were isolated to eliminate any risk of infection from the main herd.

Experimental design for adult cows

The study was performed in a dairy herd with a bTB prevalence of 49.39% located in the State of Hidalgo, México, from which, 133 single intradermal comparative cervical tuberculin (SICCT) reactors and 133 non-reactors Holstein-Friesian adult cows were analyzed to determine the effect of vaccination on tuberculin skin test. Both study populations were immunized with 10^4 CFU/1.5 ml of BCG-Phipps subcutaneously injected on right side of the neck, like

*Corresponding author. E-mail: diof0009@yahoo.com.mx.

calves. The effect on SICCT test was evaluated at six months post-vaccination (mpv) in reactors and non-reactors cows. The latter were grouped by age to evaluate the influence of this variable on development of DTH response induced by vaccination, then forming the following groups: Group 1, ≤ 1 year old (n=36); Group 2, between 1 to 2 years old (n=37); Group 3, between 3 to 5 years old (n=34); and Group 4, between 6 to 9 years old (n=26). Cows pertaining to the Groups 2, 3 and 4 remain in production stable. The cows of Group 1 were isolated from the rest of animals to avoid exposure to new infections.

Production of BCG Phipps vaccine

For elaboration of BCG Phipps vaccine (Lot number 95 001-2013-7H9), seed was cultured on Middlebrook 7H10 OADC (Oleic Albumin Dextrose Catalase) solid medium for 15 days at 37°C. Next, bacteria were transferred to Middlebrook 7H9 ADC liquid medium and they were incubated in constant swirling at 37°C. Bacilli were subcultured once in liquid medium until they reached an early exponential growth phase (OD_{600nm} 0.3) and aliquots frozen in PBS at -70°C. For bacterial enumeration, serial dilutions were plated onto modified Middlebrook 7H10 OADC. Petri dishes were incubated for 3 to 4 weeks at 37°C, and CFU/ml were calculated by the formula UFC x DF x 10 = bacteria/ml; in which DF = dilution factor, and concentration was adjusted to 10^4 CFU/ml in sterile PBS.

Single intradermal comparative cervical tuberculin test

The development of a DTH response by vaccination in study populations was determined by SICCT test, which was applied according to NOM-031-1995, in the middle third of the neck. In two different shaved and cleaned spots, 0.1 ml (3,250 IU) of bovine PPD (PPD-B) strain AN5, and 0.1 ml (3,250 IU) of avian PPD (PPD-A) strain D4 (PRONAVIBE, México) were injected. After 72 h post-inoculation skin thicknesses were measured. A positive result was considered positive if the increase in skin thickness at the bovine PPD site of injection was at least 4 mm greater than the reaction at the avian PPD injection site. The reaction was suspicious, but inconclusive, when PPD-B reaction was between 2 to 3 mm greater than PPD-A reaction. A negative result was considered when PPD-B swelling was negative or, even being positive, for no more than 2 mm greater than PPD-A reaction.

Culture filtrate protein extract

To obtain mycobaterial CFPE from *M. bovis* AN5 and *M. avium* D4, these were cultured in Dorsett-Henley medium for six weeks at 37°C. At the end of the incubation period, the bacterial mass was eliminated by filtration, using cellulose filters, followed by 1.2, 0.45 and 0.22 µm Millipore filters (Bernardelli, 2007). The proteins present on the residuals liquids were precipitated with ammonium sulfate (Sigma Aldrich, St. Louis, MO, USA) at a final saturation of 80%, under constant whirling motion for 24 h at 4°C. The precipitates were centrifuged at 4°C for 60 min at 20 000 X *g*. The CFPE were recovered and finally dialyzed through a membrane with exclusion limits from 3000 kDa (Membrane Filtration Products, Inc. TX, USA) at 4°C for 48 h with PBS. The protein content of each CFPE was determined by the Bradford method and CFPE was stored at -70°C (Bradford, 1976).

IgG ELISA

A comparative ELISA was used for the evaluation of humoral immune response in the study populations. In this ELISA, the plates (Nunclon, Roskilde, Denmark) were coated with 1 µg/well of either *M. avium* or *M. bovis* CFPE dissolved in 0.05 M carbonate-bicarbonate buffer (pH 9.6) overnight at room temperature at 4°C. Then, plates were washed three times with 0.1% Tween 20 in 0.01 M phosphate buffer at pH 7.4 (PBS-T). Free binding sites were blocked with 3% non-fat milk in PBS-T for 1 h at 37°C. Afterward, the plates were washed with PBS-T, next incubated with PBS-diluted (1:100) sera for 1 h at 37°C. After washing with PBS-T, 100 µl/well of Protein G-Peroxidase (1:10,000, in PBS) (P-8170 Sigma) were added and incubated for 1 h at 37°C. Next, the plates were washed and subsequently the chromogenic substrate solution was added; containing 0.04% O-phenylenediamine (Sigma P-3804) and 0.04% of hydrogen peroxide in citrate buffer at 37°C for 5 min. Reaction was stopped with 50 µl/well of 2 M sulfuric acid. Optical density was read at 492 nm (OD_{492nm}) in a microplate reader (Benchmark Plus, Bio-Rad, Hercules, CA, USA) (Estrada-Chavez et al., 2001).

The cut-off point was calculated as the media of the OD_{492nm} from all SICCT-negative animals before the vaccination plus two standard deviations, and animals having a value greater than this cut-off point was regarded as positives.

PCR

DNA was extracted from nasal exudate samples for detecting the presence of *M. bovis* by PCR. Briefly, the samples contained in 5 ml of sterile PBS (phosphate buffer saline 0.01 M, pH 7.4) were centrifuged at 12,000 X *g* for 5 min. The pellet was incubated with 400 µl of Tris-EDTA buffer (TE) (100 mM Tris-HCl, 10 mM EDTA, pH8.0) and 50 µl of lysozyme (100 mg/ml) 1 h at 37°C. 70 µl of 10% SDS and 5 µl of proteinase K (10 mg/ml) were added and incubated for 20 min at 65°C. Then, 100 µl of 5 M NaCl, and 100 µl of CTAB/NaCl (4.1 g of NaCl, 10 g of CTAB, 80 ml of distilled water) was added, and pre-warmed at 65°C for 10 min. After adding 750 µl of chloroform-isoamyl alcohol (24:1), mix was centrifuged at 12,000 x *g* for 5 min. After recovering the upper phase, this was mixed with 600 µl of absolute isopropyl alcohol for 30 min at -20°C. DNA was centrifuged at 12,000 x *g* for 5 min, supernatant discarded, and 1 ml of cold -20°C ethanol 70% was added to wash the DNA. Samples in microcentrifuge tubes were again centrifuged at 12,875 x *g* for 5 min; DNA was dissolved into 50 µl of sterile water, and stored at -20°C.

For PCR, primers TB1-F, 5'GAACAATCCGGAGTTGACAA3', and TB1-R, 5'AGCACGCTGTCAATCATGTA3', related to the *M. tuberculosis* Complex, were used; these primers amplify a 372 bp sequence from the gen MPB70 codifying the secreted protein MPB70 (Cousins et al., 1992).

PCR mix for a final volume of 25 µl was prepared with 0.5 µl of each primer (0.4 µM), 13.25 µl of sterile water, 2.5 µl of 10X buffer, 0.5 µl of dNTPs (250 µM), 2.5 µl of $MgCl_2$ (2.5 mM), 0.25 µl of Taq polimerase (0.5 U), and 5 µl of sample DNA (50 pg-250 ng). DNA obtained from *M. bovis* AN5, *M. tuberculosis* H36Rv, and from tuberculous lesions of diseased cows was used as positive controls. Sterile milli-Q water and DNA obtained from nasal swabs from IFN-γ and ELISA-negative calves were used as negative controls.

Cycling conditions were pre-warmed for 15 min at 96°C, and 35 cycles of denaturation for 30 s at 94°C, annealing for 30 s at 58°C, and extension for 60 s at 72°C; also a final step of extension for 5 min at 72°C (Gene Amp PCR System 9700, Applied Biosystems, Foster City, CA USA). 10 µl of each PCR product were analyzed in agarose 1.5% gels stained with ethidium bromide 1%, using 2.5 µl of molecular weight standards (Amresco K180-250 UL), and visualized with a Benchtop UV Transilluminator in a EpiChemi II Darkroom (BioImaging Systems, Upland California USA).

Table 1. Response to single intradermal comparative cervical tuberculin test (SICTT) in immunized heifers with a low dose BCG Phipp.

Group	Time post-vaccination					
	3 months (%)	**5 months (%)**	**7 months (%)**	**9 months (%)**	**11 months (%)**	**14 months (%)**
Group A, BCG (n=27)	2/27 (7.4)	-	0/27 (0)	-	0/27 (0)	-
Group B, BCG (n=27)	-	1/27 (3.7)	-	1+/-/27[a] (0)	-	0/27 (0)
Control (n=15)	0/15 (0)	0/15 (0)	0/15 (0)	0/15 (0)	0/15 (0)	1+/-/15[a] (0)

Groups of 27 heifers each were tested by SICCT alternately. Group A, calves at 0, 3, 7 and 11 months post-vaccination, and Group B, at 0, 5, 9 and 14 months; results of both groups are displayed as a whole.[a] One calf showed a reaction around the cutoff value of the test considered as suspect.

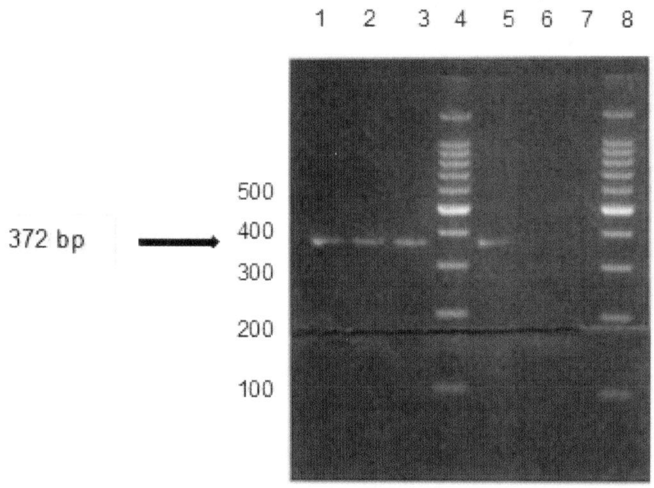

Figure 1. Products of PCR amplification from TB lesions and swabs of calves primers used were TB1-A and TB1-B which amplify a product with a length of 372 bp from the MPB70 gen of *M. bovis*. 1, *M. bovis* AN5; 2, *M. tuberculosis* H36Rv; 3, 5 DNA obtained from tuberculous lesions of diseased cows; 4, molecular weight markers (MWM); 6, DNA from swabs of a SITTC, IFN-γ and ELISA-negative calf; 7, water blank; 8, MWM. PCR showed that these calves concurrently remain negative throughout the study.

Statistical analysis

Data were analyzed with Student "*t*" test using the Statistical Analysis System software (SigmaStat Ver. 3.5) to determine significant differences between ELISA results before and after vaccination, and Xi^2 to analyze distribution of SICCT test data. A value of $p < 0.05$ was regarded as significant (Wayne, 2006).

RESULTS

SICCT test reactivity after BCG vaccination in calves

BCG vaccination in calves induced SICCT test reactivity in 2/27 (7.4%) at 3 months post-vaccination, and 1/27 (3.7%) at five months post-vaccination (Table 1); one animal alone was suspicious at 9 months; at 14 months post-vaccination, none of the animals showed reactivity. None of the control animals (n=15) was reactor at that time; however, one control animal showed a value around the cut-off point of the test. These data showed that at three months post-vaccination, the young female calves showed the greater frequency of reactivity, which diminished during the following months (Table 1). PCR analysis showed that both groups of calves concurrently remained negative all over the study (Figure 1).

ELISA in calves

The baseline levels of IgG antibodies to CFPE from *M. bovis* were similar between groups; these increased lightly in both groups without being significant at the first months post-vaccination; in the course of time, reaching a peak value of 0.34±0.24 *vs* 0.32±0.21 (OD_{492nm} ± standard error) for vaccinated group and control, respectively, at 3 months. In the subsequent two months,

Table 2. Tuberculin skin test conversion rate in adult non-reactor cows according to age, six months after having been immunized with a low dose.

Age	≤ 1 year old	1- 2 years old	3-5 years old	6-9 years old
Positive/total animals	0/36	4/37	6/34	7/26
Percentage (%)	0	10.8	17.6	26.9

levels remained without much variation for BCG vaccinated group. However, at 5 months post-vaccination the vaccinated group was higher than the control group ($P<0.05$); and at the end of the monitoring period of IgG antibodies, the values for the vaccinated group were even lower than from control group ($P<0.05$). For which, the evaluation of the humoral immune response was limited only to this period (Figure 2).

SICCT test reactivity after BCG vaccination in cows

We had the SICTT reactivities over the last three years for the dairy herd participating in this study. Figure 3 shows the bTB prevalence for 1 to 3 years in adult cows. The percentage of reactors at the beginning of the first year was 1.5% and at the end of the same year was 5.2% while for the second year, before vaccination of adult calves, it was 49.39%. As shown in Figure 3, bTB prevalence after vaccination increased from 0.9 to 50.5%, which is an insignificant increase. Because of an urgent requirement of alternative measures of bTB control, it was necessary to employ the BCG Phipps vaccine altogether with other biosafety measures to give response for the stated objectives.

Assessment of bTB prevalence in the studied dairy herd, by the SICCT test before BCG vaccination was needed with the aim to establish a reference point and from there to consider the impact of vaccination on the control of bTB prevalence. To determine the influence level of the BCG-Phipps vaccine on reactivity to the TST in adult animals, a high prevalence herd (49.39%) was chosen to analyze its effect in both reactors and non-reactors cows. Results indicate that the number of reactor cows increased slightly after BCG vaccination, and that the negative animals showed a reduction equivalent to the increase in positive ones. However, the increase in positive animals and the decrease in negative animals were not statistically significant according to the Chi-square test (Figure 4).

Related to the SICCT-non-reactor animals (n = 133), 17 animals converted to positive ones in a 12.7%. Further, a more detailed analysis showed that in older animals conversion rate was greater, as described in Table 2; conversion rates were: in animals ≤ 1 year old, 0%; between 1 to 2 years old, 10.8%; 3 to 5 years old, 17.6% and 6 to 9 years old, 26.9%. Thus, a greater conversion was observed in older cows, which could be related to a greater exposition to environmental mycobacteria considered a risk factor for bTB. These data complement those for calves, in which percentages of SICCT positive animals lesser than one month old after vaccination were low, and reactivity was diminishing during the studied period.

ELISA in cows

The prevalence of bTB was 49.39% before vaccination and antibody level was 3.15±1.01 (OD_{492nm} ± SD). Six months later, antibody level was 3.45±0.95. We found no significant differences by *t* Student test. Similarly, for isolated positive animals any differences were found.

DISCUSSION

Bovine tuberculosis is an important disease of dairy cattle, which has been difficult to control and eradicate. Incidence of this disease represents a significant problem to livestock production, because of a fast dissemination of the disease. Due to multiple factors, such as defective management, poor feeding, new infected animals in the herd, and mainly lack of adequate biosafety measures, bTB represents a risk of disease for humans (Thoen et al., 2006; Schiller et al., 2010; El-Sayed et al., 2016).

For many years, BCG vaccine effectiveness to reduce the bTB has been called into question, and a trouble that prevents its application is the interference of vaccination on tuberculin tests. However, the fundamentals of this interference and the involved factors are unknown. Considering that BCG vaccine represent an alternative for controlling bTB, and that it primes animals to give a DTH to tuberculin reaction, this results in an obstacle for using the BCG, since the TST is the primary tool in epidemiological surveys used in many countries as support for controlling bTB (OIE, 2012).

Today, conversions percentages to TST and protection effectiveness induced by BCG are unknown, as well as factors that intervene in both events. BCG strain, dose, age of vaccinated animals, role of environmental mycobacteria, and idiosyncrasy of each animal, among a number of factors, could influence in both events; conversion and protection. So our first objective was to determine the effect of BCG-Phipps vaccine in a reduced dose (10^4 CFU) on TST reactivity in bTB-free young calves of ≤ 1 month of age. The results showed a percentage of reactivity to the test in vaccinated calves

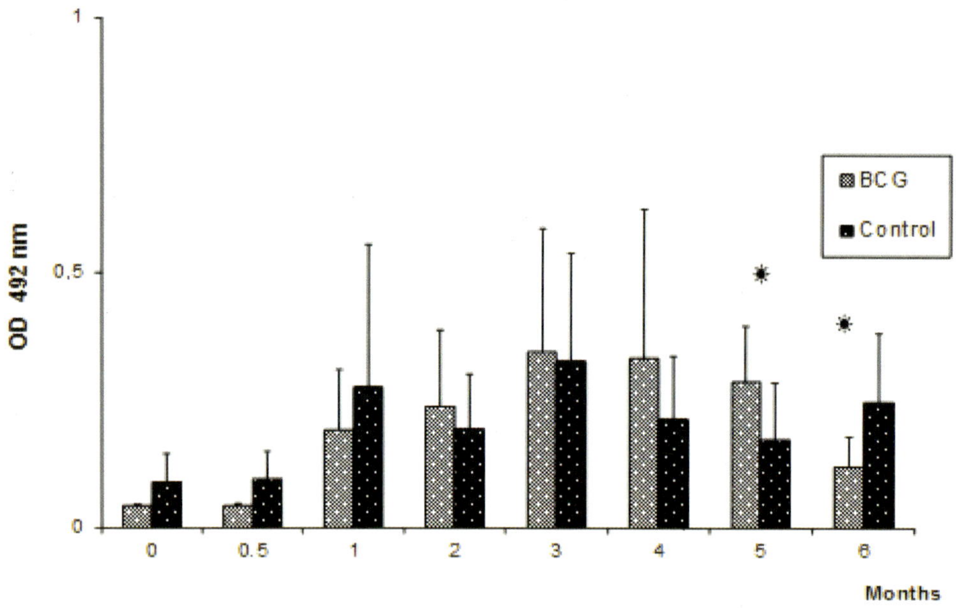

Figure 2. IgG antibody levels measured by ELISA in young female calves vaccinated with BCG Phipps compared to control non-vaccinated. Antibody levels were determined using a CFPE from *M. bovis* (see methods). Values are mean±SD; *p < 0.05; vaccinated vs non-vaccinated).

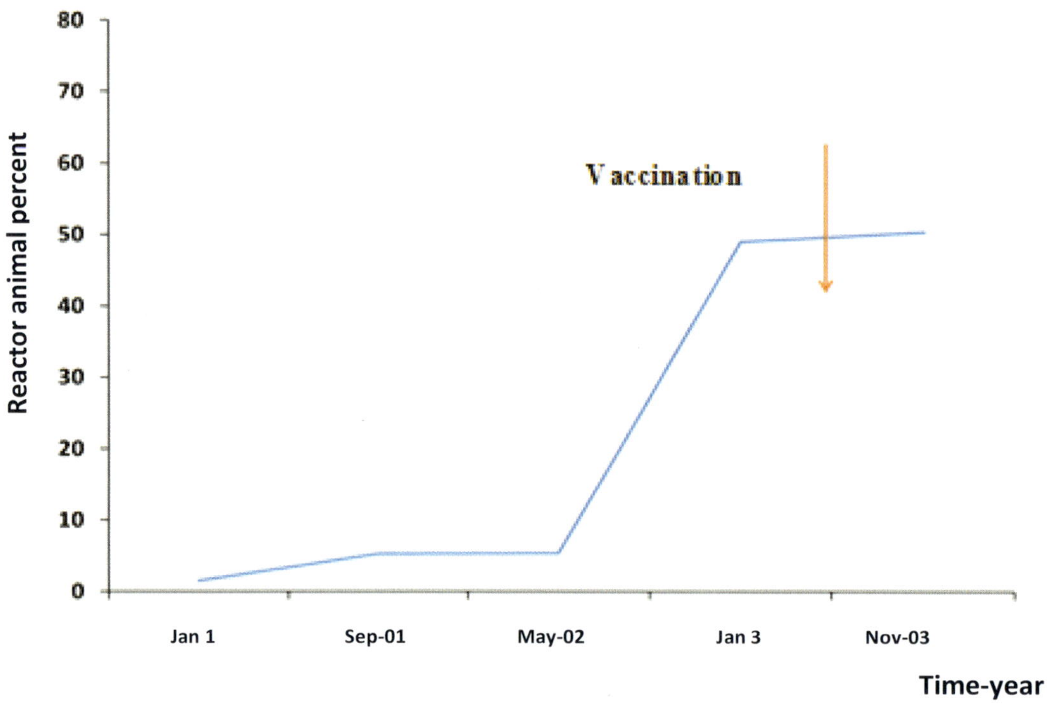

Figure 3. Historical records of bTB prevalence by SICCT test determined for the study herd three previous years vaccination, located in Hidalgo State, México. The arrow indicates the moment of vaccination of the groups of reactors and non-reactive cows to the tuberculin test

of 7.4% at three months post-vaccination, and 3.7% at five months, then wane at seven months post-vaccination. In non-vaccinated calves, there was no reactivity to TST in the first year, up to 14 months after

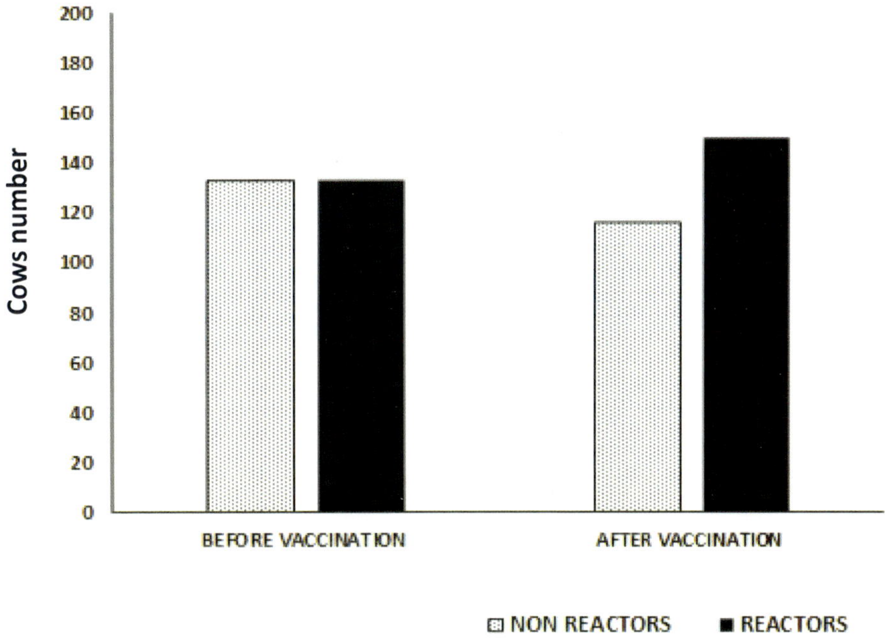

Figure 4. Number of cows that were positive or negative to the SICCT test before and after BCG-Phipps vaccination (six months post-vaccination). There were no significant differences between pre- and post-vaccination values ($p > 0.05$).

the study started in which one of them was suspicious. The percentages of reactivity observed in vaccinated calves in this study were much lower than that reported by Whelan et al. (2011). These authors, reported an 80% of TST conversion in calves vaccinated with BCG-Danish during the first six months post-vaccination, with a decay of 8% reactivity at nine months. This difference in reactivity percentages with our results could be related to the dose and strain used. Similar percentages of TST conversion have been reported in other studies using high vaccine doses between 10^6-10^8 CFU in humans, wildlife animals, and mouse model (Buddle et al., 2013; Tree et al., 2004). In addition, the protective efficacy reported in those studies was lower in vaccinated animals that showed a strong DTH response to bovine PPD than those animals that did not develop it (Skinner et al., 2001; Ritz et al., 2008). In follow-up of the possible establishment of *M. bovis* infections in vaccinated and control calves, PCR reactions performed from nasal exudates showed that both groups of calves were negative throughout this study. Even though we found no differences between vaccinated and unvaccinated groups in the detection of the DNA of *M. bovis* during time evaluated, there was concordance between TST and PCR tests after vaccination. Regarding the tuberculin conversion in vaccinated non-reactive cows, heifers less than one year old belonging to this group showed no reactivity. However, conversion percentages increased according to aging of cows, since the cows of 6 to 9 years showed a conversion percentage of 26.9% (7/26). This can be explained because cows during his long life were largely exposed to *M. bovis*, since they belonged to a herd with high prevalence of the disease. Consequently, the previous sensitizations in conjunction with the application of BCG vaccine favored the development of delayed type hypersensitivity in these animals while in the reactor group, there were no differences in the degree of reactivity or development of ulcerations and/or necrosis, at least with the dose of vaccine used. It has been mentioned that in infected cattle confirmed with at least two consecutive tests of tuberculin, as in humans, could developed an adverse reaction to vaccination with BCG (Koch phenomenon) in case of having a pathology advanced or generalized (Cardona, 2006). In this regard, Buddle et al. (2016) showed that vaccination of cattle with a high dose of BCG vaccine applied after an experimental infection with *M. bovis* increased the inflammatory response, but not tuberculosis pathology. However, all these observations should be taken with reserve and to carry out more studies, which show the benefit or prejudice resulting in the use of the BCG vaccine in infected cows. On the other hand, it has been suggested that the BCG vaccine is capable of preventing bacilli excretion. Thus, taking into account that airborne route is the most important transmission route for bovine tuberculosis, the BCG vaccine could reduce the risk of contagion among animals (López-Valencia et al., 2010).

In relation to the BCG vaccine, it is widely documented that because of the *in vitro* passage, the genome of the original strain has been modified giving rise to a series of heterogeneous strains, which show clear variations in their genomes and protective immune properties (Castillo-Rodal et al., 2006; Abdallah et al., 2015). With regards to the BCG-Phipps the main regions of differentiation (RD) lost are RD1, RD2 and nRD18. RD1 is a DNA segment comprising 9.5 kb, which was deleted in all other BCG strains, that encodes T-lymphocyte epitopes such as ESAT-6, CFP-10, Rv3873, and PPE protein among others (Okkels et al., 2003). RD2 is a 10.7 kb DNA segment that encodes many proteins including Mpt-64 and CFP-21 (Joung and Ryoo, 2013) and nRD18 is a 1.5 kb segment containing genes encoding SigI, an alternative RNA polymerase sigma factor that was only lost in the strains BCG Pasteur, Phipps, Frappier, Connaught and Tice (Da Costa et al., 2014).

In a study realized by Zhang et al. (2016) assessing the virulence and efficacy of 13 BCG strains in SCID and BALB/c, showed that BCG strains of the DU2 group IV to which BCG-Phipps belongs, showed the highest levels of virulence among strains studied. They reported that these distinct levels of virulence could be explained by strain-specific duplications and deletions of genomic DNA. There appears to be a general trend that more virulent BCG strains are also more effective in protection against challenge. Similar results were reported by Castillo-Rodal et al. (2006) whom showed that BCG-Phipps immunized mice developed lesser pneumonia areas and had lesser bacterial loads than animals vaccinated with other strains, indicating resistance establishment against disease. In addition, reactivity to tuberculin was lower compared to animals vaccinated with other BCG strains and control groups. Considering the above, our results suggest that the BCG-Phipps vaccine can be applied to neonatal calves because we observed a low and transitory DTH reaction in these animals. Besides, the results obtained in a previous study showed that the use of low dose induced the development of good immunity against *M. bovis* in vaccinated calves under field conditions (González-González et al., 2012). Thus, BCG-Phipps vaccine constitutes a good candidate for use in disease control.

On the other hand, we have not observed significant difference in antibody levels to *M. bovis* for vaccinated calves and cows compared to respective controls at first months post-vaccination which may be related to the dose of vaccine used, such as previously reported by Lyashcehnko et al. (2004), whom with a similar dose of the BCG-Pasteur strain did not observe the development of antibodies to defined antigens of *M. bovis* in vaccinated animals.

In recent years, research has expanded on the development of new vaccines in livestock and wildlife, with encouraging results for potential in the control of the disease. However, so many questions remain without response. Biomarkers to predict a protective immunity against tuberculosis is required to be studied, in order to evaluate vaccine effectiveness and reduce challenge experiments, because of controversial issues related to bioethical principles. Additional studies are needed to put into test whether cattle vaccination extends protection in function of time, or affect the results of traditional diagnostic tests. Considering progress reached in the last decade, we optimistically think answers to these questions will be found, and TB vaccination will become a valuable control measure to control this disease in human beings, livestock and wildlife.

Conclusion

BCG-Phipps vaccination with a single reduced (UFC) dose, had a minimal transient effect on development of DTH to tuberculin in neonatal calves and heifers lesser than one year, and declined in the first six months post-vaccination. In contrast, under these conditions a greater number of older cows became reactors. In addition, PCR analysis used throughout the study did not show the establishment of *M. bovis* infections in vaccinated and control groups. In vaccinated non-reactive cows, the tuberculin conversion percentages increased according to aging of cows. For additional studies, age of vaccination should be considered since bTB is a chronic disease and the exposition risk increases as the age of animals increase, hence this parameter will be a critical factor in stables where bTB vaccines are considered as a control measure. Furthermore, it remains to be tested if protective immunity and long life is induced by low doses of BCG-Phipps vaccine.

ACKNOWLEDGEMENTS

Funding for this study came from the Instituto Nacional de Investigaciones Forestales, Agrícolas y Pecuarias (INIFAP) México (No. SIGI 14294534013). Thanks go also to the farmers that provided the animals and farms for the realization of this study.

REFERENCES

Abdallah AM, Hill-Cawthorne GA, Otto TD, Coll F, Guerra-Assunção JA, Gao G, Naeem R, Ansari H, Malas TB, Adroub SA, Verboom T, Ummels R, Zhang H, Panigrahi AK, McNerney R, Brosch R, Clark TG, Behr MA, Bitter W, Pain A (2015). Genomic expression catalogue of a global collection of BCG vaccine strains show evidence for highly diverged metabolic and cell-wall adaptations. Sci. Rep. 5:15443.

Bernardelli A (2007). Producción y control de tuberculina bovina y aviar. Derivado Proteico Purificado (DPP). Servicio Nacional de Sanidad y Calidad Agroalimentaria. Buenos Aires. Argentina. Available at:

www.senasa.gov.ar/Archivos/File/File1011-tuberbov.pdf

Bradford MMA (1976). Rapid and sensitive method for the quantitation of microgram quantities of protein utilizing the principle of protein-dye binding. Anal. Biochem. 72:248-254.

Buddle BM, Hewinson RG, Vordermeier HM, Wedlock DN (2013). Subcutaneous administration of a 10-fold-lower dose of a commercial human tuberculosis vaccine, *Mycobacterium bovis* Bacillus Calmette-Guérin Danish, induced levels of protection against bovine tuberculosis and responses in the tuberculin intradermal test similar to those induced by a standard cattle dose. Clin. Vaccine Immunol. 20(10):1559-1562.

Buddle BM, Shu D, Parlane NA, Subharat S, Heiser A, Hewinson RG, Vordermeier HM, Wedlock DN (2016). Vaccination of cattle with a high dose of BCG vaccine 3 weeks after experimental infection with *Mycobacterium bovis* increased the inflammatory response, but not tuberculous pathology. Tuberculosis (Edinb). 99:120-127.

Buddle BM, Wedlock DN, Parlane NA, Corner LAL, de Lisle GW, Skinner MA (2003). Revaccination of neonatal calves with *Mycobacterium bovis* BCG reduced the level of protection against tuberculosis induced by a single vaccination. Infect. Immun. 71(11):6411-6419.

Cardona PJ (2006). RUTI: A new chance to shorten the treatment of latent tuberculosis infection. Tuberculosis (Edinb). 86(3):273-289.

Castillo-Rodal AI, Castañón-Arreola M, Hernández-Pando R, Calva JJ, Sada-Díaz E, López-Vidal Y (2006). *Mycobacterium bovis* BCG substrains confer different levels of protection against Mycobacterium tuberculosis infection in a BALB/c model of progressive pulmonary tuberculosis. Infect. Immun. 74(3):1718-1724.

Cockle PJ, Gordon SV, Lalvani A, Buddle B.M, Hewinson RG, Vordenmeier HM (2002). Identification of novel *Mycobacterium tuberculosis* antigens with potential as diagnostic reagents or subunit vaccine candidates by comparative genomic. Infect. Immun. 70:6996-7003.

Cousins DV, Wilton SD, Francis BR, Gow BL (1992).Use of polymerase chain reaction for rapid diagnosis of tuberculosis. J. Clin. Microbiol. 30(1):255-258.

Da Costa AC, Nogueira SV, Kipnis A, Junqueira-Kipnis AP (2014). Recombinant BCG: innovations on an old vaccine. Scope of BCG strains and strategies to improve long-lasting memory. Front. Immunol. 5:152.

El-Sayed A, El-Shannat S, Kamel M, Castañeda-Vazquez MA, Castañeda-Vazquez H (2016). Molecular epidemiology of *Mycobacterium bovis* in humans and cattle. Zoonoses Public Health. 63(4):251-264.

Estrada-Chavez C, Mancilla R, Arriaga-Díaz C, Pérez-González R, Díaz-Otero F (2001). Determination of anti-PPD antibodies in dairy herds with different prevalence of bovine tuberculosis in Mexico. Vet. Méx. 32:207-211.

González-González XE, Jaramillo-Meza L, Lascurain-Ledezma R, Torres-Barranca JI, Quevillon CE, Díaz-Otero F (2012). Evaluation of T lymphocyte subpopulations in cattle vaccinated against bovine tuberculosis: longitudinal comparative study. Rev. Mex. Cienc. Pecu. 3(2):137-154.

González-Salazar D, Díaz-Otero F, Jaramillo-Meza L, Pérez-González R, Padilla-Urbina J, Santillán-Flores MA, Arriaga-Díaz C, Bojórquez-Narváez L (2007). Evaluación de diferentes inmunógenos contra la tuberculosis bovina mediante la presencia de lesiones a la necropsia. Vet. Méx. 38(3):271-284.

Good M, Duignan A (2011). Perspectives on the history of bovine TB and the role of tuberculin in bovine TB eradication. Vet. Med. Int. 2011:410470.

Gupta MP, Kumar H, Singla LD (2009) Trypanosomosis concurrent to tuberculosis in black bucks. Indian Vet. J. 86:727-728.

Hope JC, Thom ML, McAulay M, Mead E, Vordermeier HM, Clifford D, Hewinson RG, Villarreal-Ramos B (2011). Identification of surrogates and correlates of protection in protective immunity against *Mycobacterium bovis* infection induced in neonatal calves by vaccination with M. bovis BCG Pasteur and *M. bovis* BCG Danish. Clin. Vac. Immunol. 18(3):373-379.

Hope JC, Thom ML, Villarreal-Ramos B, Vordermeier HM, Hewinson RG, Howard CJ (2005). Vaccination of neonatal calves with *Mycobacterium bovis* BCG induces protection against intranasal challenge with virulent *M. bovis*. Clin. Exp. Immunol. 139:48-56.

Joung SM, Ryoo S (2013). BCG vaccine in Korea. Clin. Exp. Vaccine Res. 2(2):83-91.

Kaufmann SHE, Lange C, Rao M, Balaji KN, Lotze M, Schito M, Zumla AI, Maeurer M (2014). Progress in tuberculosis vaccine development and host-directed therapies a state of the art review. Lancet Respir. Med. 2:301-320.

Lienhardt C, Fruth U, Greco, M (2012). The blueprint for vaccine research and development: Walking the path for better TB vaccines. Tuberculosis (Edinb). 92(S1):33-35.

Logan KE, Chambers MA, Hewinson RG, Hogarth PJ (2005). Frequency of IFN-γ producing cells correlates with adjuvant enhancement of bacilli Calmette-Guérin induced protection against *Mycobacterium bovis*. Vaccine 23(48-49):5526-5532.

López-Valencia G, Rentería-Evangelista T, Williams JJ, Licea-Navarro A, Mora-Valle AL, Medina-Basurto G (2010). Field evaluation of the protective efficacy of *Mycobacterium bovis* BCG vaccine against bovine tuberculosis. Res. Vet. Sci. 88(1):44-49.

Lyashchenko K, Whelan AO, Greenwald R, Pollock JM, Andersen P, Hewinson RG, Vordermeier HM (2004). Association of tuberculin-boosted antibody responses with pathology and cell-mediated immunity in cattle vaccinated with *Mycobacterium bovis* BCG and infected with *M. bovis*. Infect. Immun. 72(5):2462-2467.

Norma Oficial Mexicana NOM-031-ZOO-1995. 27 de agosto 2008. Campaña Nacional Contra la Tuberculosis Bovina (*Mycobacterium bovis*). Secretaria de Agricultura, Ganadería, Desarrollo Rural, Pesca y Alimentación. Servicio Nacional de Sanidad, Inocuidad y Calidad Agroalimentaria. Avalable at: https://www.gob.mx/senasica/documentos/norma-oficial-mexicana-nom-031-zoo-1995-campana-nacional-contra-la-tuberculosis-bovina-mycobacterium-bovis

Office International des Epizooties (OIE) (2012). Manual of diagnostic tests and vaccines for terrestrial animal. Office International des Epizooties (OIE). Chapter 2.4.7. Bovine tuberculosis, pp. 674-689. Available at: http://www.oie.int/en/international-standard-setting/terrestrial-manual/access-online/

Okkels LM, Brock I, Follmann F, Agger EM, Arend SM, T. H. M. Ottenhoff THM, Oftung F, Rosenkrands I, Andersen P (2003). PPE protein (Rv3873) from DNA segment RD1 of *Mycobacterium tuberculosis*: strong recognition of both specific T-cell epitopes and epitopes conserved within the PPE family. Infect. Immun. 71(11):6116-6123.

Ritz N, Hanekom WA, Robins-Browne R, Britton WJ, Curtis N (2008). Influence of BCG vaccine strain on the immune response and protection against tuberculosis. FEMS Microbiol. Rev. 32(5):821-841.

Schiller I, Oesch B, Vordermeier HM, Palmer MV, Harris BN, Orloski KA, Buddle BM, Thacker TC, Lyashchenko KP, Waters WR (2010). Bovine Tuberculosis: A review of current and emerging diagnostic techniques in view of their relevance for disease control and eradication. Transbound. Emerg. Dis. 57(4):205-220.

Siddiqui N, Price S, Hope J (2012). BCG vaccination of neonatal calves: potential roles for innate immune cells in the induction of protective immunity. Comp. Immunol. Microbiol. Infect. Dis. 35(3):219-226.

Skinner MA, Wedlock DN, Buddie BM (2001). Vaccination of animals against *Mycobacterium bovis*. Rev. Sci. Technol. Off. Int. Epiz. 20(1):112-132.

Thoen C, Lobue P, de Kantor I (2006). The important of *Mycobacterium bovis* as a zoonosis. Vet. Microbiol. 112(2-4):339-345.

Thom ML, McAulay M, Vordermeier HM, Clifford D, Hewinson RG, Villarreal-Ramos B, Hope JC (2012). Duration of immunity against *Mycobacterium bovis* following neonatal vaccination with Bacillus Calmette-Guérin Danish: significant protection against infection at 12, but Not 24, Months. Clin. Vaccine Immunol. 19(8):1254-1260.

Tree JA, Williams A, Clark S, Hall G, Marsh PD, Ivanyi J (2004). Intranasal bacilleCalmette–Guérin (BCG) vaccine dosage needs balancing between protection and lung pathology. Clin. Exp. Immunol. 138(3):405-409.

Waters WR, Palmer MV, Buddle BM, Vordermeier HM (2012). Bovine tuberculosis vaccine research: Historical perspectives and recent advances. Vaccine 30:2611-2622.

Wayne DW (2006). Bioestadística: base para el análisis de las ciencias de la salud. Fourth Ed., Limusa Editorial S. A. Mexico. ISBN: 978-

Study on veterinary antibiotic drugs handling and utilization in and around Holeta

Seblewongel Ayichew Megerrsa and Taddesa Bezu Ashine*

School of Veterinary Medicine, Wolaita Sodo University, Ethiopia.

A cross-sectional study was conducted to assess the antibiotics drug handling and utilization practices of the animal owners from November 2016 to April 2017. A total of 384 randomly selected animal owners in and around Holeta were interviewed using semi-structured questionnaires. Most of the respondents (animal owners) were educated (59.4%), whereas less than half of them (40.6%) were uneducated. The prevalence on the challenges faced by their animals was 25, 42.2, and 32.8% due to disease, feed shortage and both disease and feed shortage, respectively. A total of 6.5% of the respondents purchased antibiotics from private pharmacy and brought to their house by carrying them in pockets, while 3.9 and 2.9% of the respondents store drugs on the shelf and floor up to three months, respectively. Drug administration activity was performed by non-professional personnel simply by guessing. 66.1% of the respondents knew about withdrawal period of antibiotics whereas 33.9% of them did not know about withdrawal period of antibiotic drugs. At the time of drug administration, 12.8% sold the milk, 86.7% gave the milk for calf and 0.5% of them used the milk for home consumption without maintaining its withdrawal period. A few number of animal owners (2.6%) injected their animals below normal dosage resulting to resistance of the disease to the antibiotics. Majority of the animal owners (93.5%) used veterinary professional service to their diseased animals for treatment whereas a few number of the respondents (6.5%) purchased antibiotics from private pharmacy without prescription of the veterinarian for self-treatment of their animals. In conclusion, this study result revealed that there is improper handling and utilization practice of veterinary antibiotic drugs in the study area. It is recommended that training should be given for the animal owners on the appropriate handling and utilization practice of veterinary drugs and continuous follow up by the stake holders should be undertaken.

Key words: Antibiotics drug, animal owners, Holeta, veterinary.

INTRODUCTION

Ethiopia is a leading country in the number of animal population in the African continent. However, the output in terms of contributions to the improvement of the livelihood of animal owners and for the growth of the national economy is at a lower stage compared to the vast resource on hand. Poor Animal health service and

E-mail: taddesagebisa@gmail.com.

lack of properly utilizing veterinary antibiotics are among the main contributing factors for the poor utilization of the resources (Flynn, 2012).

A drug is any substance that when inhaled, injected, smoked, consumed, absorbed via a patch on the skin, or dissolved under the tongue causes a physiological change in the body. In pharmacology, a pharmaceutical drug is a chemical substance used to treat, cure, prevent, or diagnose a disease or to promote well-being (Flynn, 2012). Veterinary drugs are such substances as are made to treat, prevent or diagnosis diseases in animals that belong to different chemical classes and therapeutic areas, for example antibiotics, anti helminthics, non-steroidal anti-inflammatory drugs (NSAIDs), etc (Hirsh and Zee, 1999). An antibiotic class can be defined as a group of agents with a similar mechanism of action, regardless of chemical structure (Addah et al. 2009). Antibiotic drugs have been widely used globally in animals for more than 50 years, with tremendous benefits in animal production and economic development (Flynn, 2012).

There are many risks derived from irrational use of antibiotics resulting in environmental contamination with original substances or derivatives, indirect impact on health via resistant micro-organisms, direct organic damage and the influences on the biotic environment are a matter of concern (Thawani, 2010).

Major economic loses and animal welfare problems could arise in veterinary medicine, because antimicrobial resistance has been found to cause therapy failure and higher mortality and morbidity rate (Acar, 1997). The provision of quality animal health-care necessitates the availability of safe, effective and affordable antibiotics of the required quality, in adequate quantity at all times, and presented, dispensed and used rationally (Acar, 1997).

In and around Holeta, West Shoa Zone of Oromia Regional State, there is little information regarding, veterinary antibiotic drugs handling and utilization practice and there is no published material concerning this title.

Therefore, the objective of the study was to assess the antibiotic handling and utilization practices of the farmers and to assess the challenges that enforced the animal owners to buy antibiotics.

MATERIALS AND METHODS

Study area

The study was conducted from November 2016 to April 2017 in and around Holeta. The site is located at 9° 3' N latitude and 38° 30' E longitudes, about 33 km West of Addis Ababa along the main road to Ambo in Oromia Regional State. The study area has an altitude of 2400 m above sea level and receives an average annual rainfall of about 1000 mm.

The mean minimum and maximum temperatures are 6 and 22°C respectively. Regarding season, there are three seasons: short rainy season (March to May), long rainy season (June to September) and dry season (October to February).

Study design

Cross-sectional questionnaire - based study was carried out from November 2016 to April 2017 in and around Holeta. Data collection questionnaire format was developed and animal owners were interviewed to assess handling and utilization of veterinary antibiotic drugs used by them for treatment of animal diseases using a simple random sampling method.

Sample size determination

The sample size for collecting the questionnaire data was determined by using formula as indicated on (Thrusfield, 2005):

$$n = \frac{z^2\, p\, (1-p)}{w^2}$$

Where, Z is the confidence level, P is the estimate of the population, and W is the margin of error. (When: Z = 1.96, P = 0.5, and W = 0.05).

$$N = \frac{(1.96)^2\, (0.5)(1-0.5)}{(0.05)^2}$$

Based on the above formula the total numbers of animal owners selected for questionnaire survey was 384.

Study population

Animal owners (384) from randomly selected kebeles of in and around Holeta, were considered for this study.

Data collection and analysis

Questionnaire administration was done by local language to gather Information through semi-structured questionnaire (annex) from animal owners and the collected data from questionnaires were entered into Microsoft Excel spread sheet version 2010 and analyzed using SPSS Version 20 for descriptive statistics in percentage.

RESULTS

The present study revealed that greater than half of the respondents (59.4 %) in and around Holeta were educated whereas less than half of them (40.6%) were uneducated. The prevalence on the challenges faced by their animals was 25, 42.2, and 32.8% due to disease, feed shortage and both disease and feed shortage, respectively. A small number of farmers (6.5 %) in the study area purchased antibiotics from private pharmacy to treat their animals. 6.5% of the respondents purchased antibiotics from private pharmacy and brought to their house by carrying them in the pocket. 3.9 and 2.9% of the respondents store drugs on the shelf and floor up to three months, respectively. Drugs administration activity was performed by non-professional person simply by

Table 1. Antibiotics handling practice of animal owners.

Parameter	Category	Number	Percentage
Education level	Illiterate	156	40.6
	Below grade 8	174	45.3
	Above grade 8	54	14.1
Challenges on animal health	Disease	96	25.0
	Feed shortage	162	42.2
	Disease and feed shortage	126	32.8
Purchase of drugs	No	359	93.5
	Yes	25	6.5
Drug administered by	Not applicable	359	93.5
	Non professional	25	6.5
problem during drug administration	Not applicable	374	97.4
	Swelling of injected site	10	2.6
means of drug transportation	Not applicable	359	93.5
	Carrying in pocket	25	6.5
Store before administration	Not applicable	359	93.5
	Yes	25	6.5
Place of store	Not applicable	359	93.2
	On shelf	15	3.9
	On floor	10	2.9
Duration of drug store	Not applicable	359	93.2
	One month	10	2.6
	Two month	11	2.9
	Three month	4	1.3
Proper dose administration	Not applicable	359	93.2
	From leaflet	3	0.8
	Advice from professional	20	5.2
	By guess	2	0.5

guessing and information obtained from other professional (Table 1).

Most of the respondents (66.1%) have awareness about the withdrawal period of antibiotics whereas 33.9% of the respondents did not know about withdrawal period of drugs. Out of 384 respondents, 12.8% sold the milk, 86.7% gave milk for calf and 0.5% of them used milk for home consumption at the time of drugs administration. A few numbers of respondents (2.6%) injects their animals below the normal dosage resulting drug resistant disease to their animals (Table 2).

DISCUSSION

The handling and utilizing practice of antibiotics used in animal owners have been implicated in the development and spread of resistant bacteria phenotypes that is affecting the therapeutic efficacy of current antibiotics (Silbergeld et al., 2008; Sanford et al., 2009). This study aimed at assessing the practices of handling and utilization of veterinary antibiotics as a case study.

This study revealed that animal owners are faced with many challenges regarding their animals including feed shortage and disease. These challenges were enumerated from many sources such as lack of sufficient and standard nutrition, poor husbandry practices, inadequate animal health services such as treatment practices and disease control activity. Many of the animal owners in the study area were advised and supported by the professionally skilled person to treat their diseased animals, while some others bought antibiotics from private pharmacy and treated their animals by themselves.

Table 2. Antibiotics utilization practice of farmers.

Parameter	Category	Number	Percentage
Awareness of withdrawal period	No	130	33.9
	Yes	254	66.1
Information of withdrawal period	Not applicable	130	33.9
	From professionals	254	66.1
Use of milk after drug administration	For sell	49	12.8
	For calf	333	86.7
	For home consumption	2	0.5
Dosage below the normal	Not applicable	358	93.2
	No	22	5.7
	Yes	4	1.0
Response of below dosage	Not applicable	380	99.0
	Not cured	4	1.0
	Not available	25	6.5

The primary purpose of veterinary antibiotic drugs is to safeguard the health and welfare of animals with well diagnosed disease and well prescribed drugs under the supervision of veterinarian and professional person. Lack of practice to go to veterinary professionals, when their animals were sick and ineffective selection of veterinary drugs was the major problem of veterinary antibiotics handling and utilization. As a result, antibiotics were tried without proper diagnosis (Laxminarayan et al., 2013).

The trend of antibiotic administration by the respondents (6.5%) indicates improper practice of antibiotic utilization. The underperformance of some of the antibiotics as reported by the animal owners could be due to lack of awareness about the handling and utilization of antibiotics. The storage conditions of antibiotics in the animal owners were suboptimal because the storage environments of the antibiotics were prone to temperature fluctuations which hastens antibiotic decomposition, reducing its concentrations and efficacy (keke et al., 1999) thus promoting resistance in exposed bacteria (Laxminarayan et al., 2013; Teuber, 2001).

The major considerations for proper usage of antibiotics drugs, which are a main concern of modern medicine, are to select the optimal drugs at the proper dosage and duration, to minimize the emergence of resistance and to provide health services at a reasonable cost (Pang et al., 1994) whereas the end users of antibiotics were unable to select proper dosage and duration of treatment in the study area indicating improper utilization of antibiotic drugs. The knowledge of many animal owners concerning antibiotics withdrawal periods and dosages was found to be low. Moreover, the animal owners depended more on fellow animal owners than veterinarians for antibiotic knowledge, which resulted in the use of the same antibiotics and similar handling practices among animals in close proximity or within the same district. Poor dosing practices, for example, were common when an antibiotic failed to treat an infection. The animal owners lacked adequate measuring instruments to mete out correct dosages. In this study area there were lack of knowledge and practice concerning antibiotics dosing and withdrawal period as the same as reported earlier (Addah et al., 2009).

Ideally, good antibiotic prescribing practice should reflect the use of the most effective, least toxic, and least costly antibiotic for the precise duration of time needed to cure the infection (Gyssens, 2001) whereas the animal owners bought antibiotics without prescription in the study area that. Generally, majority of the animal owners in and around Holeta were provided veterinary professional service on animal disease treatment whereas a few number of the farmers purchased antibiotics from private pharmacy without prescription for self-treatment of their animals indicating improper handling and utilization practice of antibiotic drugs.

Abbreviations: NSAID, Non-steroidal anti-inflammatory drugs; **MICs,** minimum inhibitory concentrations; **MBCs,** minimum bactericidal concentrations; **CAFOs,** concentrated animal food operations; **HARC,** Holeta Agriculture Research Center.

CONFLICTS OF INTERESTS

The authors have not declared any conflict of interests.

REFERENCES

Acar JF (1997). Consequence of bacterial resistance to antibiotics in medical practice. Clin. Infect. Dis. 24(Supplement_1):S17-S18.

Addah W, Baah J, Tia S, Okine E (2009). Knowledge and practices of smallholder farmers and herdsmen in the use of acaricides and gastrointestinal anthelminthes in Ghana. Livest. Res. Rural Dev. 21:11.

Flynn WT (2012). The Judicious Use of Medically Important Antimicrobial Drugs in Food-Producing animal's center for Veterinary Medicine (HFV-1). Food and Drug Administration. Department Of Health and Human Services. http://www.fda.gov/downloads/animal veterinary /guidancecomplianceenforcement/.guidance for industry/ucm.21:6-9.

Gyssens IC (2009). Quality measures of antimicrobial drug use. Int. J. Antimicrobial Agents 17(1):9-19.

Hirsh DC, Zee YC (1999). Veterinary microbiology.1st ed. Blackwell Publishing Company. Colifornia. pp. 48-57.

Laxminarayan R, Duse A, Wattal C (2013). Antibiotic resistance-the need for global solutions. Lancet Infect. Dis. 13(12):1057-1098.

Okeke N, Lamikanra A, Edelman R (1999). Socioeconomic and behavioral factors leading to acquired bacterial resistance to antibiotics in developing countries. Emerging Infect. Dis. 5(1):18-27.

Pang Y, Brown BA, Steingrube VA, Wallacer RJ, Roberts MC (1994). Tetracycline resistance determinants in Mycobacterium and Streptomyces species. Antimicrobial Agents Chemother. 38(6):1408-1412.

Sanford JC, Mackie RI, Koikeetal S (2009). Fate and transport of antibiotic residues and antibiotic resistance genes following land application of manure waste. J. Environ. Qual. 38(3):1086-1108.

Silbergeld EK, Graham J, Price BL (2008). Industrial food animal production. antimicrobial resistance and human health. Ann. Rev. Public Health. 29:151-69.

Teuber M (2001). Veterinary use and antibiotic resistance. Curr. Opinion Microbiol. 4(5):493-499.

Thawani V (2010). Rational use of medicine achievements and challenges. Indian J. Pharmacol. 42:63-64.

Thrusfield M (2005). Veterinary Epidemiology, 3rd ed. Blackwell Science Ltd. Edinburgh, UK. pp. 228-247.

3

Anthelmintic resistance in gastrointestinal nematodes of goats in southern Mozambique

Alsácia Atanásio-Nhacumbe[1,2*], Maria Consuêlo Carybé Ayres[1], Sabrina Mota Lambert[1] and Bárbara Paraná Souza[1]

[1]School of Veterinary Medicine-Federal University of Bahia (UFBA), Av. Adhemar de Barros, 500, Ondina, Salvador-Bahia, CEP: 40.170-110, Brazil.

[2]National Centre for Biotechnology and Biosciences (CNBB), Ministry of Science and Technology, High Education and Vocational Training (MCTESTP), Av. Patrice Lumumba, 770, Maputo, Mozambique.

Small ruminant production is significantly constrained by gastrointestinal parasites once they cause serious production and economic losses for both small-scale and large-scale farmers in the developing world. The control of helminth parasites is most exclusively based on the use of anthelmintics for the economic production of ruminants. However, the resistance of nematodes to the commonly used groups of anthelmintics represents a threat to the production, particularly for small ruminants. The objective of this study was to assess the efficacy of albendazole, the most frequently used anthelmintic in Gaza and Maputo provinces in the southern region of Mozambique, in gastrointestinal nematodes of goats between November and December, 2016. Eleven goat farms in Gaza (n = 5) and Maputo (n = 6) were surveyed. The faecal egg count reduction test was used to assess the efficacy of the drug. The flocks were considered resistant when the reduction in eggs per gram of faeces was less than 95% and the lower limit of the confidence interval was less than 90%. Resistance to albendazole was detected in 60% (3/5) of the farms in Gaza province and 83.3% (5/6) of the farms in Maputo province. The percentage of faecal egg count reduction varied from 51 to 97% in Maputo and from 0 to 100% in Gaza in the farms surveyed. In pre-treatment coprocultures, *Haemonchus* spp., *Oesophagostomum* spp. and *Trichostrongylus* spp. were the predominant nematode species. Post-treatment larval cultures indicated that *Haemonchus* spp. and, to a lesser extent, *Oesophagostomum* spp. and *Trichostrongylus* spp., were resistant to albendazole. This study provided further evidence that anthelmintic resistance of gastrointestinal nematode parasites in goats is currently a problem of great significance in this region of the country and that appropriate measures must be taken to reverse the situation.

Key words: Albendazole, efficacy, gastrointestinal parasites, small ruminants, Mozambique.

INTRODUCTION

Small ruminants make important contributions to human livelihoods in developing countries. In 2012, about 30% of the approximately 1 billion populations of goats in the world were located in Africa (FAO, 2015; reviewed by

*Corresponding author. E-mail: alsacia.atanasio@mctestp.gov.mz.

Zvinorova et al., 2016). Gastrointestinal nematode infections of ruminant livestock cause major problems for both small-scale and large-scale farmers in the developing world, with a major impact in sub-Saharan Africa (Sissay et al., 2007; Hussain, et al., 2014; Preston et al., 2014; Pawar et al., 2017; Shija et al., 2014; Singh et al, 2017a; Wondimu and Gutu, 2017), including Mozambique with its tropical and sub-tropical areas where favourable climates for the survival and development of gastrointestinal nematodes prevail (Akkari et al., 2013; Shija et al., 2014). *Haemonchus* spp. are highly pathogenic and economically important gastrointestinal parasites affecting ruminants across the world (Chaudhry et al., 2015; Zvinorova et al., 2016). The control of helminth parasites is often essential for the economic production of animals, especially small ruminants. Current control measures rely heavily upon the use of anthelmintic drugs (Gaba et al., 2012; McArthur and Reinemeyer, 2014). However, the ability of parasites to develop quickly resistance to these drugs is spreading globally (Preston et al., 2014). Anthelmintic resistance is a globally threatening problem to sustainable livestock industry and production (Kenyon et al., 2013; Shalaby, 2013; Chaudhry et al., 2015; Singh et al., 2017b). A strain of *Haemonchus contortus* resistant to all classes of anthelmintics has been reported to have developed in South Africa, a neighbouring country of Mozambique, probably because of frequent use of anthelmintics and inappropriate dosage (Van Wyk et al., 1997). Shalaby (2013) stated also that the factors considered most significant in the development of anthelmintic resistance have been the excessive frequency of treatments and administration of inadequate anthelmintic doses.

Given that the use of anthelmintics is required for an efficient and sustainable control of helminth parasites, the knowledge of the levels of resistance to the drugs commonly used will lead to the implementation of adequate zoo technical management practices to mitigate the spread of anthelmintic resistance. The objective of this study, therefore, was to assess the efficacy of albendazole, the most frequently used anthelmintic, through the faecal egg count reduction test, in goats in Maputo and Gaza provinces, two of the 11 provinces of Mozambique.

MATERIALS AND METHODS

Study locations and animals

The study was carried out between November and December 2016, in seven districts of the southern region of Mozambique, namely, Xai-Xai (farms G1 and G2), Chibuto (farms G3 and G4) and Chókwe (farm G5) in Gaza province, and in Magude (farm G6), Namaacha (farm G7), Boane (farms G8 and G9) and Moamba (farms G10 and G11) in Maputo province. Mozambique is located on the eastern coast of Africa, between Latitudes 10° 20' S and 26° 50' S. The study areas were located between Latitudes 24° 38' S and 26° 02' S, and between Longitudes 33° 39' E and 32° 07' E (Figure 1). The study areas were characterized by a tropical dry climate influenced by the motions of the Indian Ocean, with a hot rainy season from October to March and a cool dry season from April to September. The average maximum temperature is 30°C in January/February, with a maximum of 43°C in January, and the minimum average temperature is 15°C in June/July. The mean maximum precipitation is 152 mm in January, and the minimum average precipitation is 10 mm in June/August (Diniz et al., 2012).

Eleven farms, five in Gaza province and six in Maputo province comprising 1,040 goats, were selected. The number of goats in each of the flocks varied from 26 to 180 animals, and three flocks, two in Gaza (G1 and G3) and one in Maputo (G8), were kept extensively on communal grazing without supplementation throughout the year. The rest of the flocks were kept semi-intensively on private delimited pasture areas with supplementation during the dry season. For the study purpose, only 26 to 30 goats were randomly allocated to two groups of 13 to 15 animals in each flock; thus, a total of 355 goats were surveyed. In order to assess the profile of the zoo technical management systems, a questionnaire was administered to the owners or managers of the farms.

Faecal examination

Faecal collection was done directly from the animals' rectal bulb in order to avoid contamination, and the samples were kept cooled in Coleman thermoelectric cooler until the determination of the eggs per gram of faeces (EPG) was performed at the Central Veterinary Laboratory, Animal Sciences Directorate of the Agricultural Research Institute of Mozambique (IIAM) in Maputo province, and at the Provincial Veterinary Laboratory in Gaza province, respectively.

Reinecke's (1961) modification of the McMaster technique was used for the quantitative determination of nematode eggs in the faecal samples. The number of nematode EPG was calculated using the formula: $EPG = Te_1 + Te_2 \times 100$, where Te_1 is the number of eggs in chamber 1 and Te_2 is the number of eggs in chamber 2 of the McMaster slide (Ueno and Gonçalves, 1998).

One hundred larvae per culture were identified (Gupta and Singla 2012), unless there were fewer than 100 in which case all were identified, using the descriptions of Georgi et al. (1985) and Ueno and Gonçalves (1998).

Determining anthelmintic resistance

The efficacy of oral suspensions of albendazole (5 mg/kg body weight; Albenol-100®, Interchemie, Holland), which is frequently used in Mozambique, was assessed using the faecal egg count reduction test (FECRT). The latter was performed according to the methods recommended by the World Association for the Advancement of Veterinary Parasitology (Coles et al., 1992), described and updated by Coles et al.(2006) and interpreted using RESO® to determine anthelmintic resistance.

Once a flock was selected, 26 to 30 goats were randomly allocated to two groups of 13 to 15 animals each, identified with coded ear tags, and weighed. On each of the 11 farms, an untreated control group was formed to monitor the changes in the nematode egg counts during the test period and a treated group that received oral administration of albendazole (5 mg/kg body weight). Individual faecal egg counts and pooled larval cultures were performed from samples collected on the day of treatment and 14 days after the anthelmintic treatment.

Goats with less than 100 nematode EPG in their pre-treatment samples and those with missing values for either the pre- or post-treatment EPG were excluded from the analyses.

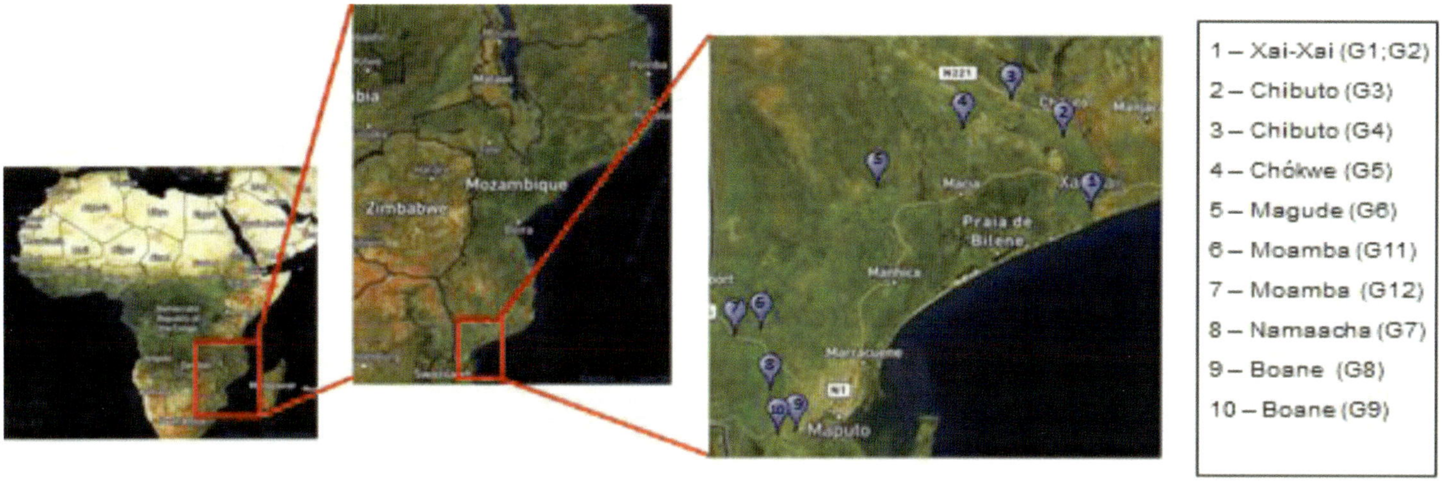

Figure 1. Map of Mozambique indicating the study locations, namely Xai-Xia (G1;G2) and Chokwe (G5) districts in Gaza province and Magude (G6), Namaacha (G7), Boane (G8;G9) and Moamba (G10;G11) districts in Maputo province.

The percentage faecal egg count reduction (%FECR) was calculated, as *100 × (1 - T2/C2)*, where *T2* was the mean egg count of the treated group at day 14, and *C2* was the mean EPG count of the untreated control group 14 days after treatment. The flocks were considered resistant when the EPG reduction percentage was less than 95% and the CI's lower limit was less than 90%. They were considered suspicious if the flock only complied with some of the aforementioned criteria. Flocks that did not comply with any of the required criteria were considered susceptible (Coles et al., 1992, 2006; Canul-Ku et al., 2012).

Statistical analysis

The Pearson's Chi-square test was performed to check for possible differences between the animals surveyed with reference to an association between EPG and factors such as age, sex, and goat breeds. The comparison of susceptibility and resistance of gastrointestinal nematodes to albendazole between farms relating to the frequency of anthelmintic use, grazing system, location at provincial, district, and locality levels was also performed using the Pearson's Chi-square test with 95% confidence interval (CI). All statistical analyses were performed using SPSS version 21, and $p < 0.05$ was considered significant.

RESULTS

Questionnaire

The analysis of the zoo technical management information as per the questionnaire administered indicated that the main objective in all of the flocks (100%) was to produce goat meat. The animals were kept either in communal or private pastures during day hours and shared the pastures with cattle and/or sheep. The animals were reared under extensive systems in communal pastures during the day and kept in corrals at night in 27.3% of the farms (flocks G1 and G3 in Gaza and flock G7 in Maputo). In the rest of the flocks (72.7%), goats were reared under semi-intensive systems in private pastures and kept in cement or metal slabs at night.

Drenching of animals with anthelmintics was based on visual estimative weight in 90.9% (10/11) of the farms except in flock G7 in Maputo, where animals were weighed to determine the adequate anthelmintic dosage. In 81.8% (9/11) of the farms, all animals were drenched with anthelmintics on each occasion, and no EPG tests were performed to decide which animals should be drenched in all farms. Anthelmintics were chosen without any criteria, no drug combination was used, and no quarantine was undertaken in case of acquiring animals from other countries or from other locations within the country in all the studied farms. The data from the questionnaire indicated also that most of the farms had poor management practices, including inadequate disease control measures, inadequate nutrition during the dry season, and face disease challenges, mainly gastrointestinal parasitism.

Faecal egg counts, percentage faecal egg count reduction, statistical analysis, and larval cultures

The arithmetic means of the faecal egg counts before and after treatment for each of the eleven flocks surveyed in Gaza and Maputo provinces and the %FECR are presented in Tables 1 and 2, respectively. According to Coles et al. (1992), flocks are considered resistant when %FECR is less than 95. Resistance to albendazole was detected in 60% (3/5) of the farms in Gaza and 83.3% (5/6) of the farms in Maputo. The %FECR varied from 0 to 100% in Gaza and from 51 to 97% in Maputo.

Possible differences between the animals surveyed with reference to the EPG and factors such as age, sex and goat breeds were assessed using the Pearson's Chi-square test. No statistical difference was found between

Table 1. The arithmetic means of faecal nematode egg counts before and after treatment and %FECR of five farms (G1 to G5) in Gaza province.

Farm no.	Control			Albendazole			% FECR
	No. of goats	Before treatment	After treatment	No. of goats	Before treatment	After treatment	
G1	12	425	567	10	560	20	96
G2	13	846	1885	14	707	593	0[R]
G3	12	658	1092	11	786	0	100
G4	11	355	500	12	708	375	34[R]
G5	11	1345	1218	13	1138	577	0[R]

R, Resistant.

Table 2. The arithmetic means of faecal nematode egg counts before and after treatment and %FECR of six farms (G6 to G11) in Maputo province.

Farm no.	Control			Albendazole			% FECR
	No. of goats	Before treatment	After treatment	No. of goats	Before treatment	After treatment	
G6	12	417	500	12	492	183	68[R]
G7	11	391	245	13	400	108	81[R]
G8	11	245	245	11	209	18	97
G9	12	908	2025	14	886	279	51[R]
G10	10	250	360	11	218	182	68[R]
G11	10	240	290	10	580	160	72[R]

R, Resistant.

Table 3. The percentages of gastrointestinal nematode species found in pre-treatment and post-treatment larval cultures on five flocks tested in Gaza province.

Farm no.	*Haemonchus* spp. (%)		*Oesophagostomum* spp. (%)		*Trichostrongylus* spp. (%)		*Strongyloides* spp. (%)	
	Pre-treatment	Post-treatment	Pre-treatment	Post-treatment	Pre-treatment	Post-treatment	Pre-treatment	Post-treatment
G1	37	0	4	0	59	0	0	0
G2	40	84	26	1	31	6	3	9
G3	65	0	24	0	6	0	5	0
G4	95	100	1	0	2	0	2	0
G5	88	100	10	0	0	0	2	0

the animals surveyed in terms of an association between EPG and all analysed factors (p>0.05).

In the pre-treatment larval cultures, *Haemonchus* spp. (37 to 95% in Gaza and 19 to 100% in Maputo) and *Oesophagostomum* spp. (up to 26%) were the predominant nematode species, while *Trichostrongylus* spp. And *Strongyloides* spp. (except flock G9) were present in small numbers, except in two flocks (G1 and G2) in Gaza province where *Trichostrongylus* spp. appeared in large numbers (31 and 59%) as indicated in Tables 3 and 4. Post-treatment faecal cultures indicated that *Haemonchus* spp., and to a lesser extent *Oesophagostomum* spp. and *Trichostrongylus* spp., were resistant to albendazole. However, *Strongyloides* spp. appeared in large numbers in the post-treatment larval cultures of three flocks, one in Gaza (G2) and two in Maputo (G7 and G9).

DISCUSSION

The present study demonstrated that goats from all the flocks surveyed in seven districts of Gaza and Maputo provinces were infected with gastrointestinal nematodes,

Table 4. The percentages of gastrointestinal nematode species found in pre-treatment and post-treatment larval cultures on four of the six flocks tested in Maputo province.

Farm No.	*Haemonchus* spp. (%)		*Oesophagostomum* spp. (%)		*Trichostrongylus* spp. (%)		*Strongyloides* spp. (%)	
	Pre-treatment	Post-treatment	Pre-treatment	Post-treatment	Pre-treatment	Post-treatment	Pre-treatment	Post-treatment
G6	58	50	26	50	0	0	16	0
G7	88	100	8	0	4	0	0	9
G8	*	*	*	*	*	*	*	*
G9	19	7.5	2	0	2	0	79	92.5
G10	100	100	0	0	0	0	0	0
G11	*	*	*	*	*	*	*	*

*The larvae collected from coprocultures of the two flocks were reserved for molecular diagnostics since the numbers of larvae were too small.

and eight of the flocks were considered resistant to albendazole.

Knowledge about the species of the gastrointestinal nematodes present and the anthelmintic resistance status of the farms is important for performing control and treatment strategies, and to identify where alternative control measures should be used (Burgess et al., 2012). Laboratory analyses should include knowledge on the reality in the field to make the application of intervention strategies feasible for the farmers (Salgado and Santos, 2016). The faecal egg counts are the most used *in vivo* techniques for detecting infections by nematode parasites, and they help farmers decide when and whether or not to drench animals (Lira, 2005). The chief method for the detection of resistance remains the FECRT, which can be used for all anthelmintic groups. The FECRT estimates anthelmintic efficacy of one or more drugs by comparing the faecal egg counts of animals at the time of treatment and at defined times after treatment, depending on the anthelmintic group used (Coles et al., 1992; Pena-Espinoza et al., 2014). Although the test is considered reliable only if more than 25% of the worms are resistant (Martin et al., 1989; Coles et al., 2006), the FECRT is still the most widely used and most feasible test and is considered the gold standard for detecting anthelmintic resistance *in vivo*.

On all the farms where resistance of the worms to albendazole was detected in both provinces, albendazole had been used over long durations, and the owners had been complaining of the failure of this drug to control nematode infections. Therefore, some of them have dismissed albendazole and used ivermectin or moxidectin to drench animals. According to Van Wyk (2001) and Pena-Espinoza et al. (2014), frequent anthelmintic treatments, use of anthelmintics with similar mode of action for several years, and underdosing are some of the factors that contribute to the development of resistance. Thus, inappropriate use of anthelmintic drugs in small ruminants has led to failures in their effectiveness, leading to a global constraint of anthelmintic resistance (Salgado and Santos, 2016).

On the three farms (G2, G4 and G5) in Gaza province, where resistance to albendazole was detected, most of the goats (mainly Boer breed) were imported from Zimbabwe and South Africa, while the goats (Kalahari red breed) were imported from South Africa in farm G11 in Maputo province. An important feature to note in the referred farms is that animals were neither kept in quarantine nor dewormed after they had been imported before introducing them to their new farms. Shalaby (2013) indicated that introducing newly acquired animals to a farm without prior quarantine and deworming constitutes a faster way to spread resistance of gastrointestinal nematodes.

Indiscriminate use of anthelmintics to treat the entire flocks was observed in the surveyed farms, and this may have probably contributed to the higher levels of anthelmintic resistance in the present study. Das Neves et al. (2014) suggested that the low cost and practicability of anthelmintic administration encourage farmers to treat entire flocks irrespective of the individual's needs, thus resulting in the emergence and rapid spread anthelmintic resistance of gastrointestinal nematodes. Geary et al. (2012) also suggested that, although unsustainable with regard to selection for anthelmintic resistance, routine treatment of the entire flock rather than selective treatment of individuals has become a common practice. Therefore, refugia-based drenching regimes have been widely recommended to slow down the development of anthelmintic resistance (Van Wyk, 2001; Kenyon et al., 2013). Based on the levels of resistance to albendazole detected in the farms studied, "refugia" should be explored to prevent and delay the development of anthelmintic resistance, and even to reverse the situation in flocks where resistance levels are already high.

The occurrence of different levels of resistance to benzimidazoles in gastrointestinal nematode parasites, as evidenced by the FECRT results, is in agreement with other studies undertaken elsewhere, including Denmark (Pena-Espinoza et al., 2014), India (Chaudhry et al. (2015), Mexico (Herrera-Manzanilla et al., 2017), North Ireland (McMahon et al., 2013) and Scotland (Kenyon et al., 2013), where resistance of *H. contortus*, *Trichostrongylus* spp. and *Oesophagostomum* spp. to benzimidazoles was registered. Kumsa and Abebe (2009) reported anthelmintic resistance in *Haemonchus* spp. to albendazole and tetramisole in goats in Southern Ethiopia. Chagas et al. (2013) reported the presence of a multiple-resistant strain of *H. contortus* in Southeast Brazil. Borges et al. (2015) reported the occurrence of resistance of *Haemonchus* spp. and *Trichostrongylus* spp. to albendazole in the northeast Bahia State in Brazil.

In the present study, resistance to albendazole was detected in eight (72.7%) of the 11 farms surveyed. The results indicated high levels of resistance to the tested anthelmintic, and demonstrated that there was an alarming increase in the resistance rate compared to the results reported by Atanásio et al. (2002).

Any viable eggs in post-treatment coprocultures indicate that some resistant worms may have been present in the animals at the time of treatment. Evidence of small percentage of survivors may indicate a resistance problem that could develop with further rounds of treatments, and should be monitored (Pena-Espinoza et al., 2014). Since large numbers of infective larvae of *Strongyloides* spp. in the post-treatment larval cultures compared with the pre-treatment larval cultures were observed only in three of the flocks (G2, G7, and G9), it was not possible to determine whether the resistance of this species to albendazole has occurred.

Conclusion

This study provided evidence that anthelmintic resistance of gastrointestinal nematode parasites in goats is currently a problem of great significance and imposes severe constraints on the production of small ruminants in this region of the country. Our findings were in agreement with previous studies that indicated the resistance to benzimidazoles as an emerging problem in southern Mozambique. Different control strategies or appropriate measures including sustainable control strategies using integrated approaches and an alternation strategy of drug groups in order to minimize the pressure for parasite adaptation must be taken to reverse the situation. Refugia-based anthelmintic treatments are recommended to slow down the development of resistance to drugs, and target selective treatments to extend the efficiency of anthelmintics mainly in the farms where the levels of resistance are low or anthelmintic drugs are still effective must be applied. Adoption of strict quarantine procedures should be instituted for all newly acquired animals to prevent the importation of resistant nematodes to the farms.

ACKNOWLEDGMENTS

This study was financed by the Ministry of Science and Technology, High Education and Technical Vocational Training (MCTESTP) through HEST Project-World Bank. The author gratefully acknowledges the technical assistance provided by Dr Aida Cala, Mr Carlos Sitoe, and Mrs Ana Paula from the Parasitology Laboratory at Animal Sciences Directorate (DCA) of the Agricultural Research Institute of Mozambique (IIAM) and Mr Gedeão Macanze from the Provincial Veterinary Laboratory in Gaza. Sincere appreciation is extended to the IIAM General Director, Dr Olga Fafetine and the DCA Director, Dr Zacarias Massango, for logistical support during the field work, and to Dr Muller Ribeiro for generating the study locations map. The authors would like to thank reviewers for proof reading the manuscript. The authors express special acknowledgements to Editage for professional editing and English review of the manuscript.

REFERENCES

Akkari H, Jebali J, Gharbi M, Mhadhbi M, Awadi S, Darghouth MA (2013). Epidemiological study ofsympatric *Haemonchus* species and genetic characterization of *Haemonchus contortus* in domestic ruminants in Tunisia. Vet. Parasitol.193:118-125.

Atanásio A, Boomker J, Sitoe C (2002). A survey on the occurrence of resistance to anthelmintics of gastrointestinal nematodes of goats in Mozambique. Onderstepoort J. Vet. Res. 69:215-220.

Borges SL, Oliveira AA, Mendonça LR, Lambert SM, Viana JM, Nishi SM, Julião FS, Almeida MAO (2015). Anthelmintic resistance in goat flocks from Caatinga and Mata Atlântica biomas.Pesq. Vet. Brasileira. 35:643-648.

Burgess CGS, Bartley Y, Redman E, Skuce PJ, Nath M, Whitelaw F, Tait A, Gilleard JS, Jackson F (2012). A survey of the trichostrongylid nematode species present on UK sheep farms and associated anthelmintic control practices. Vet. Parasitol. 189:299-307.

Canul-Ku HI, Rodriguéz-Vivas RI, Torres-Acosta JFJ, Aguilar-Caballero AJ, Perez-Cogollo LC, Ojeda-Chi MM (2012). Prevalence of cattle herds with ivermectin resistant nematodes in the hot sub-humid tropics of Mexico. Vet. Parasitol. 183:292-298.

Chagas ACS, Katiki LM, Silva IC, Giglioti R, Esteves SN, Oliveira MC, Junior WB (2013). *Haemonchus contortus:* A multiple-resistant Brazilian isolate and the costs for its characterization and maintenance for research use. Parasitol. Int.62:1-6.

Chaudhry U, Redman EM, Ramen M, Gillead JS (2015). Genetic evidence for the spread of a benzimidazole resistance mutation across southern India from a single origin in the parasite nematode *Haemonchus contortus*. Int. J. Parasitol. 45:721-728.

Coles GC, Bauer C, Borgsteede FHM, Geerts S, Klei TR, Taylor MA, Waller P (1992). World Association for the Advancement of Veterinary Parasitology (W.A.A.VP) methods for the detection of anthelmintic resistance in nematodes of veterinary importance. Vet. Parasitol. 44:35-44.

Coles GC, Jackson F, Pomroy WE, Prichard RK, von Samson-Himmelstjerna G, Silvestre A, Taylor MA, Vercruysse J (2006). The detection of anthelmintic resistance in nematodes of veterinary importance. Vet. Parasitol.136:167-185.

Das Neves JH, Carvalho N, Rinaldi L, Cringoli G, Amarante AFT (2014). Diagnosis of anthelmintic resistance in cattle in Brazil: A comparison of different methodologies. Vet. Parasitol. 206:216-226.

Diniz MA, Bandeira S, Eurico S, Martins ES (2012). Flora and Vegetation of Maputo province: Its appropriation by populations. Proceedings of International Congress on Tropical Knowledge in Mozambique: History, Memory and Science, IICT-JBT:1-2. Available at: https://2012congressomz.files.wordpress.com/2013/08/t10c01.pdf

FAO (2015). The Second Report on the State of the World's Animal Genetic Resources for Food and Agriculture [Scherf, B.D. and Pilling, D. (eds)]. FAO Commission on Genetic Resources for Food and Agriculture Assessments. Rome. Available at: http://www.fao.org/3/a-i4787e.pdf.

Gaba S, Cabaret J, Chylinski C, Sauve C, Cortet J, Silvestre A (2012). Can efficient management of sheep gastrointestinal nematodes of sheep be based on random treatment? Vet. Parasitol.190:178-184.

Geary TG, Hosking BC, Skuce PJ, von Samson-Himmelstjerna G, Maeder S, Holdsworth P, Pomroy W, Vercruysse J, (2012). World Association for the Advancement of Veterinary Parasitology (W.A.A.V.P.) Guideline: Anthelmintic combination products targeting nematode infections of ruminants and horses. Vet. Parasitol.190:306-316.

Georgi JR, Theodorides VJ, Georgi ME (1985). Parasitology for Veterinarians. 4th Edition, Philadelphia: W.B. Saunders Company. Available at: https://www.abebooks.com/booksearch/isbn/9780721611761/

Gupta SK, Singla LD (2012) Diagnostic trends in parasitic diseases of animals. In: *Veterinary Diagnostics: Current Trends.* Gupta RP, Garg SR, Nehra V and Lather D (Eds), Satish Serial Publishing House, Delhi. pp: 81-112.

Herrera-Manzanilla FA, Ojeda-Robertos NF, González-Garduño R, Cámara-Sarmiento R, Torres-Acosta JFJ (2017).Gastrointestinal nematode populations with multiple anthelmintic resistance in sheep farms from the hot humid tropics of Mexico. Vet. Parasitol. 9:29-33.

Hussain T, Periasamy K, Nadeem A, Babar ME, Pichler R, Diallo A (2014). Sympatric species distribution, genetic diversityand population structure of *Haemonchus*isolates from domestic ruminants in Pakistan. Vet. Parasitol.206:188-199.

Kenyon F, McBean D, Greer AW, Burgess GS, Morrison AA, Bartley DJ, Bartley Y, Davin L, Nath M, Jackson F (2013). A comparative study of the effects of four treatment regimens on ivermectin efficacy, body weight and pasture contamination in lambs naturally infected with gastrointestinal nematodes in Scotland. Int. J. Parasitol. Drugs Drug Resist. 3:77-84.

Kumsa B, Abebe G (2009). Multiple anthelmintic resistance on a goat farm in Hawassa (southern Ethiopia). Trop. Anim. Health Prod. 41:655-662.

Lira CMD (2005). 'Willow fodder blocks for growth and sustainable management of internal parasites ingrazinglambs', MSc Thesis, Massey University, New Zealand.

Martin PJ, Anderson N, Jarrett RG (1989). Detecting benzimidazole resistance with faecal egg count reduction tests and in vitro assays. Aust. Vet. J. 1989 66:236-240.

McArthur MJ, Reinemeyer CR (2014). Herding the U.S. cattle industry towards a paradigm shift in parasite control. Vet. Parasitol. 204:34-43.

McMahon C, Barley JP, Edgar HWJ, Ellison SE, Hanna REB, Malone FE, Brennan GP, Fairweather I (2013). Anthelmintic resistance in Northern Ireland II: Variations in nematode control practices between lowland and upland sheep flocks. Vet. Parasitol. 192:173-182.

Pawar PD, Khasnis MW, Hong CD, Khole RP, Mhase PP, Singla LD (2017). Coproprevalence and successful management of parasitic infections in sheep in Pune district of Maharastra.. Proceedings of 25th National Congress of Veterinary Parasitology and International Symposium on Current Concepts in Diagnosis & Control of Parasitic Diseases to Combat Climat Change (15-17 February, 2017) at Veterinary College, Shimoga. P 56.

Pena-Espinoza M, Thamsborg SM, Demeler J, Enemar KH (2014). Field efficacy of four anthelmintics and confirmation of drug-resistant nematodes by controlled efficacy test and pyrosequencing on a sheep and goat farm in Denmark. Vet. Parasitol. 206:208-215.

Preston SJM, Sandeman M, Gonzalez J, Piedrafita D (2014). Current status for gastrointestinal nematode diagnosis in small ruminants: where are we and where are we going? J. Immunol. Res. 2014:1-12.

Reinecke RK (1961). Helminth research in South Africa III. The diagnosis of nematode parasites in ruminants for worm survey purposes. J. South African Vet. Assoc.37:27-31.

Salgado JA, Santos CP (2016). Overview of anthelmintic resistance of gastrointestinal nematodes of small ruminants in Brazil. Rev. Brasileira Parasitol. Vet. 25(1):3-17.

Shalaby HA (2013). Anthelmintic resistance; How to overcome it? Iranian J. Parasitol. 8:18-32.

Shija DSN, Kusiluka LJM, Chenyambuga SW, Shayo D, Lekule FP (2014). Animal health constraints in dairy goats kept under smallholder farming systems in Kongwa and Mvomero Districts, Tanzania. J. Vet. Med. Anim. Health 6(11):268-279.

Singh E, Kaur P, Singla LD, Bal MS (2017a). Prevalence of gastrointestinal parasitism in small ruminants in western zone of Punjab, India. Vet. World 10(1):61-66.

Singh R, Bal MS, Singla LD, Kaur P (2017b). Detection of anthelmintic resistance in sheep and goat against fenbendazole by faecal egg count reduction test. J. Parasitic Dis. 41(2):463-466.

Sissay MM, Uggla A, Waller PJ (2007). Prevalence and seasonal incidence of nematode parasites and fluke infections of sheep and goats in eastern Ethiopia. Trop. Anim. Health Prod. 39:521-531.

Ueno H, Gonçalves PC (1998). Handbook for diagnosis of helminthoses of ruminants. 4th Edition, Tokyo, JP: Japan International Cooperation, P 143. Available at: https://r1.ufrrj.br/adivaldofonseca/wp-content/uploads/2014/06/manual_helmintoses-UENO-site-do-CBPV.pdf

Van Wyk JA (2001). Refugia-overlooked as perhaps the most potent factor concerning the development of anthelmintic resistance. Onderstpoort J. Vet. Res.68:55-67.

Van Wyk, JA, Malan, FS, Randles, JL (1997). How long before resistance makes it impossible to control some field strains of *Haemonchus contortus* in South Africa with any of the modern anthelmintics?. Vet. Parasitol. 70:111-122.

Wondimu A, Gutu S (2017). Gastrointestinal nematodes of small ruminants in Guto Gida District, East Wolloega, Ethiopia. J. Vet. Med. Anim. Health 9:83-87.

Zvinorova PI, Halimani TE, Muchadeyi FC, Matika O, Riggio V, Dzama K (2016). Breeding for resistance to gastrointestinal nematodes- the potential in low-input/output small ruminant production systems. Vet. Parasitol. 225:19-28.

4

Epidemiological investigation of Middle East respiratory syndrome corona virus (mers-cov) among dromedary camels in selected areas of Afar and Oromia region, Ethiopia

Getnet Fekadu[1], Gelagay Ayelet[2] and Fufa Abunna[3]*

[1]College of Veterinary Medicine, Haramaya University, P. O. Box, 138, Dire Dawa, Ethiopia.
[2]National Veterinary Institute, P. O. Box, 19, Bishoftu, Oromia, Ethiopia.

[3]College of Veterinary Medicine and Agriculture, Department of Clinical Studies, Addis Ababa University, P. O. Box 34, Bishoftu, Oromia, Ethiopia.

A cross-sectional study was conducted between October 2014 and May 2015, to determine the sero-prevalence, assess the presence of active cases through isolation and identify possible risk factors for the Middle East Respiratory Syndrome Corona Virus (MERS-CoV) in camels, in selected areas of Oromia and Afar regional states of Ethiopia. A total of 569 dromedary camel sera were collected and screened with two serological tests: Pseudo particle neutralization for screening and Micro-neutralization test for confirmation. The overall prevalence of MERS-CoV in the study area was 93% (n=529). Higher prevalence (93.9%) was recorded in female dromedary camels compared to males (91.3%) but the difference was not significant (Chi-Square=1.323 and P=0.250). Age wise prevalence was higher in adult camels (94.6%) than young ones (90.8%), however the difference was statistically insignificant (Chi-Square=3.068 and P=0.080). Similarly, higher prevalence was recorded in larger herds (93.4%) than small herds but the difference observed was not statistically significant (Chi-Square=0.220 and p=0.639). Also, no significant (Chi-Square 0.525 and P=0.469) difference was observed in prevalence between the two regions (Oromia=93.3% and Afar=93.3%). However significant difference was observed in the lower administrations of the regions (Zones, District and Kebeles) in which the highest prevalence recorded in East Shoa, Fentale district of Adis Ketema kebele (99.3%). From total of 100 swabs collected, MERS-CoV was detected in seven (1 Fentale, 4 Amibara and 2 Dubti) districts by Real-time reverse transcription polymerase chain reaction (RT-PCR). Generally, this study showed the existence of high seroprevalence of MERS-CoV among Ethiopian dromedary camels, which was also confirmed by RT-PCR. Therefore further study is required to determine its significance from both animal and public health perspectives and further research should focus on identifying similarity between MERS-CoV viral isolates in neighboring countries and clinical isolates from the Middle East and elsewhere.

Key words: Dromedary camel, MERS-CoV, serum, swab, Real-time reverse transcription polymerase chain reaction (RT-PCR), Ethiopia.

INTRODUCTION

More than 60% of the world population of one-humped dromedary camels (Camelus dromedarius) lives in the Greater Horn of Africa. Their role as one of the most important livestock species for nutrition in arid and semi-arid areas of Eastern Africa is likely to increase since the predicted climate change is in favour of this drought resilient species. Camel milk, for domestic consumption or sale, is often the most important product for female and male pastoralists alike (Marshall et al., 2014). In 2012, a novel coronavirus called Middle East Respiratory Syndrome Coronavirus (MERS-CoV) emerged on the Arabian Peninsula. Human cases have been reported from 25 countries, with the most recent outbreak in the Republic of Korea (which itself originated in the Middle East). MERS-CoV has caused at least 1,200 laboratory confirmed cases of severe respiratory infection, including more than 400 deaths. Several studies have demonstrated that dromedary camels can act as a source of human MERS-CoV infection (Reusken et al., 2015).

In June 2012, a novel beta corona virus, associated with severe respiratory disease in humans, emerged in the Middle East (Zaki et al., 2012), which is closely related to beta corona viruses, circulating in bats (Anthony et al., 2013). The first isolate of Middle East respiratory corona virus (MERS-CoV), HCoV-EMC/2012, was obtained from a patient with a fatal pneumonia and acute renal failure. To date, 107 additional human cases have been identified, of which 49 were fatal (WHO, 2013). Aside from cases in Saudi Arabia, Qatar, Jordan, and the United Arab Emirates, imported cases have been identified in the United Kingdom, Germany, France, Tunisia, and Italy.

Although no information is available on the source or route of primary transmission of MERS-CoV, human-to-human transmission has been recorded (Assiri et al., 2013). The severity of disease distinguishes MERS-CoV from other corona viruses, circulating in the human population HCoV-229E, HCoV-OC43, HCoV-NL63, and HCoV HKU1, which are generally associated with upper respiratory tract infections. Instead, MERS-CoV appears to be more similar to the severe respiratory disease, caused by severe acute respiratory syndrome (SARS)-CoV. *In vitro* studies have shown that MERS-CoV replicates efficiently in non-ciliated cells in the primary human airway epithelium (Kindler et al., 2013), and in *ex vivo* human lung cultures, MERS-CoV replicated in bronchial, bronchiolar, and alveolar epithelial cells (Chan et al., 2013). The MERS-CoV virus is thought to be an animal virus that has sporadically resulted in human infections, with subsequent limited transmission between humans. The evidence for the animal origin of the virus is circumstantial.

Nevertheless, the alternative explanation to explain sporadic appearance of severe human cases with long periods of time between them, and the wide geographical area over which the virus was apparently distributed, is unrecognized ongoing transmission in people. Surveillance efforts, since the discovery of the virus and retrospective testing of stored respiratory specimens suggest this is not the case (Gautret et al., 2013). In August, 2013, the possible source of MERS-COV virus was traced to an Egyptian tomb bat found in a building, in close proximity to an index patient home. The virus genome fragment isolated from the bat was a 100% genetic match to the virus, isolated from the index patient (Jobs, 2013). There had been speculation that, bats might be the source of the virus (Abedine and Saad, 2013). On 9th August, 2013 a report in the journal "The Lancet Infectious Disease" showed that 50 out of 50 (100%) blood serum from Omani camels and 15 out of 105 (14%) from Spanish camels had protein specific antibodies against MERS- COV spike protein and also in Egypt (between 94 and 98% of a total of 110 camels tested positive). A further study on dromedary camels from Saudi Arabia published in December 2013, revealed the presence of MERS–COV in 90% of the evaluated dromedary camels (310), suggesting that dromedary camels not only could be the main reservoir of MERS–COV, but also the animal source of MERS–COV (Hemida et al., 2013).

The Arabian Peninsula remains the site of primary human infection from the zoonotic source of human cases as reported so far and dromedary camels in other parts of North, West and East Africa appear to have serological evidence of MERS infection. The full geographic range of MERS CoV circulation has not been established so far in the above sites including Ethiopia. Sero-prevalence of MERS-CoV in Ethiopia was 97% in adult camels, 93% in young camels and overall prevalence of 96% (Reusken et al., 2013). Therefore the objectives of this study were to determine the seroprevalence of MERS-CoV, to assess the presence of active cases through isolation of MERS-CoV and to identify possible risk factors for theMERS-CoV in

*Corresponding author. E-mail: fufa.abunna@aau.edu.et.

the study areas.

MATERIALS AND METHODS

Study area and animals

This study was conducted between November 2014 and May 2015 in pastoral areas of Afar (Dubti, Ayssaita, Chifra, Ewa and Amibara districts) and Oromia (Yabello and Fentale districts) regions where camels are populated. Camels of all age and both sexes were randomly selected and included in the study for determination of antibody prevalence against MERS-COV. For the purpose of virus isolation and characterization, nasal swab was taken from 100 camels (Yabelo, Amibara, Fentale and Dubti), 25 from each district. Geographically, the Afar Regional state is located in the northeastern part of Ethiopia. The total geographical area of the region is about 270,000 km^2 (CSA, 2008). It is geographically located between 39°34' and 42°28' East Longitude and 8°49'and 14° 30'North Latitude. The region shares common international boundaries with the State of Eritrea in the north-east and Djibouti in the east, as well as regional boundaries with the Regional States of Tigray in the north-west, Amhara in the south-west, Oromia in the south and Somali in the south-east. Afar is characterized by an arid and semi-arid climate with low and erratic rainfall. Rainfall is bi-modal throughout the region with a mean annual rainfall below 500 mm in the semi-arid western escarpments, decreasing to 150 mm in the arid zones to the east. Afar is increasingly in drought prone and the region receives three rainy seasons. The main rain karma accounts for 60% of annual rainfall and occurs from mid-June to mid-September. This is followed by rainy showers in mid-December called dadaa and a minor rainy season during March to April called sugum. Disruptions on the performance of any rainy season will impact on the availability of pasture and water as well as the overall food security situation of the pastoral and agro-pastoral communities (ANRSP, 2010).

Study design and sampling technique

A cross sectional study was conducted for serological investigation of MERS-CoV among dromedary camels found in the study area. Multi stage cluster sampling technique was used to select specific cluster (kebele) for all sites found in the study areas. Finally samples were taken randomly from each selected cluster. Dromedary camels found in Afar and Oromia region of both age groups (young 1 to 3 years and adults > 3 years of age), both sex groups (male and female) and two categories of herd size (large herd size=herd having above 50 camels and small herd size = herd having less than or equal to 50 camels) were included in the study.

Sample size

Based on Thrusfield (2007) formula, the sample size of study animals was calculated.

$$n = \frac{1.96^2 (Pexp) (1 - Pexp)}{d^2}$$

$$n = \frac{1.96^2 (0.96) (1 - 0.96)}{0.0025}$$

n = 59 and the sample size multiplied by the cluster number to get the final sample size 59 x 8 sites = 472 (Total sample size required).

But additional 97 samples were taken to increase the precision of the study and the final sample size became 569. Where n = required sample size, Pexp = expected prevalence (96%) and d = desired absolute precision (95%)

Sample collection, transportation and storage

The samples were taken from randomly selected dromedary camels from each cluster (kebeles) of randomly selected Zones and woredas of Afar and Oromia. Then 10 mm of blood sample was collected from jugular veins of the animals using needle and plain test tube (without anticoagulants). The blood was allowed to clot for2 h at room temperature, stored overnight at 4°C and then, serum was separated from the clot standing for 20 min at room temperature, to allow for clot formation.

Serum was separated from the clot by centrifugation at 3000rpm for 10 min and transferred to crayovial tubes. Then the separated serum was labeled and kept under refrigeration (–20°C) until transported to National Veterinary Institute (NVI) for storage, before taken to the University of Hong Kong for analysis.

The collected 569 sera samples were transported in the icebox to National Veterinary Institute serology laboratory and kept under refrigeration (–20°C) until transported to University of Hong Kong for serological analysis. Hundred swabs were collected by using cotton swab from randomly selected sites (Borena and Metehara) from Oromia region (Dubti and Melka werer). Twenty five swabs were taken from each site mentioned above. The swabs were preserved in buffer solution until transported to NVI virology section for deep freezing at -80°C. Finally the swabs transported to Hong Kong University for analysis.

Laboratory analysis

The blood samples collected were analyzed by two serological tests MERS-CoV spike, pseudoparticle neutralization assay (screening test) and Micro neutralization tests (confirmatory test).

The swabs collected undergo extraction of DNA and Polymerase Chain Reaction (PCR) to identify the presence of MERS-CoV in the sample.

Serology

MERS-CoV spike pseudo particle neutralization assay

A codon-optimised spike gene was designed according to published MERS-CoV genome sequence (GenBank accession number: JX869059.1), synthesised by GeneCust (Luxembourg) and subcloned into pcDNA3.1+ vector to generate pcDNA-S. To produce HIV/MERS spike pseudoparticles, 10 µg pNL Luc E- R- and 10 µg pcDNA-SS were co-transfected into 4x106 293T cells. Supernatants of transfected cells were harvested 48 h later and quantified for HIV p24 viral protein using a p24 ELISA Kit (Cell Biolabs, San Diego, United States).

For ppNT assay, HIV/MERS pseudoparticles containing 5 ng p24 were used to infect Vero E6 cells (ATCC CRL-1586) in a single well (96-well plate format; 1x104 cells/well). Infected cells were lysed in 20 µl lysis buffer and 100 µl of luciferase substrate at 2days postinfection (Promega Corporation, Madison, United States).

Luciferase activity was measured in a Microbeta luminometer (PerkinElmer, Waltham, United States). For ppNT, HIV/MERS pseudoparticles (5 ng of p24) were pre-incubated with serially diluted sera for 30 min at 4°C and then added to cells in triplicate. Residual virus replication was assayed at 2days post infection, as described above. The highest serum dilution giving a 90% reduction of luciferase activity was regarded as the ppNT antibody titre.

Viruses and virus titration

MERS-CoV (strain EMC) virus was obtained from Dr R Fouchier (Erasmus University Medical Center, Rotterdam, and the Netherlands). SARS-CoV (strain HKU-39849) was taken from the virus repository at Hong Kong University. Virus stock for MERS-CoV was prepared in Vero cell culture (ATCC CCL-81) in minimal essential medium containing 2% fetal bovine serum, 100 units/mL penicillin and 100 µg/mL Streptomycin. Virus aliquots were stored at -80°C. Virus was titrated in serial half-log10 dilutions (from 0.5 log to 7 log) to obtain 50% tissue culture infectious dose (TCID50) on 96 well tissue culture plates of Vero cells. The plates were observed in a phase contrast microscope for cytopathic effect (CPE) daily, for three days. The endpoint of viral dilution leading to CPE in 50% of inoculated wells was estimated, by using the Reed Muench method and designated as one TCID50. SARS-CoV was grown and titrated in the same manner with the exception that Vero E6 cells (ATCC CRL-1586) were used.

Micro-neutralization tests

Serial two fold dilutions of heat inactivated sera (56°C for 30 min) were made, starting with a dilution of 1:10. The serum dilutionswere mixed with equal volumes of 200 TCID50 of MERS-CoV or SARS-CoV as indicated. After 1 h of incubation at 37°C, 35 µL of the virus serum mixture was added in quadruplicate to Vero or Vero-E6 cell monolayers for MERS-CoV and SARS-CoV, respectively, in 96 well microtiter plates. After 1 h of adsorption, an additional 150 µL of culture medium were added to each well and the plates was incubated for three more days at 37°C in 5% CO_2 in a humidified incubator. A virus back-titration was performed without immune serum to assess input virus dose. CPE was read at three days post infection. The highest serum dilution that completely protects the cells from CPE in half of the wells was taken as a neutralizing antibody titre and was estimated using the Reed-Muench method. Positive and negative control sera were included to validate the assay.

Extraction of RNA and Polymerase Chain Reaction (PCR)

Real-time reverse transcription PCR (RT-PCR) targeting upstream of E gene of MERS-CoV was used for screening. The open reading frame (ORF) 1a gene was used for confirmation as recommended by the World Health Organization. We also used a previously described pan-CoV nested PCR, targeting the viral RNA-dependent RNA polymerase (RdRp) region (*13*), and PCR products were analyzed by sequencing (online Technical Appendix, wwwnc.cdc.gov).
EID/article/20/6/14-0299-Techapp1.pdf). We detected MERS-CoV RNA in (n=7/100) (7%) of 100 nasal swab specimens from dromedary camels with the upstream of E gene assay (cycle threshold [Ct] 23.2–36.8), confirmed by the ORF1a assay (Ct 23.2–39.1), fulfilling the World Health Organization criteria for diagnosis of MERS-CoV infection. PCR was repeated from a fresh RNA extract to confirm positive results.

Data analysis

Data obtained from the investigations was coded and stored in Excel spread sheets. The independent variables age, sex, herd size and origin (kebele) of the dromedary camels have been compared to evaluate their effect on the magnitude of the disease. The collected data was analyzed using SPSS version 20 software. Descriptive statistics was used to determine the frequency of proportion (prevalence) and chi square, and logistic regression was used to check the association between the sero-prevalence and the independent variables. The precision level used was 5% with the level of significance differences set at $p < 0.05$, chi square(x^2) > 3.841 for association and logistic regression with odds ratio >1 for the magnitude of the risk(effect) of exposure variables.

RESULTS

Seroprevalence of MERS-CoV

From the total of 569 camel sera tested, 93% (n=529/569) were positive for MERS-COV specific antibody with MERS-CoV spike pseudoparticle neutralization assay and Microneutralisation tests. Out of 238 sera tested from young Dromedary, camels (n=216/238) (90.8%) were positive and from 331 adult, camels (n=313/331) (94.6%) were also positive and the difference seen was not significant (Pearson Chi-Square=3.068 and P=0.080) (Table 1).

From 569 dromedaries camel sampled 361 were Female and 208 were Male. (n=339/361) (93.9%) and (n=190/208) (91.3%) of Female and Male were positive respectively. The difference seen between the two sex groups was insignificant (Pearson Chi-Square=1.323 and P=0. .250) (Table 2).Out of 222 Camels tested from small herd sized group (n=205/222) (92.3%) were positive and from 347 large herd sized camels (n=324/347) (93.4%) were positive but the difference observed was not statistically significant (Pearson Chi-Square=0.220and P=0.639 (Table 3).Out of 230 camels tested from Oromia region (n=216/230) (93.9%) were positive and 339 samples from Afar (n=313/339) (92.3%) were positive but the difference was not statistically significant (Pearson Chi-Square =0.525 and P=0.469) (Table 4).

Among Zones included in the study highest prevalence recorded in East Shoa (n=136/137) (99.3%) and the lowest at Borena (n=80/93) (86.0%).The prevalence difference among Zones was highly statistically significant (Pearson Chi-Square=24.285 and P=0.000) (Table 5). Out of 7 districts included in the study the highest prevalence was observed in Fentale (n=136/137) (99.3%) and the lowest in Yabello (n=80/93) (86.0%) with

Table 1. Seroprevalence of MERS-CoV in the two age groups (Young and adult dromedary camels).

Variable	Negative	Positive	Total
Young	22(9.2%)	216(90.8%)	238
Adult	18(5.4%)	313(94.6%)	331
Total	40(7%)	529(93%)	569
	Pearson Chi-Square=3.068	df=1	P=0.080

Table 2. Sero prevalence of MERS-CoV in the two sex groups of dromedary camels.

Variable	Negative	Positive	Total
Female	22(6.1%)	339(93.9%)	361
Male	18(8.7%)	190(91.3%)	208
Total	40(7%)	529(93%)	569
	Pearson Chi-Square=1.323	df=1	P=0. .250

Table 3. Sero prevalence of MERS-CoV in the herd size categories of dromedary camels.

Herd Size	Negative	Positive	Total
Small	17(7.7%)	205(92.3%)	222(100%)
Large	23(6.6%)	324(93.4%)	347(100%)
Total	40(7%)	529(93%)	569(100%)
	Chi-Square=0.220	df=1	P=0.639

Table 4. Sero prevalence of MERS-CoV in the two regions (Afar and Oromia) Ethiopia.

Variable	Negative	Positive	Total
Oromia	14(6.1%)	216(93.9%)	230(100%)
Afar	26(7.7%)	313(92.3%)	339(100%)
Total	40(7%)	529(93%)	569(100%)
	Pearson Chi-Square =0.525	df=1	P=0.469

Table 5. Sero prevalence of MERS-CoV in different zones of the study area among dromedary camels.

Variable	Negative	Positive	Total
Borena	13(14.0%)	80(86.0%)	93(100%)
East Shoa	1(0.7%)	136(99.3%)	137(100%)
Zone 1(Afar)	20(10.4%)	172(89.6%)	192(100%)
Zone 3(Afar)	1(1.1%)	94(98.9%)	95(100%)
Zone 4(Afar)	5(9.6%)	47(90.4%)	52(100%)
Total	40(7%)	529(93%)	569(100%)
	Pearson Chi-Square=24.285	df=4	P=0.000

Table 1. Sero prevalence of MERS-CoV among Dromedary camels in different districts of Afar and Oromia.

Variable	Negative	Positive	Total
Ayssaita	4(6.2%)	61(93.8%)	65(100%)
Chifra	8(13.6%)	51(86.4%)	59(100%)
Dubti	8(11.8%)	60(88.2%)	68(100%)
Ewa	5(9.6%)	47(90.4%)	52(100%)
Amibara	1(1.1%)	94(98.9%)	95(100%)
Fentale	1(0.7%)	136(99.3%)	137(100%)
Yabelo	13(14.0%)	80(86.0%)	93(100%)
Total	40(7%)	529(93%)	569(100%)
	Pearson Chi-Square=27.173[a]	df=6	P=0.000

Table 7. Seroprevalence of MERS-CoV among Dromedary camels in different kebeles of Afar and Oromia.

Variable	Negative	Positive	Total
Surupha	13(14%)	80(86%)	93(100%)
Adis Ketema	1(0.7%)	136(99.3%)	137(100%)
Badule	5(9.6%)	47(90.4%)	52(100%)
Galifage	1(4%)	24(96%)	25(100%)
Geriro	4(17.4%)	19(82.6%)	23(100%)
Gurmudale	8(11.8%)	60(88.2%)	68(100%)
Heladegi	1(1.1%)	94(98.9%)	95(100%)
Jarakontola	4(11.1%)	32(88.9%)	36(100%)
Urmaytu	3(7.5%)	37(92.5%)	40(100%)
Total	40(7%)	529(93%)	569(100%)
	Pearson Chi-Square=28.308	df=8	P=0.000

Table 8. Isolation and Identification MERS-CoV among dromedary camels from selected sites (Yabelo, Fentale, Dubti and Amibara) of the study areas.

Variable	Negative	Positive	Total
Yabelo	25(100%)	0(0.00%)	25(100%)
Fentale	24(96%)	1(4%)	25(100%)
Dubti	23(92%)	2(8%)	25(100%)
Amibara	21(84%)	4(16%)	25(100%)
Total	93(93%)	7(7%)	100(100%)

Pearson Chi-Square=27.173 and P=0.000 value) (Table 6). Among the kebeles (n=136/137) (99.3%) prevalence was the highest prevalence from Adis Ketema of Metehara and the lowest Geriro (n=19/23) (82.6%) of Afar with Pearson Chi-Square=28.308 and P=0.000 values (Table 7).

Molecular identification of MERS-CoV

From the 100 swab randomly sampled (n=7/100) (7%) of them evident circulation of MERS-CoV in the study area 2 from Dubti, 1 from Fentale and 4 from Amibara (Table 8).

DISCUSSION

The overall high prevalence (n=529/569) (93%) evident in this study completely agree with study done in Ethiopia by (Reusken et al., 2013). The prevalence recorded in Young Dromedary camel (n=216/238) (90.8%) and Adult (n=313/331) (94.6%) was also similar with work of the same author (93% in young Dromedary and 97% in Adult). The higher prevalence observed in the Adult Dromedary camel, may be due to their access to MERS-CoV infected animal at common watering place found in the study area. The overall prevalence of MERS-CoV in this study also agree with study done in Egypt by (Chu et al., 2014), (n=48/52) (92.3%) using the same pseudoparticle neutralization assay as the current study. The slight lower prevalence recorded in Female dromedary camels of this study (n=339/361) (93.9%) compared to the Males (n=190/280) (91.3%) may be due frequent interaction of female camels with humans and their calves.

The two herd size categories in the current study have little variation in their prevalence. Camels in the larger herd size have slightly higher prevalence (n=324/347) (93.4%) than the small herd sized (n=205/222) (92.3%), but the difference between the herds categories was not statistically significant. This may be related with the possibility of increment of an infected animal in the herd which further facilitate transmission of the virus. The prevalence observed in Oromia region was higher (n=216/230) (93.9%) as compared to Afar (n=313/339) (92.3%), this may be because of the high contact rate of the camels in each other during watering in Oromia as compared to the Afar camels. Among the five Zones included in the study, the highest prevalence was evident in East Shoa (n=136/137) (99.3%) and the lowest in Borena zone (n=80/93) (86.0%).The difference observed among the zones was highly significant (p=0.000).

Fentale was the district where the highest prevalence of MERS-CoV recorded (n=136/137) (99.3%) the lowest in Yabelo district (n=80/93) (86.0%) both from Oromia regional state of Ethiopia. Nine kebeles were included in the study with highest prevalence from Adis Ketema (136/137) (99.3%) and the lowest from Geriro (n=19/23) (82.6%).The difference observed was statistically significant (P=0.000). Hundred nasal swabs were used for identification of MERS-CoV from Yabelo, Fentale, Dubti and Amibara district by RT-PCR. Twenty five swabs from each district except Yabelo MERS-CoV was recovered from all the districts sampled. From the overall 7 identified MERS-CoV cases, Amibara district account the highest (n=4/100) (4%) this may relate with the highest seroprevalence recorded in the area (n=94/95) (98.9%).

Chu et al. (2014) reported identification of MERS-CoV (n=4/110 swabs) (3.6%) from dromedary camels of Egypt using RT-PCR, the same molecular technique used in the current study except MERS-CoV strain (variant) was not identified.

Conclusion

There was high seroprevalence of MERS-CoV evident in the study area (Afar=92.3% and Oromia =93.9%), regional states of Ethiopia. The seroprevalence evidence was supported by identification of the virus by RT-PCR, which indicates existence of active infection of MRS-CoV in the study area. Among 569 Dromedary camel sampled, highest prevalence was observed in East Shoa, Fentale district and the lowest in Borena, Yabelo district both from Oromia regional state of Ethiopia.

The study also implies the probability of circulation of MERS-CoV in human being in the study areas, due to the zoonotic nature of the virus and is transmissibility between Dromedary camel and human. Therefore, further study should be conducted to identify which specific factors favor the high prevalence observed, identify the strain (variant) of MERS-CoV in the area and serological and molecular characterization to check the status of the disease in human beings in Ethiopia.

ACKNOWLEDGEMENTS

The authors acknowledge Addis Ababa University, Haramaya University and National Veterinary Institute for their financial support. The authors are also very grateful to the camel owners and field staff who gave their time to this research.

REFERENCES

Abedine, Saad (2013). Death toll from new SARS-like virus climbs to 9. CNN news March 13, 2013 NRSP (2010): Semera, Ethiopia. P 67.

Assiri A, McGeer A, Perl TM (2013). Hospital outbreak of Middle East respiratory syndromecoronavirus. N. Engl. J. Med. **369**(5):407-416.

Chan RW, Chan MC, Agnihothram S, Chan LL, Kuok DI, Fong JH, GuanY, Poon LL, Baric RS, Nicholls JM, Peiris JS (2013). Tropism of innate immune responses to the novel human betacoronavirus lineage C virus in human ex vivo respiratory organ cultures. J. Virol. **87**(12):6604-6614.

Chu DKW, Poon LLM, Gomaa MM, Shehata MM, Perera RA, Zeid DA (2014). MERS coronaviruses in dromedary camels, Egypt. Emerg. Infect. Dis. 20(6):1049-53.

CSA (2008). Agricultural sampling survey report on area and crop production, Addis Ababa.

Gautret P, Charrel R, Belhouchat K, Drali T, Benkouiten S, Nougairede A, Zandotti C, Memish ZA, al Masri M, Gaillard C, Brouqui P, Parola P, (2013). Lack of nasal carriage of novel coronavirus (HCoV-EMC) in French Hajj pilgrims returning from the Hajj 2012, despite a high rate of respiratory symptoms. 29(7):E315-E317.

Hemida MG, Perera RA, Wang P (2013). Middle East respiratory syndrome (MERS) coronavirus Seroprevalence in domestic livestock in Saudi Arabia, 2010 to 2013. Eurosurvill.50, 200659.

Marshall K (2014). The Complex and Gender Differentiated Objectives of Livestock Keeping for Somali Pastoralists. Proceedings of the 10th World Congress of Genetics Applied to Livestock Production, Vancouver, Canada.

Reusken CB (2015). Occupational Exposure to Dromedaries and Risk for MERS-CoV Infection, Qatar, 2013-2014, Emerg. Infect. Dis. 21(8):1422-1425.

Reusken CBEM, Haagmans BL, Muller MA, Ashenafi F, Fufa D, Endrias Z, Lilia M, Hussaini U, Simenew M, Gert-Jan G, Yusuf W, Marion PG (2013). Middle East respiratory syndrome coronavirus neutralising serum antibodies in dromedary camels: a comparative serological study. Lancet Infect. Dis. 13(10):859-866.

Thrusfield M (2007). Veterinary Epidemiology, 3rd Edition, University of Edinburgh, Scotland UK.

WHO (2013). Coronavirus infections. Available at: http://www.who.int/csr/don/archive/%20Disease%20coronavirus_infections/en/

Zaki AM, van Boheemen S, Bestebroer TM, Osterhaus AD, Fouchier RA (2012). Isolation of a novel coronavirus from a man with pneumonia in Saudi Arabia. N. Engl. J. Med. 367(19):1.

5

Composition, prevalence and abundance of Ixodid cattle ticks at Ethio-Kenyan Border, Dillo district of Borana Zone, Southern Ethiopia

Golo Dabasa[1], Wubishet Zewdei[1], Tadelle Shanko[1], Kula Jilo[2*], Gete Gurmesa[1] and Garu Lolo[1]

[1]Yabello Regional Veterinary Laboratory, P.O. Box 169 Yabello, Ethiopia.
[2]School of Veterinary Medicine, College of Agriculture and Veterinary Medicine, Jimma University, Jimma, Ethiopia.

Ixodid ticks are common and a major obstacle to development and utilization of animal resource in tropical countries like Ethiopia. Ethiopia shares long international frontiers with adjacent countries, tick dynamics and influx of ticks across the border are major obstacles of tick control and management. Thus, border-oriented epidemiological surveys are of paramount importance to identify a potential port of cross border diseases, particularly ticks and to formulate complimentary bilateral policies. The current study was therefore, designed with the objectives to assess prevalence, abundance and to identify genera and species of major ixodid tick of cattle circulating at Ethio-Kenyan border. A cross-sectional study was conducted from November 2016 to January 2017 in purposively selected four Pastoral Associations of Dillo district, Southern Ethiopia. A total of 7524 adult ticks were randomly collected from 384 cattle and examined with a stereomicroscope. Logistic regression was used to determine the association of risk factors with positivity for Ixodid ticks. The study revealed an overall prevalence of 98.2% of Ixodid ticks of cattle. Three genera of ticks, *Rhipicephalus* (including the subgenus *Boophilus*), *Amblyomma* and *Hyalomma* and seven species of ticks were identified and found to be abundant with overall mean burdens of 40 ticks/head. The association of age and body condition of animals to tick infestation were statistically significant but there was no significant association between sex and tick infestation (OR=3, P=0.007). Animals in poor body condition were twice more likely to be infested with tick than animals with good body condition (OR=2, P=0.031) and animals with medium body condition were also found more prone to tick infestation than animals in good body condition (OR=1.7, P=0.043). Ixodid ticks that were less abundant in most parts of the country were encountered as well adapted and widely distributed in this area. Uncontrolled animal movement across the border may play a great role in high density and diversification of tick in Dillo district. Therefore, collaborative nationwide studies was done to have the country-wide distribution figures and to identify a potential port of cross border diseases particularly ticks and to formulate complimentary bilateral policies for prevention and control of ticks.

Key words: Ixodid, tick, cattle, Dillo, Borena, cross border disease.

INTRODUCTION

Ethiopia is endowed with a very large and diverse livestock resource, composed of approximately 56.71 million cattle, 29.33 million sheep, 29.11 million goats, 2.03 million horses, 7.43 million donkeys, 0.4 million mules, 1.16 million camels, 56.87 million poultry and 5.88 million bee hives (CSA, 2016). The livestock subsector contributes to 12 and 33% of the total and agricultural GDP, respectively, and accounts for 12 to 15% of the total export earnings, second in order of importance (Ayele et al., 2003; Minjauw and Mcleod, 2003; Argaw, 2014). Nevertheless, cattle productivity is low, with hide represents a major source of foreign exchange earnings for the country that accounts for 14 to 16% of the total export revenue. In addition to a large contribution to the export earnings, hides and skins also contribute much to the domestic leather industry (Argaw, 2014).

Despite the relatively large animal population with a high potential for production, its utilization is far lower than could be expected due to cattle production in Ethiopia is constrained by the compound effects of animal diseases, poor management and low genetic performance (Dabassa et al., 2013; Abdela and Jilo 2016; Jilo and Tegegne 2016; Jilo and Adem 2016; Jilo et al., 2016; Jilo 2016; Jilo et al., 2017; Dabasa et al., 2017). External parasites are common and a major obstacle to development and utilization of animal resources in tropical countries because of the favorable climatic conditions for their development and the poor standards of husbandry practices (Solomon et al., 1998; Mungube et al., 2008; Yalew et al., 2017; Dabassa et al., 2017). In Ethiopia, ticks occupy the first place amongst the external parasites that cause serious economic loss to small holder farmers, the tanning industry and the country as a whole through mortality of animals, decreased production, downgrading and general rejection of skins and hides (Tikit and Addis, 2011; Dabassa et al., 2017).

Beside direct effect of irritation, discomfort, tissue damage, blood loss, toxicosis, allergies and dermatitis ticks are the most important ecto-parasites of the livestock in tropical and sub-tropical areas due to their ability to transmit protozoan, rickettsial and viral diseases of livestock, which are of great economic importance world-wide (Jaswal et al., 2014; Salih et al., 2015; Dabassa et al., 2017). The most economically cover important ixodid ticks of livestock in tropical regions belong to the genera of *Hyalomma*, *Rhipicephalus* and *Amblyomma* (Jongejan and Uilenberg, 2004). Several tick genera are widely distributed in Ethiopia. The major tick genera recorded are *Amblyomma*, *Haemaphysalis*, *Hyalomma* and *Rhipicephalus*. Over 60 tick species are known to exist in Ethiopia and the most economically important and wide spread ticks are *A. variegatum* and *R. pulchellus*. In Ethiopia, more than half of total ticks are confined to arid and semi-arid areas at periphery for advantage of suitable climate condition and abundance of hosts (livestock) while tick densities are usually greater in lowland than highland areas (Pegram et al., 1981). In addition to the climatic advantages and adequacy of host animals, insufficient veterinary extension services combined with extensive management systems have exacerbated tick burdens in arid and semi-arid parts of the country (Jilo et al., 2016). Given the long international borders (mainly covered by lowlands) that Ethiopia shares with adjacent countries, tick dynamics and influx of ticks from neighboring countries are major obstacles of tick control and management.

Although, a number of studies have attempted to know burden, distribution and abundance of tick species in different parts of the country, they were largely restricted to central highlands for accessibility and availability of infrastructures. However, the most infested peripheral lowlands bordering adjacent countries are not yet studied well to have the country wide distribution figures, to identify a potential port of cross border diseases particularly ticks and to formulate complimentary bilateral policies for prevention and control of ticks. Thus, the current study was designed to be conducted at the arid area of Southern lowland at the Ethiopia-Kenya border in Dillo district, possessing a large livestock population and where no single study from any scientific discipline has been conducted before, with the objectives of assessing prevalence and abundance, identifying genera and species of major ixodid tick of cattle circulating at the border and to recommend formulation and implementation of joint policy for prevention and control of tick and tick induced losses.

MATERIALS AND METHODS

Description of study area

The study was conducted in Dillo district located at 695 km at South of Addis Ababa, the capital city of Ethiopia. Dillo district is one of the entirely pastoral areas in Borana zone located at the South most part of the country and bordered on the south and southwest (Kenya), Northwest (Teltelle district), Northeast (Yabello district) and East (Dubluk and Dirre districts). Agroecologically, its characterized by an arid climate with altitude ranging from 521 to 1420 m above sea level and temperatures from 22 to 40°C. The area receives low, erratic and bimodal with a mean annual rainfall about 450 mm. There is considerable spatial and temporal variability in quantities and distribution of rainfall, where about 60% is covered by long rainy season (*Ganna*) extending from mid-March to May and erratic short rain season (*Hagayya*) is received from mid-September through mid-November.

Study design and study population

Cross-sectional study design was used to determine the tickspecies, population dynamics and mean burden of adult tick species in different predilection site, age groups and sex of animal. The study animal was cattle from four purposively selected PAs of

*Corresponding author. E-mail: kula.jilo1@gmail.com. Tel: +25116323883.

Dillo district based on distribution of tick as told by woreda animal health experts and indigenous knowledge of the community. Accordingly, lowland areas with reddish brown fragile soil, locally called "*Golbo*" like Arbale and Kadim are relatively free of tick, while Northern and Northeastern part of Dillo covered by dark cracking soil (clay), locally called "*Koticha*" are pointed out for study as severe infestation of ticks is found abundant. Likewise, four PAs from *Koticha* land (Goray, Liso, Kancharo and Magole) were selected and adult ticks were randomly sampled from 384 indigenous cattle by considering age, sex and body condition as risk factors. Body conditions were determined as described previously by Eversole et al. (2005). For convenience, animals <1.5 and ≥1.5 year were considered as young and adult, respectively.

The desired sample size for the study was calculated using the formula given by Thrusfield (2005) with 95% confidence interval and 5% absolute precision. $N = 1.96^{2} * P_{exp}(1\text{-Pexp})/D^{2}$ Where; n = sample size, Pexp = expect prevalence and D = absolute precision (5%). There was no previously published and documented prevalence in the study area and therefore, sample size was calculated using expected prevalence of 50% by substituting the value, the required sample size was calculated and found to be 384 (Thrusfield, 2005). Study was conducted during short rainy season in November, the collected ticks were transported to Yabello Regional Veterinary Laboratory for acaroscopy. Counting and identification of ticks were done using hand lens and stereomicroscope according to standard taxonomic identification procedure described by (Keirans et al., 1999).

Data management and statistical analysis

All collected data were entered to Micro-Soft Excel sheet 2010 and analyzed by SPSS version 20. Descriptive statistics was used to determine the frequency and percentage of both dependent and independent variables. The prevalence was calculated as percent of infested animals from the total number of animals examined. Logistic regression was applied to assess association of risk factors and strength of the association. For statistical analysis, a confidence level of 95% and a *P*-values less than 5% were judged as significant.

RESULTS

Overall prevalence and distribution of ticks in the different PAs in the study area

From this study, Ixodid ticks of cattle were found highly prevalent in Dillo district with overall prevalence of 98.2% (377/384) and within different PAs of current study area 100, 97.9, 97.7 and 97% prevalence of Ixodid ticks of cattle were recorded in Kancharo, Liso, Magole and Goray, respectively (Table 3). *Rhipicephalus* (including *Rhipicephalus Boophilus*), *Amblyomma*, *Hyalomma* and *Boophilus* were the four important genera of ticks identified with a total prevalence of 98.2, 96.8, 64.3 and 42.4%, respectively. While eight species of ticks with their total prevalence were *Rhipicephalus pulchellus* (68.7%), *Rhipicephalus decoloratus* (42.4%) *Rhipicephalus pravus* (29.4%), *Ambylomma* (65.8%), *Ambylomma lepidum* (30.9%), *Hyalomma truncatum* (19.2%), *Hyalomma* rufipes (25.7) and Hyalomma impeltatum (19.2%) (Table 6 and 7).

Relative abundance of tick genera and species

A total of 7524 adult ixodid ticks were collected from different body regions of 377 cattle that were found to be positive for tick infestation and consequently sampled. Generally, three Ixodidae tick genera and eight species were identified from the study area. The genera *Rhipicephalus* (81.1%, of which 1.1% belonged to the subgenus *Boophilus*), *Ambylomma* (16.5%) and *Hyalomma* (3.2%) were abundant in this study area (96.2%) (Table 2). Regarding tick species distribution, *R. pulchellus* was the most abundant tick species, representing 75.2% of the total ticks in Dillo district, followed by *R. pravus* (35.5%), *Ambylomma gemma* (11.6%) and *A. lepidium* (4.8%), respectively. In contrast, *H. rufipes* (1.8%), *R. decoloratus* (1.1%) and *H. impeltatum* (0.09%) were the least abundant Ixodid species in the study district (Table 4 and 5).

Male to female ratio for tick genera and species

Male to female ratio for tick genera of this result indicates higher number of males for most species except genus *Boophilus* that have higher ratio of female tick. Similarly, at the level of species of ticks higher ratio of male to female was obtained except, *R. decoloratus* (Table 6 and 7).

Tick distribution

The spatial distribution of tick genera and species on the body of the animal was considered in this study. As a result, ticks were found widely distributed in different parts of the hosts' body such as ear, sternum, dewlap, scrotum, udder, anal-vulval area and tail. Ear (13 ticks/head), scrotum (10 ticks/head), udder (10 ticks/head), sternum (8 ticks/head), dewlap (8 ticks/head), anal area (6 ticks/head) and vulvar regions (6 ticks/head) were heavily infested but the tail (3 ticks/head of animal) was lightly infested with ticks (Tables 5 and 6). Among three genera of Ixodid ticks, *Rhipicephalus* was found as the only genus infesting the ear of the animal while the other two genera were spread on different body parts of the animal, except the ear.

Risk factors

Age of the animal was found statistically significant for infestation of Ixodid tick and from two age groups prevalence of tick were relatively higher in adult (100%) than the young (92%) and multivariable logistic regression revealed that adults are about three times more likely to be prone to tick infestation than young animals (OR=3, P =0.007) (Table 1). Regarding sex of animal, the tick prevalence was 98.6 and 96.7% in

Table 1. Logistic regression analysis (univariable and multivariable) output of risk factors associated with Ixodid ticks in cattle in Dillo district.

Risk factor		No. of animal examined	No. of animal positive	Prevalence	Univariable regression		Multivariable	
					COR (95% CI)	P-value	AOR (95% CI)	P-value
Age	<1.5year	87	81	92%	4(11.8-83.21)	0.000	10.23(1.89-55.19)	0.007
	≥1.5year	297	297	100%				
Sex	Male	91	88	96.7%	0.8(0.586-1.578)	0.77	0.34(0.063-1.87)	0.914
	Female	293	289	98.6%				
Body condition	Poor	201	201	100%	3.2(2.82-5.84)		2(2.55-4.67)	0.331
	Medium	149	148	99.3%	2.12(1.27-7.52)	0.032	1.7(1.25-6.73)	0.043
	Good	34	28	82.4%	Ref*		Ref*	

Table 2. Distribution and prevalence of tick genera among age, sex and body conditions of cattle in Dillo district.

Parameters		Tick genera identified, Total animal examined(n=384)									
		Rhipicephallus		*Ambylomma*		*Hyalomma*		*Rhipicephallus (Boophilus)*		Multispecies	
		Examined/+ve animal	% from total	Examined /+ve animal	% from total	Examined /+ve animal	% from total	Examined /+ve animal	% from total	Examined /+ve animal	% from total
Age	<1.5	87/80	20.8	87/76	19.7	87/53	13.8	87/47	12.2	87/76	19.7
	≥1.5	297/297	77.3	297/296	77.0	297/194	50.5	297/116	30.2	297/296	77.0
Sex	M*	91/88	22.9	91/84	21.8	91/64	16.7	91/57	14.8	91/84	21.8
	F	293/289	75.2	293/288	75.0	293/183	47.6	293/106	27.6	293/288	75.0
BCS	P	201/201	52.3	201/200	51.5	201/103	26.8	201/71	18.5	201/198	51.5
	M	149/148	38.5	149/146	37.2	149/118	30.7	149/80	20.8	149/143	37.2
	G	34/28	7.3	34/26	6.7	34/26	6.7	34/12	3.1	34/31	8.0

Table 3. Prevalence of Ixodid tick of cattle among PAs in Dillo district.

PA	Animal examined	Prevalence
Goray	100	97(97%)
Liso	96	94(97.9%)
Kancharo	98	98(100%)
Magole	90	88(97.7%)
Total	384	377(98.2)

Table 4. Distribution of tick genera on the animal.

Genus	No. of animal positive	Prevalence	Mean burden
Rhipicephallus	377	98.2%	31.6
Ambylomma	372	96.8%	6.6
Hyalomma	247	64.3%	2
Rh.(Boophilus)	163	42.4%	1
Multispecies	372	96.2%	6.6

Total animal examined (n=384).

Table 5. Distribution of major Ixodid ticks of cattle on predilection sites of animal body in Dillo district.

Body region	*Rhipicephallus*	*Ambylomma*	*Hyalomma*	*Boophilus*	Total	Mean burden
Ear	2383	0	0	6	2389	13
Sternum/dew	894	555	11	21	1481	8
Scrotum/udder	1488	495	5	24	2012	10
Ano-vulva	714	181	224	3	1122	6
Tip of Tail	477	8	3	32	520	3
Total	5956	1239	243	86	7524	40
Mean burden	31.6	6.6	2	1	40	

Table 6. Male to female ratio and percentages of identified genera of Ixodid ticks of cattle and their predilection site on the animal body in Dillo district, Southern Ethiopia.

Genus	Male : Female (Male/Female)	Percentage of total tick	Predilection sites
Rhipicephallus	2.3:1(4167/1783)	79%(5950/7524)	Ear
Ambylomma	2.6:1(899/346)	16.5%(1245/7524)	Sternum,dew,scrotum,udder, ano-vulva and tail
Hyalomma spp.	3.4:1(188/55)	3.2%(243/7524)	Sternum,dew,scrotum,udder, ano-vulva and tail
Boophilus spp.	0.4:1(24/62)	1.1%(86/7524)	Sternum,dew,scrotum,udder, ano-vulva and tail

female and male. There was no statistical (P=0.914) significance between the two sexes (Table 1). Out of the 384 animals examined, 34 were in good body condition, of which 28 (82.4%) were positive to tick infestation, 149 (38.8%) were in medium body condition and 148 (99.3%) were positive for tick infestation and the remaining 201 animals were of poor body condition and all of them, 201 (100%) were positive to tick infestation. Tick prevalence among body condition of animal varies and it was statistically significant. By multivariable logistic regression analysis animal with poor body condition was twice more likely to be infested with tick than animal with good body condition (OR=2, P=0.031) and animal with medium body condition was also found more prone to tick infestation than the animal in state of good body condition (OR=1.7, P=0.043) (Table 1).

DISCUSSION

A number of researchers have reported that different tick genera are widely distributed in Ethiopia (Solomon et al., 2001). In the present study, a total of 7524 adult ticks were sampled from 384 cattle and overall prevalence of tick infestation was found to be 98.2%. To the best of the authors' knowledge, this finding is the highest report ever reported from Ethiopia. For instance, lower prevalence of 16.0% in Benchi Maji Zone, Southern Ethiopia (Tesfahewet and Simeon, 2013), 33.21% in Haramaya district, Eastern Ethiopia (Kassa and Yalew, 2012), 40.26% in and round Haramaya town, Eastern Ethiopia (Yalew et al., 2017), 81.25% in Dembia district, Northern Ethiopia (Alemu et al., 2014), 82% in Borena province of southern Oromia (Regassa, 2001), 88.8% in Jimma district, Western Ethiopia (Chali *et al.,* 2017), 89.4% from Western Amhara Region, Northern Ethiopia (Nigatu and Teshome, 2012) and 95.2% in Bedelle district, Southwestern Ethiopia (Abera et al., 2010), were reported from different parts of the country. The highest prevalence in the current study area could be largely by presence of wide range of cracking soil that helps larva of ticks to stay long and survive, season of study (wet season), short and sticky grasses used for adherence of adult ticks and their transmission to grazing animals, large livestock population and herd size may also contribute as ticks can easily get access to host and complete their life cycle to perpetuate rapidly. Furthermore, arid agro-ecology, poor veterinary extension service, sedentary management practice employed by herders might also pave the way for the highest tick infestation. Ecto-parasites are common in tropical countries because of the favorable climatic conditions for their development and the poor standards of husbandry practices (Mungube et al., 2008).

Rhipicephalus (including ticks of the subgenus *Boophilus*), *Amblyomma* and *Hyalomma* were the three important genera of ticks identified with a total prevalence of 98.2, 96.8, 64.3 and 42.4%, respectively. While eight species of ticks have total prevalence of: *R. pulchellus* (68.7%), *R. pravus* (29.4%), *R. decoloratus* (42.4%) *A. gemma* (65.8%), *A. lepidium* (30.9%), *H. truncatum* (19.2%), *H. rufipes* (25.7%) and *H. impeltatum* (19.2%). Among the total, *R. pulchellus* (68.7%) was found to be highly prevalent in this area and this finding was higher

Table 7. Male to female ratio, percentages and prevalence of identified species of Ixodid ticks of cattle and their predilection site on the animal body in Dillo district, Southern Ethiopia.

Species	Male : Female	Percentage of tick	N(Prevalence)	Predilection sites
Rhipicephalus pulchellus	2.4:1(3994/1665)	75.2%(5659/7524)	264(68.7%)	Ear
Rhipicephalus pravus	1.46:1(173/118)	35.5%(291/7524)	113(29.4%)	Ear
Ambylomma gemma	2.47: 1(621/251)	11.6%(872/7524)	253(65.8%)	Sternum, dew, scrotum, udder, ano-vulva and tail
Ambylomma lepidium	2.8:1(278/95)	4.8%(373/7524)	119(30.9%)	Sternum, dew, scrotum, udder, ano-vulva and tail
Hyalomma truncatum	4.2:1(75/18)	1.2%(93/7524)	74(19.2)	Sternum, dew, scrotum, udder, ano-vulva and tail
Hyalomma marginatum rufipes	3.25:1(108/34)	1.8%(142/7524)	99(25.7)	Sternum, dew, scrotum, udder, ano-vulva and tail
Hyalomma impeltatum	2:1(5/3)	0.09%(8/7524)	74(19.2%)	Sternum, dew, scrotum, udder, ano-vulva and tail
Boophilus decolaratus	0.38:1(24/62)	1.1%(72/7524)	163(42.4%)	Sternum, dew, scrotum, udder, ano-vulva and tail

than 5.46% in East Hararghe (Bedasso et al., 2014), or 6.4% from East Hararghe (Yalew et al., 2017). This could be due to arid climate condition and savanna and steppe vegetation in thr current study area. *R. pulchellus* is prevalent in the arid and desert climatic regions with savanna and steppe grasses (Pegram et al., 1981; Feseha, 1983).

On the other hand, *A. gemma* (65.8%) was the second most prevalent tick species in the present study which was by far more than 2.42% from Jimma high land (Chali et al., 2017) and 8.3% from Mizan Teferi (Tadesse et al., 2012). Higher prevalence of *A. gemma* in Dillo district could be due to the arid climate condition which as reported by many scholars are very suitable for *A. gemma*. Pegram et al. (1981) stated that *A. gemma* is confined to semi-arid lands due to humidity of highland which is not favorable to their survival. As a result, this tick species was collected from restricted area of arid, semi-arid plain and bush land receiving 100 to 800 mm rainfall annually (Morel, 1980). Morel (1980) also stated that *A. gemma* is widely distributed in woodland, bush land, wooded and grassland in arid and semiarid area between altitude 500 and 1750 m above sea level and receiving 350 to 750 mm annual rain fall.

Rhipicephalus (Boophilus) decolaratus was third abundant tick species in the current study area with prevalence of 42.4%. Similar finding has also been reported from Rift Valley (Solomon et al., 2001) and in Girana valley of North Wollo (Zenebe, 2001) and Western Ethiopia (Amante et al., 2014). Contrary to our results, Morel (1980) stated that *R. decoloratus* is often collected in Ethiopia and does not seem really abundant anywhere. Pegram et al. (1981) also added that this tick species is abundant in wetter highlands and sub-highlands receiving more than 800 mm rainfall annually and has similar distribution to *A. variegatum*. *R. (Boophilus) decolaratus* can transmit *Babesia bigemina* and *Anaplasma marginale* to cattle and severe tick infestation can lead to tick problem, anorexia and anemia (Singh et al., 2000; Silashi et al., 2001).

A. lepidium (30.9%), and *R. pravus* (29.4%), was also a prevalent species collected from this study area. Regassa (2001) reported that *R. pravus* (about 8%) is from Southern Ethiopia which disagrees with the current result on *R. pravus*. Wasihun and Doda (2013) reported lower finding of 6.68% *A. lepidum* from Humbo district. It was also reported that *A. lepidum* was common but not abundant in Wolaita zone according to Dessie and Getachew (2006). It is limited by semi-desert conditions (Morel, 1980). It is also known as the "East African bont tick" and is common in many of the semi-arid regions of East Africa (Walker et al., 2003). This is also similar with the findings of Mesele et al. (2010) in Bedelle district. In southwest of Ethiopia including Gambella region and western Oromiya, this tick species was also reported with less abundance by several workers (Pegram et al., 1981) which agrees with the current result. In Gambella region, *A. lepidum* transmits *Rickettsia. ruminantium*, the organism that causes cowdriosis. *A. lepidum* was irregularly dispersed throughout most of the country and was collected from Tigray, Amhara, Oromiya, SNNP and Harare Regional States (Sileshi et al., 2007).

H. rufipes was the sixth most prevalent tick with prevalence of 25.7%. This result was higher than 2.5% report from Asella (Tessema and Gashaw, 2010). This tick species was restricted to warm, moderately dry mid lands areas between altitudes of 1800 and 1950 masl (Tessema and Gashaw, 2010). Hoogstraal (1956) stated that *H. rufipes* is widely distributed in the most arid parts of tropical Africa, receiving 250 to 650 mm annual rainfall and his results concur with the current study findings.

Risk factors (age, sex and body condition) were also

involved in the variations of the prevalence of ticks in the study area. Statistically significant association of tick infestation with age and body condition score of study animal was found. However, association of tick infestation and sexes of study animal were not statistically significant. Multivariable logistic regression analysis revealed that adults are about three times more likely to be prone to tick infestation than young animals (OR=3, P =0.007). These results were lined with findings of Bossena and Abdu (2012), Gedilu et al. (2014) and Admassu et al. (2015) but different from that of Kassa and Yalew (2012) and Tesfaheywet and Simeon (2013). This variation could be due to management; animals in different age groups were managed differently. In the current study area, younger animals (<1.5 year) are kept indoor for 1.5 to 2 years in a small separate housing locally called "dokoba" and as a result, unlike adult animals, younger animals have no access to harbor ticks from the field. Young animals are affected less than adult animals due to the less exposure to field grazing with other animals in the field and adults are exposed due to the communal grazing habit (Admassu et al., 2015).

By multivariable logistic regression analysis, animal with poor body condition was twice more likely to be infested with tick than animal with good body condition (OR=2, P=0.031) and animal with medium body condition was also found more prone to tick infestation than the animal in the state of good body condition (OR=1.7, P=0.043). This may due to the fact that ticks have contributed to emaciation of infested animals by causing anemia and stress. Insignificant association obtained between sex of animals and tick infestation concurred with the results of Kassa and Yalew (2012) and this might be due to equal opportunities of oxen and cows to tick infestation since they are kept extensively under similar agro-ecology and management condition.

Concerning predilection sites of ticks on the host body, different tick species were found to be having preference for predilection sites in this study. Accordingly, *R. pulchellus* and *R. pravus* had strong preference for ear, while *Ambylomma, Hyalomma* and the *Boophilus* subgenus were distributed on sternum, dewlap, scrotum, udder, ano-vulva and tail. This result was in line with the results of Stachurski (2000) and Tesgera et al. (2017), who stated that short hypostome ticks like *Rhipicephalus* usually prefer soft tissues like ear while, long hypostome ticks like *Amblyomma* attaches to lower parts of the animal body which is also the case in the current study. Cattle in this study were heavily infested and mean burden of tick was high (mean = 40 ticks/head). This finding was higher that reports of Alemu et al. (2014) from North west Ethiopia with mean = 13.1 tick/head. This variation in mean burden could be justified as tick densities are usually greater in lowland than highland areas (Pelgram, 1981).

The male to female sex ratio of the ticks were higher and similar to previous reports (Solomon et al., 2007; Chali et al., 2017). In all cases, except *R. decoloratus,* males outnumbered females. This is due to fully engorged female ticks drop off on the ground to lay egg while the male tends to remain on the host before dropping off and hence males normally remain on the host longer than females (Solomon et al., 2001).

CONCLUSION AND RECOMMENDATIONS

From this study Ixodid ticks of cattle were found to be highly prevalent in Dillo district with overall prevalence of 98.2%, the highest prevalence ever reported in Ethiopia to the best of the authors' knowledge. Three important genera of ticks, *Rhipicephalus* (including the subgenus *Boophilus*), *Amblyomma* and *Hyalomma* were identified and were found to be highly prevalent and abundant with overall mean burden of 40 ticks/head which was again highest burden of tick in Ethiopia. Eight species of Ixodid tick that were less abundant in most parts of the country were encountered as well as adapted and widely distributed in this area. Climatic advantage and adequacy of host animals for ticks, insufficient veterinary extension service combined with extensive management system may have contributed to the highest tick burden in the current study area. Additionally, Since, Ethiopia shares border of about 600 km with Kenya at this district and animal movement across the border during shortages of pasture and water may play a great role in high density and diversification of tick genera and species circulating around Dillo district. Therefore, both countries need to conduct collaborative nationwide studies to show the country wide distribution figures and to identify a potential port of cross border diseases particularly ticks and to formulate complimentary bilateral policies for prevention and control of ticks. Moreover, researchers in this regard should pay more attention on neglected lowland areas at peripheries that are at risk of tick and tick-borne diseases than any other part of the country.

REFERENCES

Abdela N, Jilo K (2016). Impact of Climate Change on Livestock Health: A Review. Glob. Vet. 16(5):419-424.

Abera M, Mohammed T, Abebe R, Aragaw K, Bekele J (2010) "Survey of ixodid ticks in domestic ruminants in Bedelle district, Southwestern Ethiopia. Trop. Anim. Health Prod. 42(8):1677-1683.

Admassu B, Yeneneh H, Shite A, Haile B, Mohammed S(2015). Prevalence and identification of major ixodid Tick genera of Ccttle in Dangila District, Awi Zone, North West Ethiopia. Acta Parasitol. Glob. 6(2):129-135.

Alemu G, Chanie M, Mengesha D, Bogale B (2014). Prevalence of ixodid ticks on cattle in Northwest Ethiopia. Acta Parasitol. Glob. 5(2):139-145.

Amante M, Alelgn Z, Hirpa E (2014) Prevalence of ixodid ticks on cattle in and around Diga Town, West Ethiopia. European J. Biol. Sci. 6(1):25-32.

Argaw D (2014).Marketing chain and quality management of hide and skin in Tiyo and Digelu-Tijo woreda, East Arsi zone, oromia reginal state, Ethiopia, MSc. Thesis, Department of Animal Production Studies, College of Veterinary Medicine and Agriculture, Addis Ababa University, Bishoftu, Ethiopia.

Ayele S, Assegid W, Jabbar M, Ahmed M, Belachew A (2003). A Review of Structure, Performance and Development Initiatives, Working Paper No. 52, Addis Ababa, Ethiopia. pp:1-14.

Bedasso M, Abebe B, Degefu H (2014). Species composition, prevalence and seasonal variations of ixodid cattle ticks in and around Haramaya town, Ethiopia. J. Vet. Med. Anim. Health 6(5):131-137.

Bossena F, Abdu M (2012). Survey on the Distribution of Tick Species in and Around Assosa Town, Ethiopia. Res. J. Vet. Sci. 5:32-41.

Chali E, Melaku M, Negero J (2017). Study on cattle tick species frequency distribution in and around Jimma province of Ethiopia. J. Parasitol. Vect Biol. 9(4):34-38.

Central Statistical Agency (CSA) (2016).Federal democratic republic of Ethiopia. Central statistical agency. Agricultural sample survey, Volume II, Report on livestock and livestock characteristics. Statistical bulletin 583, Addis Ababa, Ethiopia.

Dabassa G, Addis M, Tefera M (2013).Small ruminants Brucellosis: Serological survey in Yabello district. Asian J. Anim. Sci. 7(1):14-21.

Dabassa G, Shanko T, Zewdei W, Jilo K, Gurmesa G, Abdela N (2017). Prevalence of small ruminant gastrointestinal parasites infections and associated risk factors in selected districts of Bale zone, south eastern Ethiopia. J. Parasitol. Vect. Biol. 9(6):81-88.

Dessie S, Getachew A (2006). Cattle tick dynamics in different agro-ecological zones of Wolaita, Southern Ethiopia. Ethiop. Vet. J. 10(2):85-99.

Eversole DE, Browne MF, Hall JB, Dietz RE (2005).Body condition scoring in beef cows. Virginia polytechnic and state university, Verginia, USA.

Feseha G (1983). Notes on tick species and tick borne diseases of domestic animals in Ethiopia, FVM, AAU, Ethiopia. pp: 1-64.

Gedilu M, Mohamed A, Kechero Y (2014).Determination of the Prevalence of Ixodid Ticks of Cattle Breeds, Their Predilection Sites of Variation and Tick Burden Between Different Risk Factors in Bahir Dar, Ethiopia. Jimma University College of Agriculture and Veterinary Medicine, Jimma, Ethiopia. Glob. Vet. **13**(4):520-529.

Hoogstraal H (1956). African Ixodoidea. Vol. I. Ticks of the Sudan (with special reference to Equatoria Province and with Preliminary Reviews of the Genera Boophilus, Margaropus, and Hyalomma). Afr. Ixodoidea. Vol. I. Available at: https://www.cabdirect.org/cabdirect/abstract/19572901469

Jaswal H, Bal MS, Singla LD, Amrita Kaur P, Mukhopadhyay CS, Juyal PD (2014) Application of msp1β PCR and 16S rRNA semi nested PCR-RFLP for detection of persistent anaplasmosis in tick infested cattle. Int. J. Adv. Res. 2(8):188-196.

Jilo K (2016). *Peste Des Petits Ruminants (PPR):* Global and Ethiopian Aspects. A standard review. Glob. Vet.17(2):142-153.

Jilo K, Abdela N, Adem J(2016).Insufficient Veterinary Service as a Major Constrants in Pastoral Area of Ethiopia: A Review, J. Biol. Agric. Healthcare **6**(9):94-101.

Jilo K, Abdela N, Dabasa G, Elias M, (2017). Camel Trypanosomiasis: A Review on Past and Recent Research in Africa and Middle East American-Eurasian J. Sci. Res. 12(1), 13-20

Jilo K, Adem J (2016). Toxoplasmosis and its Current Status in Ethiopia: A Review. Glob. Vet. 17(2):135-141.

Jilo K, Tegegne D, (2016). Chemical composition and medicinal values of camel milk. Intern. J. Res. Stud. Biosci. 4:13-25.

Jongejan F, Uilenberg G (2004).The global importance of ticks. Parasitology 129(S1):S3-S14.

Kassa SA, Yalew A (2012). Identification of Ixodide ticks of cattle in and around Hararamaya district, Eastern Ethiopia. Sci. J. Crop Sci. 1(1):32-38.

Keirans JE, Needham GR, Oliver Jr, JH (1999).The Ixodes ricinus complex worldwide: diagnosis of the species in the complex, hosts and distribution. Acarology IX 2:341-347.

Mesele A, Mohammed T, Abebe R, Aragaw K, Bekele J (2010).Survey of Ixodids ticks in Domestic ruminants in Bedelle district, south western Ethiopia. Trop. Anim. Health Prod. 42:1677-1683.

Minjauw B, Mcheod A (2003). Tick-born disease and poverty. The impact of ticks and tick-borne disease on the live hood of small-scale and marginal livestock owners in India and Eastern and Southern Africa. Research Report, DFID Animal Health Programme, Center for Tropical Veterinary Medicine, University of Edinburgh, UK. pp:1-116.

Morel P (1980). Study on Ethiopia ticks (Argasidae, Ixodidae) Republic of France, Ministry Of foreign affairs, French Vet Mission, Addis. C. J. E. V. T. pp:12: 332.

Mungube E, Bauni S, Tenhagen B, Wamae W, Nzioka M, Mohammed L, Nginyi M (2008). Prevalence of parasites of the local scavenging chickeni selected semi-arid zone of Eastern Kenya. Trop. Anim. Health Prod. Bull. 40:101-109.

Nigatu K, Teshome F (2012). Population dynamics of cattle ectoparasite in western Amhara National Regional State Ethiopia. J. Vet. Med. Anim. Health 4: 22

Pegram RG, Hoogstral H, Wassef HY (1981). Ticks (acarida ixodidae) of Ethiopia. I. Distribution, ecology and host relationship of species infesting livestock. Bull. Entomol. Res. 71:339-359.

Regassa A (2001). Tick infestation of Borana cattle in the Borana Province of Ethiopia. Onderstepoort J. Vet. Res. 68:41-45.

Wasihun P, Doda D (2013). Study on prevalence and identification of ticks in Humbo district, Southern Nations, Nationalities, and People's Region (SNNPR), Ethiopia J. Vet. Med. Anim. Health 5(3):73-80.

Salih DA, Hussein AM El and Singla LD (2015). Diagnostic approaches for tick-borne haemoparasitic diseases in livestock. J. Vet. Med. Anim. Health **7**(2):45-56

Silashi M, Hussein I, Bedane B (2001). The distribution of ixodid ticks in central Ethiopia. On Derstepoort J. Vet. Res. 68(4):243-251.

Singh AP, Singla LD, Singh A (2000). A study on the effects of macroclimatic factors on the seasonal population dynamics of *Boophilus micropus* (Canes, 1888) infesting the cross-bred cattle of Ludhiana district. Int. J. Anim. Sci. 15(1):29-31.

Solomon G, Nigist M, Kassa B (2001). Seasona variation of ticks on calves at Sebeta in western Shewa Zone. Ethiop. Vet. J. 7(1&2):17-30.

Solomon G, Silashi M, Niguist M, Thomas C, Getachew T, Abebe M, Genet B, Demeke S, Ejigu Z (2007). Distribution and seasonal variation of ticks on cattle at Ghibe Tolly in Central Ethiopia. Ethiopian Vet. J. 11:121-139.

Solomon G, Kassaye GP, Feseha G, Teferi G, Getachew T (1998). Ticks and tick borne diseases associated with indigenous cattle in Didtuyura Ranch, southern Ethiopia. Int. J. Trop. Insect Sci. 18(1):59 66.

Stachurski F (2000). Invasion of West African cattle by the tick Amblyomma variegatum. Med. Vet. Entomol. 14(4):391-399.

Tadesse F, Abadfaji G, Girma S, kumsa B ,Jibat T(2012). Identification of tick species and their preferred site on cattle's body in and around Mizan Teferi, Southwestern Ethiopia. J. Vet. Med. Anim. Health 4(1):1-5.

Tesfahewet Z ,Simeon H (2013). Prevalence of ectoparasite infestations of cattle in Bench Maji zone, southwest Ethiopia. Vet. World 6(6):291-294.

Tesgera T, Regassa F, Giro B, Mohammed A (2017). Study on prevalence and identification of ixodid ticks in cattle in Gursum district, East Hararghe Zone of Oromia Regional State, Ethiopia. J. Parasitol. Vect. Biol. 9(4):27-33.

Tessema T, Gashaw A (2010). Prevalence of ticks on local and crossbred cattle in and around Asella town, southeast Ethiopia.
Ethiopian Vet. J. 14(2):79-89.

Thrusfield M (2005).Veterinary Epidemiology. 3rd ed. UK: Black well science ltd. P 233.

Tikit B, Addis M (2011). Distribution of Ixodid Ticks on Cattle in and Around Holeta Town, Ethiopia. Glob. Vet. 7(6):527-531.

Walker AA, Bouatour A, Camicas JL, Estadapena AA, Harok IG, Hatif AA, Pegram RG, Preton PM (2003).Ticks of domestic animals in Africa: A guide to identification species. The University of Edinburgh, UK pp:67-80.

Yalew A, Adugna S, Keffale M (2017). Identification of Major Ixodid Ticks on Cattle in and Around Haramaya Town, Eastern Hararghe,

6

Prevalence of bovine of schistosomosis in and around Nekemte, East Wollega zone, Western Ethiopia

Abriham Kebede[1]* Jiregna Dugassa[1], Geremew Haile[1] and Berhanu Wakjira[2]

[1]School of Veterinary Medicine, College of Medical and Health Science, Wollega University, P. O. Box, 395, Nekemte, Ethiopia.
[2]School of Veterinary Medicine, College of Agriculture and Veterinary Medicine, Jimma University, Ethiopia.

A cross-sectional study was conducted from March 2016 to May 2016 at Guto Gida District, Nekemte, Ethiopia to determine the prevalence of bovine schistosomosis. Simple random sampling method was used to select the study animals and sedimentation technique was applied for finding *Schistosoma* eggs from fresh fecal samples. Out of 384 fecal samples examined, 22 were found positive indicating an overall prevalence of 5.7% schistosomosis in the study area. The prevalence of bovine schistosomosis was higher in Jirenga kebele (9.1%) than Gaarii kebele (4.6%) and Dalo kebele (3.7%). However, no statistically significant difference in the prevalence of bovine schistosomiasis in relation to origin was found. Similarly, there was no statistically significant difference observed between both sexes (P>0.05). The prevalence in body condition category was reported relatively higher in poor body condition (8.4%) and lower in good body condition (3.8%). However, no statistically significant differences appreciated among the three body condition categories (P>0.05). The finding indicated that, schistosomosis should be taken into consideration as one of the major limiting factor to livestock productivity at Guto Gida District. The control measures against schistosomosis must be designed to target either the parasite or the snail intermediate host.

Key words: Bovine, *Guto Gida,* prevalence, schistosomiasis

INTRODUCTION

Schistosomosis is an infection which occurs due to trematodes of genus *schistosoma.* The disease, characterized by its chronic nature, affects the productivity and production performances and predisposes animals to other diseases in the World (Mc-Cauley et al., 2000), and it is endemic in the tropical and subtropical countries of Africa, Asia and Southern Europe (Lawerence, 2001).

Epidemiological studies on bovine schistosomosis are suggestive of the endemicity of the infection particularly in areas with large permanent water bodies and marshy pasture areas. In Ethiopia, the optimum range for distribution of *S. mansoni* has been reported as 1500 to 2000 m above sea level (masl) (Gashaw, 2010). *Schistosoma* bovis has a localized distribution found commonly in Northern, Eastern, South Western and

*Corresponding author. E-mail: abrahamkebede2016@gmail.com

central parts of Ethiopia (Fekade et al., 2002); It is affecting all ages of animals and mainly prevalent in cattle kept around lakes and rivers (Dwight et al., 2003; Pitchford, 2006).

Schistosomosis is transmitted by using snails as an intermediate host; the immature infective form penetrates the skin of the host and may also infect cattle by ingestion through drinking water (Allen et al., 2002; Lindbergh et al., 2006). Animals affected by the disease show different clinical signs such as diarrhea, sometimes blood stained and containing mucus, and also anorexia, thirst and emaciation is the sign shown by animals with disease (Gutierrez, 2004).

Diagnosis of the disease is primarily based on the history of schistomosis in the area and the identification of snail habitats with history of access to natural water bodies (Bedarkar et al., 2000; Pawar et al., 2016). Postmortem examination, hematological tests and examination of feces for *schistosoma* eggs are also useful. The clinical signs alone will not be sufficient to arrive at definitive diagnosis but, it should be used to indicate the necessity of feces examination, which reveals the eggs of parasites mixed with blood and mucous (Thrusfied, 2005).

For treating the disease, older drugs include antimonial preparation, tartar emetic, antimosan and stibophen, and niridirozole and trichlorphon. The praziquantel, which is a drug of choice for treatment of human schistosomosis is also effective in ruminant at 15-29 mg/kg, peros (Gracia and Bruckner, 2007).

The effective control of the disease is to prevent contact between the animals and the parasite by fencing of infected waters and supplying clean water and also by the destruction of intermediate host or snails (Hansen and Perry, 2004). Even though, schistosomiasis is an economically important disease of livestock leading to huge economical losses, due to morbidity and mortality and thereby contributing to productivity loss, there is no considerable work done on the prevalence of the disease in and around Nekemte.

Therefore, the objective of this study was to determine the prevalence of Schistosomiasis in cattle in Nekemte area.

MATERIALS AND METHODS

Study area

The study was conducted from March to May, 2016 in Guto Gida district, Nekemte town, East Wollega Zone of Oromia Regional State, Ethiopia. The district is about 331 km from Addis Ababa to the West. The area has average temperature of 20°C and mean annual rainfall of 21500 mm. The altitude of the area ranges from 1300 – 3140 m a. s. l. According to the Nekemte District Agricultural Office, livestock population of cattle in head is 85,584, sheep 14,702, Goat 11,861, Equine 98,674, chicken 94,276 and mixed crop and livestock farming system is the mode of agriculture in the district in which cattle and sheep operate as major livestock, highly important for livelihood of the local population (NWAROD, 2016).

Study population

The study population was cattle with different age groups, body condition and sex. The age of animal was determined based on dentition (Pope, 2008) and the body condition of the animals was classified into three groups:- poor, medium and good based on visibility of skeleton by inspectional examination (Debont et al., 2005).

Study design

A cross sectional study was used to determine the prevalence of bovine schistosomosis and its risk factors at Nekemte area from March to May, 2016.

Sampling and sample size determination

From area of Nekemte town the Kebeles (Jirenga, Gaari and Dalo) were selected by purposive sampling based on animal population of the Kebeles and consideration of the representativeness.

The desired sample size was determined by using the formula given by Thrushfield (2004); also, with 95% confidence level and 5% desired absolute precision, and since there was research conducted in this area, 50% expected prevalence was taken.

$$N = \frac{1.96 * P\exp(1 - \mathrm{Exp})}{d^2}$$

where
n = required sample size
$p_{exp=}$ prevalence
d^2 = Desired absolute precision.

$$N = \frac{1.96 * 0.5(1 - 0.5)}{(0.05)}$$

=384

Accordingly, animals were selected randomly to estimate the prevalence of the infection in the study area.

Study method and sample collection

Coproscopic examination

The fresh fecal sample was collected directly from rectum of randomly selected animals and preserved in 10% formalin in universal bottle to prevent hatching of miracidia. Then eggs were examined by fecal sedimentation techniques and observed under microscope in the laboratory (Ash and Orihel, 2004).

Data management and analysis

The data was entered into MS excel Database, coded, thence analyzed using SPSS 20.0 version statistical software program. The prevalence was calculated by dividing number of positive animals by total number of animals tested. Pearson's chi square (x^2) was used to evaluate the association between the prevalence the disease with related risk factors. P value < 0.05 was considered as significant in the analysis.

RESULTS

Overall prevalence

Among 384 cattle examined using coproscopical

Table 1. Prevalence of bovine schistosomosis based on PAs or kebeles.

PAs or Kebeles	No. examined	No. infected	Prevalence (%)	X^2	P value
Garii	129	6	4.6		
Jirenga	120	11	9.1	0.928	0.055
Dalo	135	5	3.1		
Total	**384**	**22**	**5.7**		

Table 2. Prevalence of bovine schistosomosis based on sex.

Sex	No. examined	No. infected	Prevalence (%)	X^2	P value
Male	187	13	6.9	1.009	0.382
Female	197	9	4.5		
Total	**384**	**22**	**5.7**		

Table 3. Prevalence of bovine schistosomosis based on body condition.

Body condition	No. examined	No. infected	Prevalence (%)	X^2	P value
Poor	119	10	8.4		
Medium	135	7	5.1	0.503	0.073
Good	130	5	3.8		
Total	**384**	**22**	**5.7**		

examination, 5.7% (22/384) were found to be positive for bovine schistosomosis or infected.

Prevalence based on origin

According to the present study, the prevalence of bovine schistosomosis was higher in Jirenga kebele (9.1%) than Gaarii kebele (4.6%) and Dalo kebele (3.7%). However, there was no statistically significant difference on the prevalence of bovine schistosomosis based on three PAs ($p>0.05$) as indicated in Table 1.

Prevalence based on sex

The study indicated that, the prevalence of bovine schistosomosis in male and female was 6.9% and 4.5%, respectively. Although the prevalence was relatively higher in female as indicated in Table 2 the difference was not statistically significant ($P>0.05$).

Prevalence based on body condition

Prevalence of bovine schistosomosis on poor body condition animals was 8.4% and medium body condition (5.1%). However, animals with good body condition showed prevalence of 3.8%. As described in Table 3, significant difference ($P > 0.05$) was not observed among body condition of the study animals for the occurrence of schistosomosis.

Prevalence based on age

According to the age of animal, the prevalence of schistosomosis varied. Low prevalence was observed in young (4.9%), and highest prevalence was observed in adult (6.2%). However, there was no significant difference ($P > 0.05$) among age groups (Table 4).

DISCUSSION

The overall prevalence of bovine schistosomosis infection of the study area was found to be 5.7%. When this result is compared with the prevalence of other authors in the country it is much lower than the finding of Mersha et al. (2012) which was 13.7% in Fogera. Similarly, 22.06% was reported in and around Bahir Dar (Solomon, 2008) and 27.13% in Dembia (Alemseged, 2010). The difference in prevalence may be due to the variation in the study seasons, sample size, humidity, management and climate change between various agro ecologies. The present study is nearly similar with that of Mihret and

Table 4. Prevalence of bovine schistosomosis based on of animal age.

Age	No. examined	No. infected	Prevalence (%)	X^2	P value
Young	161	8	4.9	0.297	0.661
Adult	223	14	6.2		
Total	**384**	**22**	**5.7%**		

Samuel (2015) (7.6%) in and around Debre Tabor town, South Gondar Zone of Amhara region, Northwestern Ethiopia, which can be due to similar management in the areas.

The relatively greater prevalence of the disease was in Jiregna and Gaarii PAs maybe due to swampiest and moisture nature of most of the grazing areas in these PAs. Similarly, many authors also reported that water lodged and poorly drained areas with acidic soils are often endemic for schistosomosis (Almaz, 2007). Mihret and Samuel (2015) also reported that there was difference of bovine schistosomosis prevalence based on origin but there was no significant difference between origin and the infection.

The higher prevalence of bovine schistosomosis was in adult animals in this study and agrees with the work of (Alemseged, 2010) who reported a prevalence of 17.6% in young animals and 30.10% in adults in Dembia district, disagreeing with the work of Taylor et al. (2007) who reported highest prevalence in young animals.

The variation in the prevalence was found in male (6.9%) and in female (4.5%) revealing no statistically significant ($P>0.05$) difference. This variation is similar with previous study which was 29.61% in male and 19.54% in female (Solomon, 2008), in and around Bahir Dar and 30.70% in male and 23.30% in female (Alemseged, 2010) in Dembia district. The study disagrees with the study conducted by Mihret and Samuel (2015) and found higher prevalence in female (33.1%), and lowers in male (27.1). The results indicated that both sexes have the same risk to acquire disease. This is because of equal exposure to the risk factors since there were no restrictions on movement for grazing and contact with the parasite and animals in terms of sex.

This exacerbates the multiplication of *Schistosoma* and increases the epidemiology of the disease. It was also reported that the increased contact time with *Schistosoma* infested habitat increases the rate and endemicity of schistosomosis.

Schistosoma infection rate in relation with body condition score in the present study varied in cattle. Animals with poor body condition score were more affected than other groups of animals. Similarly, Merawe et al. (2014) affirmed that the infection rate increase with animals which have poor body condition score. This could be due to the acquired immunity status of poor body condition and weak animals becoming more suppressed and susceptible possibly due to malnutrition and other parasite infection. Thus, infected animals may require long period of time to respond against *Schistosoma* infection. This gives suitable time for establishment and fecundity of the parasite in animals. This finding also coincides with the work of Belayneh and Tadesse (2014) that accounted the prevalence of *Schistosoma* as more common in animals with poor body score animals than medium and good body condition.

CONCLUSION AND RECOMMENDATION

According to the present study, the overall prevalence of bovine Schistosomosis was found to be 5.7% in and around Nekemte. The study also revealed that the prevalence of schistosomosis is high in Jirenga and followed by Gari peasant associations. The prevalence of the disease is also closely linked with environmental factors that are suitable for the development and multiplication of snail which is intermediate hosts and the parasite. Therefore, depending on the result of the study, the following recommendations are forwarded:

(i) There should be initiation and awareness creation on the prevention and control of snails.
(ii) Further epidemiological investigations should be conducted to assess the *Schistoma* infection and its associated risk factors.
(iii) There should be regular deworming and veterinary service in the study area.
(iv) Grazing management should be involved to avoid grazing around marshy area in which snail population is high.

ACKNOWLEDGEMENTS

The authors are grateful to Wollega University, the whole staff of School of Veterinary Medicine, for their inspiration to complete this work. Also, thanks are due to the respondents (farmers and animal health workers) of in and around Nekemte for their collaboration in allowing their animals for collection of fecal sample.

REFERENCES

Alemseged G (2010). Prevalence of bovine schistosomosis in Dembia District North west Ethiopia. Dvm thesis, Faculty of Veterinary Medicine. Gondar, Ethiopia.

Allen GP, Adrian GS, Richard OG, Gail MW, Donald PM (2002). Schistosomiasis. New Engl. J. Med. 346:1212-1220.

Almaz H (2007). Pathology of naturally occurring *Schistosoma* infection in cattle slaughtered at Bahir Dar municipal abattoir North West Ethiopia. MSc thesis, Faculty of Veterinary medicine, Addis Ababa University, Debere Zeit, Ethiopia.

Ash LA, Orihel TC (2004). Parasites: A guide to Laboratory Procedures and Identification. ASCP Press, American Society of Clinical Pathologists, USA.

Bedarkar SN, Narladkar BW, Despande PD (2000). Seasonal prevalence of snail borne fluke infections in ruminants of Maratwada region. J. Vet. Parasitol.14:51-54.

Belayneh L, Tadesse G (2014). Bovine schistosomiasis: A Threat in Public Health perspective in Bahir Dar Town, Northwest Ethiopia. Acta. Parasitol. Glob. 5:1-6.

Debont J, Vercruysse J, Sabbe F, Southgate VR, Rollinson D (2005). *Schistosoma bovis* infection in cattle: changes associated with season and age. Vet. Parasitol. 57:299-307.

Dwight D, Bowman k, George A (2003). Parasitology for Veterinarians, 1st ed. USA: Elsevier, pp. 129-133.

Fekade D, Woldemichael TA, Tadele S (2002). Pathogenesis and pathology of shistosomiasis, 5th edition. Addis Ababa University printing press, Addis Ababa. P 34

Gracia LS, Bruckner DA (2007). Diagnostic Medical Parasitology. Elsevier Science Publishing Co. Inc., New York, USA.

Gashaw A (2010). Epidemiology of intestinal schistosoma in Hayk town, North East Ethiopia. Addis Ababa.

Gutierrez Y (2004). Diagnostic Pathology of Parasitic infections with clinical correlation.

Hansen J, Perry B (2004). The epidemiology, Diagnosis and control of Helminthes parasite of ruminants. A hand book of Animal Production parasite. Immunology 26:167-175.

Lawerence JA (2001).Bovineschistosomiasisin Southern Africa. Helminthologic abstracts. pp: 261-270.

Lindbergh R, Johansen M, Nitsson C, Nansen P (2006). An immunohistological study of phenotypic characteristics of cells of the inflammatory response in the intestine of Schistosoma bovis-infected goats. Parasitology 118(1):91-99.

Mc-Cauley EH, Majid AA, Tayed A (2000). Economic evaluation of the production impact of bovine Schistosomiasis. pp: 735-754.

Merawe M, Amsslu K, Hagos Y, Afera B (2014). Intestinal schistosomosis of Bovine and Ovine in Fogera district, South Gondar Zone, Amhara National Regional State, Ethiopia. Acta Parasitol. Glob. 5:87-90.

Mersha C, Belay D, Tewodros F (2012). Prevalence of Cattle schistosomosis and Associated Risk Factors in Fogera Cattle, South Gondar Zone and Amhara National Regional State, Ethiopia. J. Adv. Vet. Res. pp: 53-56.

Mihret T, Samuel D (2015). Prevalence of Bovine Schistosomosis and its Associated Risk Factor in and Around Debre Tabor Town, North West of Ethiopia. Eur. J. Biol. Sci. 7(3):108-113.

NWAROD (Nekemte woreda Agricultural and Rural Development office), (2016). Annual progress report.

Pawar PD, Singla LD, Kaur P, Bal MS (2016). Caprine Schistosomosis: Prevalence and associated host factors in Barnala District of Punjab State. Proceedings of *15th* Convocation of National Academy of Veterinary Sciences India and National Symposium on “Sustainable Livestock Development for Food and Nutritional Security: Way Forward” (22-23 October 2016) P. 16.

Pitchford RJ (2006). A check list of definitive host exhibiting evidence of the genus Schistosoma Weinland-1858 acquired naturally in Africa and Middle East. J. Helminthol. 51:229-252.

Pope GM (2008). Determining the age of cattle by their teeth. Farmers' Bulleitin1066 USA departement of Agriculture. pp. 1-12.

Solomon O (2008). Observations on the prevalence of Schistosoma Bovis infection in Bahir Dar area. North central Ethiopia. DVM Thesis, Faculty of veterinary Medicine, Mekele University, Ethiopia.

Taylor MA, Coop RL, Wall RL (2007). Veterinary parasitology 3rd edition, Blackwell publishing, Oxford. pp. 201-208.

Thrushfield M (2004). Veterinary epidemiology, 2nd edition. UK, Black well sciences.

Thrusfied M (2005). Survey in veterinary epidemiology 2 ed. Cambridge: Blackwell science. Ltd. pp. 182-189.

Prevalence of bovine trypanosomiosis in Gamogoffa Zone, Ouba Debrestahay District, Southern Ethiopia

Migbaru Keffale Bezabih[1]* and Mabure Shille Bisho[2]

[1]Department of Biomedical Science, College of Veterinary Medicine, Haramaya University, P. O. Box 38, Haramaya, Ethiopia.
[2]Debre-Tsehay District Agricultural Office, Southern Nations Nationalities and Peoples Region, Ethiopia.

This cross-sectional study was conducted in Ouba Debre-Tsehay District, Gamogoffa Zone, Southern Ethiopia from October 2013 to July 2014 with the objectives of estimating the prevalence of bovine trypanosomiasis and to assess the possible risk factors. Blood samples were collected from 384 randomly selected cattle from purposefully selected peasant associations with consideration of different age groups and both sexes. Buffy coat method was employed for parasitological survey and packed cell volume (PCV) determination was done. From the examined animals, 58 (15.1%; 95% CI: 11.7-19.6) were positive for trypanosome infection. In the area, *Trypanosome congolense* and *Trypanosome vivax* were the two identified *Trypanosoma* species with proportion of 60.3 and 27.6% , respectively and 12.1% mixed infection. Trypanosomiasis was observed as 13.8% in males and 15.9% in females out of these, 4.9 (95% CI: 1.0-13.7), 11 (95% CI: 5.8-18.4) and 20.1% (95% CI: 14.9-26.1) were found in animals <1year, between 1 and 3 years and above 3 years of age, respectively. Significant difference was observed between <1 year and >3 years of age (p<0.05). Based on body condition category, 8 (95% CI: 4.7-13.8), 16 (95%CI: 10.2-23.5) and 26.1% (95%CI: 17.3-36.6) were good, medium and poor conditioned animals, respectively and there was a significant association between good and poor condition animals (p<0.05). The recorded overall mean PCV in parasitaemic and aparasitaemic animals was 20.4 and 25.6%, respectively; it significantly varied (t=12.28, p = 0.00). Out of the parasitaemic and aparasitaemic animals, 77.6 and 16.6% were anemic, respectively (with PCV < 24%).

Key words: Cattle, Ouba Debre-Tsehay, prevalence, Trypanosoma, trypanosomosis.

INTRODUCTION

Cattle population of Ethiopia is estimated at about 49.3 million heads (CSA, 2009). Despite its huge population size, cattle productivity remains marginal due to various diseases, malnutrition and management constraints. Parasitism represents a major obstacle to the development of sub-sector of which trypanosomiasis plays a great role (FAO, 2005). Animal trypaposomosis is a protozoan parasitic disease of domestic animals resulting from infection with different *Trypanosoma* species transmitted by tsetse fly and other haematophagous flies, mechanically (Sharma et al., 2013). It is a chronic, debilitating disease, which occur in some 240,000 km^2 area of Ethiopia. About 10-14 million heads of cattle and a significant number of

*Corresponding author. E-mail: migkafe@gmail.com.

small ruminants and equines are under serious risk of contracting the disease of which 20,000 heads die every year (Solomon, 2006). Animals affected with trypanosomiasis become anaemic and weak; lose weight and have reduced productivity, and often, mortality rates are high due to pathology induced by trypanosomes (Urquhart et al., 1996; Bal et al., 2012).

In Ethiopia, there are five economically important animal *Trypanosoma* species; however, *T. congolense* is responsible for the most important form of animal trypanosomosis in domestic animals and also the most prevalent trypanosome species in tsetse-infested areas of the country (Leak, 1999).

Trypanosomosis in Africa is mainly restricted to areas in which the vector, tsetse fly species like *G. m. submorsitans*, *Glossina pallidipes, Glossina fuscipes fuscipes* and *Glossina tachinoides* can survive. These species of tsetse flies are distributed along the lowlands of western, southern and southwestern part of Ethiopia. The disease is also found outside the tsetse belt areas transmitted mechanically by biting flies of the genus *Tabanus*, *Haematopota*, *Chrysops* and *Stomoxys*. This type of transmission has caused the spread of *Trypanosoma evansi* and *Trypanosoma vivax,* outside tsetse infested areas (Abebe, 2005). In very acute infections with highly susceptible exotic animals, infection with *T. vivax* can also pass through the placenta and into the fetus in pregnant animals. As a result, some cows abort and some calves are born before birth time (Abebe and Jobre, 1996).

Trypanosoma congolense and *T. vivax* exert their effect mainly by causing severe anemia and mild to moderate organ damage. The onset and severity of the anemia is directly related to the appearance of the parasite in the blood and to the level of the parasitaemia. The rapid decline in the hemoglobin concentration, red blood cell number and PCV and the clear clinical sign of pallor of the mucus membrane reveals that the animal is infected with trypanosome (OIE, 2008).

Animal Trypanosomosis in and around Arbaminch has socio-economic impact due to debilitation and death of untreated animals and reduces production and productivity of affected animals (Waldeyes and Aboset, 1997); but the disease had not yet been assessed and there is no documented baseline data in Ouba Debre-Tsehay district. Therefore, this study was done with the objectives of estimating the prevalence of bovine trypanosomiasis, to identify the predominant species of trypanosomes and to estimate the risk factors for the occurrence of the disease in the study area.

MATERIALS AND METHODS

Study area

Ouba Debre-Tsehay district is found in southern Ethiopia at 549 km from Addis Ababa, and 285 km from Arbaminch. The altitude of the selected PAS varies from 1001 to 1600 m.a.s.l. The rainfall pattern is bimodal; a short rainy season runs from March to May and long rainy season runs from June to September and the average annual rain fall ranges from 600 to 1800 mm. The mean temperature varies from 27- 40°C. The land is covered by different vegetation types mainly savanna grassland forest, and bush lands predominated by acacia tree. The district has a livestock population of 218732 cattle, 90670 sheep and goat, 3947 equines and 250600 poultry (MARDO, 2011).

Study population

The study population was local breed zebu cattle which are kept in traditional management system. The animals in the area mainly depend on communal grazing fields and crop residues as feed source and watering paints are the tributaries of Lomat and Bezo Rivers which is infested with tsetse flies predominantly by *G. pallidipes* and Tabanus (Amenu et al., 2008).

Sampling method and sample size determination

A cross-sectional study using simple random sampling technique was employed to determine the prevalence of bovine trypanosomiasis in the study area. The 8 PAs (Shele-bune, Yela-shabo, Galada, Zeka –zelto, Hoshele- shambara, Shala-Tito-Tife, Beto and Bala) were selected purposively based on the availability of transportation and logistics as well as their agroecological representativeness for the district was considered. From each selected PA, the farmers as well as the study animals were selected randomly in each household. During sampling, PAs, age, sex and body condition score (BCS) of the animal were recorded. The body condition score was grouped into good, medium and poor conditioned animals based on the appearance of ribs and dorsal spines applied for zebu cattle (Nicholson and Butterworth, 1986). Age of the animal was estimated by dentition (De-lahunta and Habel, 1986) and owner's information. The desired sampling size was calculated according to the formula given by Thrusfield (2005) with the expected prevalence of 50%, 95% confidence level and 5% absolute desired precision; as a result, the maximum sample size (384) was taken.

Trypanosome survey

Parasitological and hematological techniques were employed to detect the trypanosome and determine blood PCV, respectively. Accordingly, blood samples were obtained by bleeding marginal ear veins of cattle using a sterile lancet and drawing the blood into the heparinized capillary tube up to 3/4th of the length. The collected blood was sealed with crystal sealant and centrifuged for about 5 min with 12,000 rpm. After centrifugation, the packed cell volume (PCV) level was measured using hematocrit capillary reader and the length of the packed red cells column was expressed as a percentage of the total volume of blood. Animals with PCV below 24% was designated to be anemic (OIE, 2008).

Blood smears were made via cutting the centrifuged blood containing capillary tube 1 mm above and below the buffy coat layer using a diamond tipped pencil so as to include plasma and red blood cell (RBC) in the blood smear. The blood then expanded onto the clean glass slide, mixed well and covered with a clean cover glass. Examination was done under 40x objective lenses and 10x eye piece magnification, and the parasites were identified based on their morphology and movement in wet film preparation (Radostits et al., 2007). When the presence of the parasite was determined, a small drop of blood from a micro-haematocrit

Table 1. Prevalence of bovine Trypanosomosis in Ouba Debre-Tsehay district and proportion of the disease in the eight PAs.

PAs	Number of animals examined	*Trypanosoma* species			Total positives (%)	(95% CI)	X^2 (P-value)
		T. congolense (%)	T. *vivax* (%)	Mixed (%)			
Shele-bune	56	6(60)	3(30)	1(10)	10 (17.9)	8.9-30.4	
Yela-shabo	49	4(50)	3(37.5)	1(12.5)	8 (16.3)	7.3-29.7	
Galada	48	4(57.1)	2(28.6)	1(14.3)	7 (14.6)	6.1-27.8	
Zeka –zelto	46	5(71.4)	1(14.3)	1(14.3)	7 (15.2)	6.3-28.9	4.1 (1.00)
Hoshele- shambara	48	5(71.4)	2(28.6)	-	7 (14.6)	6.3-27.8	
Shala-Tito-Tife	51	5(62.5)	2(25)	1(12.5)	8 (15.7)	7.0-28.6	
Beto	42	2(40)	2(40)	1(20)	5 (11.9)	4.0-25.6	
Bala	44	4(66.7)	1(16.7)	1(16.7)	6 (13.6)	5.2-27.4	
Total	384	35(60.3%)	16(27.6%)	7(12.1%)	58(15.1%)	11.7-19.1	

capillary tube was applied to a clean slide and spread by using another clean slide at an angle of 45°. The smear was dried by moving it in the air and fixed for 2 min in methyl alcohol. The thin smear was flooded with Giemsa stain (1:10 solution) for 30 min. Excess stain was drained and washed by using distilled water. Then, it was allowed to dry and examined under the microscope (100x) oil immersion objective lens (OIE, 2008).

Data management and analysis

The collected raw data and the results of parasitological and hematological examination were entered into a Microsoft excel spread sheet. Then, the raw data was summarized using SPSS version 20.

The prevalence of trypanosome infection was calculated as the number of positive animals as examined by Giemsa stain of thin blood film and buffy coat method divided by the total number of animals examined at the particular time. Pearson's Chi-square (χ^2) was used to evaluate the association of different variables with the prevalence of trypanosome infection and independent t-test was used to compare the mean PCV value between parasitaemic and non parasitaemic animals. P-value less than 0.05 was considered as significant.

RESULTS AND DISCUSSION

This study show that the overall prevalence was 15.1% (95% CI: 11.7-19.1) which is in agreement with the reports of Feyissa et al. (2011) in Humbo District, Southern Ethiopia, but higher than the reports of Ayana et al. (2012) and Achenef and Admas (2012) in Amhara region. The higher prevalence might be due to the presence of frequent tsetse fly challenge as a result of high density in the study area (Amenu et al., 2008).

T. congolense and *T. vivax* were the two trypanosome species identified. However, higher proportion of T. *congolense* (60.3%) was observed than *T. vivax* (27.6%) and also 12.1% mixed infection (Table 1) which is in agreement with the reports of Feyissa et al. (2011). This might be due to the absence of significant variation in vector density and agro-climatic difference (Dagnachew, 2004).

In the present study, higher prevalence was observed in females (15.9%) than males (13.8%) which is in agreement with the reports of Feyissa et al. (2011) who reported 15 and 13.7% in female and males, respectively but there was no significant difference ($P > 0.05$) (Table 2). This was inconsistent with the report of Abrham and Tesfaheywot (2012). The possible explanation for relative increment of prevalence in female animals might be due to physiological differences (Torr et al., 2006).

Based on age category, 4.9, 11 and 20.1% prevalence was observed in animals less than one year, between one and three years and above three years of age, respectively which revealed significant variation ($P<0.05$) (Table 2). This might be due to young animals slightly protected by maternal antibodies (Fimmen et al., 1999).

The overall prevalence of trypanosome infection was significantly associated with the body condition of the study animals ($P<0.05$) (Table 2). The prevalence was higher in poor body condition score animals (26.1% [95%CI: 17.3-36.6]) than the medium (16% [95% CI: 10.2-23.5]) and good (8.5% [95%CI: 4.7-13.8]) score animals. This is comparable with the finding of Feyissa et al. (2011). This is because Trypaosomosis is a chronic wasting disease characterized by slow progressive loss of condition (Uilenberg, 1998).

In this study, out of the total animals examined, 25.8% were anemic having PCV <24% and 74.2% were not anemic (PCV ≥24). On the other hand, out of the total 58 parasitaemic animals, 77.6%

Table 2. Prevalence of Trypanosomosis based on sex, age and body condition score of examined animals.

Variables		Number of examined	Number of positive (%)	(95% CI)	χ^2 (p-value)
Sex					
	Male	145	20 (13.8%)	8.6-20.5	0.31 (0.6)
	Female	239	38 (15.9%)	11.5-21.2	
Age					
	≤1 year	61	3 (4.9%)	1-13.7	
	1-3 years	109	12 (11%)	5.8-18.4	10.5 (0.005)
	>3 years	214	43 (20.1%)	14.9-26.1	
BCS					
	Good	165	14(8.5%)	4.7-13.8	
	Medium	131	21 (16%)	10.2-23.5	14.1 (0.001)
	Poor	88	23 (26.1%)	17.3-36.6	
Total		384	58 (15.1%)	11.7-19.1	

Table 3. Comparison of mean PCV between parasitaemic and aparasitaemic cattle.

Condition	Total examined	Number of PCV <24%	Number of PCV ≥24%	Mean PCV	[95% CI]	t-test (p-value)
Parasitaemic	58	45(77.6%)	13 (22.4%)	20.4	19.6-21.3	12.28 (0.001)
Aparasitaemic	326	54 (16.6%)	272(83.4%)	25.6	25.28-25.9	
Total	384	99(25.8%)	285 (74.2%)	24.8	24.5-25.2	

were anemic (PCV<24) and only 22.4% were not; whereas, from 326 aparasitaemic animals, only 16.6% were anemic (PCV<24) but 83.4% were not anemic. There was significant difference between the mean PCV values of parasitaemic and aparasitaemic animals ($t=12.28$, $p<0.05$) (Table 3). This lower PCV was reported in previous studies in different parts of the country (Nigatu, 2004; Abraham and Tesfaheywet, 2012).

CONCLUSION AND RECOMMENDATIONS

Trypanosomosis is an important disease and a potential threat to health and productivity of cattle in Ouba Debre-Tsehay district. The result revealed that *T. congolense* is the most prevalent species in the study area and the infections significantly affect the PCV values and body condition. Therefore, economical and environment friendly community based tsetse fly and typanosomosis control program should be designed and implemented in the area.

ACKNOWLEDGMENTS

The researchers thank Southern Tsetse Eradication Project (STEP) professionals, especially John "the bush man" who spent countless dedicated hours in complex and challenging laboratory process of parasitological and hematological techniques.

REFERENCES

Abebe G (2005). Trypanosomiasis in Ethiopia. Ethiopia J. Biol. Sci. 4(1):75-121.
Abebe G, Jobre Y (1996). Trypanosomosis: A threat to cattle production in Ethiopia. Revue de Medecine Veteterinaire 147(12):896-902.
Abraham Z, Tesfaheywet Z (2012). Prevalence of bovine trypanosomosis in selected district of Arba Minch, SNNPR, Southern Ethiopia. Glob. Vet. 8(2):168-173.
Achenef M, Admas A (2012). Bovine Trypanosomosis and Its Vector Type and Density at Debre Elias District, North-western, Ethiopia. J. Advan. Vet. Res. 2:247-251.
Amenu A, Sheferaw D, Wossene A, Fekadu A (2008). Prevalence of bovine trypanosomosis and tsetse density in selected woredas of SNNPS, Ethiopia. Ethiopian Vet. J. 12(2):131-139.
Ayana M, Tesfaheywet Z, Getnet F (2012). A cross-sectional study on the prevalence of bovine Trypanosomosis in Amhara region, Northwest Ethiopia. Livest. Res. Rural Dev. 24(8).
Bal MS, Singla LD, Kumar H, Ashuma, Gupta K, Juyal PD (2012). Pathological studies on experimental Trypanosoma evansi infection in swiss albino mice. J. Parasit. Dis. 36:260-264.
Central Statistical Agency (CSA) (2009). Livestock and livestock characteristics 2008–09 (Private peasant holdings). Statistical Bulletin No. 446. Addis Ababa, Ethiopia: CSA.
Dagnachew S (2004). Epidemiology of Bovine Trypanosomosis in the Abbay Basin Areas of Northwest Ethiopia. MSc thesis, Addis Ababa University, Faculty of Veterinary Medicine, Debrezeit, Ethiopia.
De-lahunta A, Habel RE (1986). Teeth, applied veterinary anatomy. W.B. Saunders Company. pp. 4-6.

FAO (2005). The influence of trypanosomosis on African animal production. Animal Zootechnica. pp. 1-2.

Feyissa B, Samson A, Mihreteab B (2011). Bovine Trypanosomosis in Selected Villages of Humbo District, Southern Ethiopia. Glob.Vet. 7(2):192-198.

Fimmen HO, Mehlitz D, Horchiners F, Korb E (1999). Colostral antibodies and Trypanosome Congolese infection in calves.Trypanotolerance research and application GTZ, 116:173-178.

Leak SGA (1999). Tsetse biology and ecology. Their role in the epidemiology and control of trypanosomosis. CABI publishing in association with International Livestock Research Institute (ILRI). Nairobi, Kenya.

Ministry of Agriculture Rural Development Office (MARDO) (2011). Annual report on general agricultural activities, MARDO (Ouba Debre-Tsehay district Agricultural and Rural Development Office), Ouba Debre-Tsehay.

Nicholson MJ, Butterworth MH (1986). A guide to scoring of zebu cattle, International Livestock Centre for Africa, Addis Ababa.

Nigatu SD (2004). Epidemiology of bovine trypanosomosis in the Abbay Basin areas of Northwest Ethiopia. MsSc thesis, FVM, AAU, Debre Zeit.

OIE (2008). Standardized techniques for the diagnosis of tsetse transmitted trypanosomiasis, in OIE Terrestrial Manual, OIE, Rome, Italy. P 49.

Radostits OM, Blood DC, Gay CC, Hinchicliff WK, Constable PD (2007). Veterinary medicine. A textbook of the diseases of cattle, sheep, pigs, goats and horses, 10th edn., Saunders Ltd, Edinburgh.

Sharma A, Singla LD, Tuli A, Kaur P, Batth BK, Javed M, Juyal PD (2013). Molecular prevalence of Babesia bigemina and Trypanosoma evansi in dairy animals from Punjab, India, by duplex PCR: A step forward to the detection and management of concurrent latent infections. BioMed Res. Int. Aug 29; 2013.

Solomon M (2006). Tsetse control or eradication (strategy action plan of the SNNPRS. In Tsetse and trypansomosis control approaches and southern Tsetse and trypansomosis control actor's forum establishment, proceeding of the regional work shop, Hawassa, August 22-23, pp. 61-63.

Thrusfield M (2005). Veterinary Epidemiology. 3rd ed., UK, Blackwell science Ltd, pp. 233-250.

Torr SJ, Mwangwiro TNC, Hall DR (2006). The effects of host physiology on the attraction of tsetse (Dipteral: Glossinidae) and Stomoxys (Dipteral: Muscidae) to cattle. Bull. Entomol. Res. 96(1):71-84.

Uilenberg G (1998). A field guide for the diagnosis, treatment and prevention of African animal trypanosomosis. Food & Agriculture Org. ISBN: 9251042381.

Urquhart GM, Armour J, Duncan JL, Dunn AM and Jennings FW (1996). Veterinary parasitology. 2nd Edition, Blackwell Science, Oxford. pp. 212-230.

Waldeyes G, Aboset G (1997). Tsetse and Trypanosomiasis distribution, identification and assessment of socio-economic viability of new vector control approaches in Arbaminch zuria woreda. Ethiopian veterinary association proceeding of the 11th conference, pp. 143-154.

8

A study on the sero epidemiology of African horse sickness in three woredas of Sidama Zone, Hawassa, Ethiopia

Getaw Yeshitila and Dejene Bekele*

Ministry of Livestock and Fisheries, Ethiopia.

A cross-sectional study was conducted in the three woredas of Sidama zone, Southern Nations, Nationalities and Peoples' Region (SNNPRS) with the aim of determining the overall prevalence of African horse sickness (AHS) in equines and the effect of putative risk factors on the prevalence of AHS. A total of 230 equines (66 donkeys, 161 horses and 3 mules) were included. Serological examination was conducted using blocking enzyme linked immuno sorbent assay (blocking ELISA) revealing a point prevalence of 46.97, 13.66 and 33.33% AHS in donkeys, horses and mules, respectively. The overall prevalence of AHS in equines in Sidama zone of the three districts was 23.47%. The prevalence at Dale, Hula and Wonsho woreda' was 52.72, 10.47 and 17.98%, respectively. Statistical analysis of the result showed significance difference in prevalence among donkeys, horses and mules (P< 0.05). The prevalence of 52.72% in midland and 14.28% in highland revealed statistically significant difference (P<0.05). The difference observed between Dale and Hula, and Dale and Wonsho was seen to be statistically different, but no difference was seen between Wonsho and Hula. Among the hypothesized risk factors, agro ecology is the predominant risk for the prevalence of AHS and this was asserted by P-value (P<0.05).

Key words: African horse sickness, enzyme linked immuno sorbent assay (ELISA), equines, sero-epidemiology, Sidama, prevalence.

INTRODUCTION

African horse sickness (Peste equina Africana, Peste equine) is an insect born viral disease characterized by severe pyrexia, wide spread hemorrhage and edematous exudations (OIE, 2008). AHS virus affects all species of Equidae family (horses, mules, donkeys and zebras) and transmitted by a biting midge belonging to the genus *Culicoides* (Maclachlan and Guthrie, 2010). This devastating disease is endemic in sub- Saharan African (OIE, 2008). In the late 1980s, AHS spread out side its endemic region reaching Spain and Portugal (OIE, 2008; Ferhandey et al., 2012).

African horse sickness virus (AHSV) belongs to the family *Reoviridac*, and genus *Orbivivus* (OIE, 2008). Like other *Orbiviruses*, AHSV virions are double-stranded

*Corresponding author. E-mail: dejenebekele52@yahoo.com. Tel: +251 920966749.

with their genomes composed of 10 double stranded RNA (dsRNA) segments (Cetre-Sossah et al., 2008). Nine serologically distinct AHS virus serotypes (AHSV-1 to AHSV-9) have been identified with the evidence of cross-neutralization among them (Cetre- Sossah et al., 2008; OIE, 2004).

The disease confined to sub-Saharan Africa although periodic epizootics have caused severe outbreaks of the disease outside enzootic regions like North Africa, Middle East, and Southern Europe (Rodriguez-Sanchez et al., 2008; Torrecuadrada et al., 2011). The nine known virus serotypes of AHSV have been isolated from clinical cases of the disease in Kenya (Binepal et al., 2013). The most important factor in the epizootology of AHS is the host.

The existence of the reservoir of infection is suggested by the fact that the disease passes from one season to another in a particular area. An outbreak mostly occurs during rainy season and quickly disappears during dry and cool periods before it appears when wet and warm weather returns.

Many factors can contribute to the poor performance of equines, among which viral diseases characterized by high morbidity and mortality rates are the first. Clinically, the disease is characterized by an acute pulmonary form, a cardiac form or sub-acute form, mixed form and a mild form know as horse sickness fever (Upadhyaya, 2011). Hence, African horse sickness is one of the viral diseases characterized by up to 95, 50 and 10% mortality rates in horses, mules and donkeys, respectively (OIE, 2008).

According to the Central Statistical Authority of Ethiopia (2009) there are 5. 42 million donkeys, 1.78 million horses and 373, 519 mules. It has the largest equine population, probably with the highest density per square kilometer in the world (Mulualem et al., 2012). An important but often overlooked aspect is that in most cases, donkeys and mules are reared by land less and marginal farmers and are the means of subsistence for millions in the least privileged parts of the world. These beasts of burden receive little care and are subjected to intensive work throughout their lives.

Like most parts of the country, in Sidama zone as well, the attention given to these animals was very poor despite their enormous role in the economy and they are subjected to arrays of management constraints and diseases.

Among the reported diseases, African horse sickness has been known for years (Sidama Zone Agricultural and Rural Department (SZARD), 2011). However, to the authors' knowledge, in the last decades, no systemically collected information are available pertinent to the disease in the study area. Hence, the research work aimed to estimate the prevalence of African Horse sickness and to identify some of the hypothesized risk factors in three woredas' of Sidama zone, Hawassa, Ethiopia.

MATERIALS AND METHODS

Study area

This study was carried out in the Sidama zone of Southern Nations, Nationalities and Peoples Region (SNNPRs). The zones is located in the northern part of SNNPRs, with its capital town at Hawassa, which lies about 275 km south of Addis Ababa. Geographically, the zone lies between 4°27′and 8°30′ N latitude and 39°1′E longitude [Sidama Zone Planning and Economic Development Department (SZPEDD), 2004]. Like most parts of Ethiopia, the relief configuration of Sidama ranges from very high mountains to lowland plains, where the altitude varies between 1001 and 3200 m above sea level (m.a.s.l.). It has an annual rainfall and temperature ranging from 960 to 1100 mm and 18.1 to 20°C, respectively (SZPEDD, 2004).

Study animals

The study animals were equines, namely: horses, donkeys and mules above 4 years of age and non-vaccinated for AHS were considered from two ecological zones of midland (Dale) and highland (Wonsho and Hula) of Sidama zone. A total of 230 equines were selected, of which 66 were females and 164 males. Most of the equines in the area are used for pack, race and cart pulling.

Study design

The study was an observational one made in two distinct agro ecological zones namely midland and highland of the study area. As animals of the same village are usually kept in a communal grazing land, list of pass of respective district was used to represent primary sampling unit (epidemiological unit) and individual animals (secondary unit) using two stage cluster sampling technique. To this effect, a cross sectional study design was employed. Blood samples were collected using plain vacationer tube and information (data) relevant to the epidemiology was collected using semi-structured questionnaire format.

Sample size

A two-stage cluster sampling techniques was used to calculate the actual sample size having the following parameters predetermined: CL= 90%, desired level of precision =5%, expected total clusters prevalence and in between cluster variance (Thrusfield, 2005). Average number of equines per peasant association (n) is estimated to be ten (10), using the formula:

$$g = \frac{1.96^2(nVc+Pexp(1-Pexp)}{nd^2} = 21$$

Where, n = hard size; Vc = in between cluster variance; D= desired level of precision; Pexp= expected prevalence; g = number of clusters needed. In order to get the total sample size,

$$Ts = \frac{1.96^2 * g * Pexp(1-Pexp)}{gd^2 - 1.96^2 Vc} = 230$$

A total of 230 equines in 21 clusters were picked randomly

Table 1. Prevalence of AHS in the three districts

Location	Equines		
	Number mined	Number seropositive	Prevalence (%) 95%CI
Dale	55	29	52.72 (39.10-66.35)
Hula	86	9	10.47 (3.86-17.07)
Wonsho	89	16	17.98 (9.84-26.11)
Total	230	54	23.47

considering 10 clusters from midland and 11 clusters from highland agro ecological zones.

Diagnostic test

Serum was collected from three selected sites and targeted species; to this effect, 10 ml of blood using non-haparinized vacutainer tube were collected and sera were harvested from the clotted blood that was kept for 30 min at 37°C (OIE, 2004). Each serum sample was given an identification code and kept at -20°C until assayed in the laboratory. At the National Veterinary Institute (NVI), ELISA was used to detect the presence of specific antibody against the AHS virus in the sera samples collected.

Test procedure

All reagents were brought to room temperature before use. 100 µl of diluted samples was dispensed into appropriate wells (dilution 1/5). Running the samples in duplicate was recommended. 100 µl of positive control was dispensed into two wells and 100 µl of negative control into two wells. The plate was covered and incubated for 1 h at 37°C and washed 5 times. Then, 100 µl/well of conjugate was added and incubated for 30 min at 37°C.

Again, it was washed 5 times. 100 µl/well of substrate solution was dispensed using a multichannel pipette and incubated for 10 min at room temperature. 100 µl/well of stop solution was dispensed, taking care to avoid dispensing of bubbles. Finally, it was read at 405 nm (OIE, 2004).

Data analysis

The result was analyzed in relation to location, agro ecology, species, sex and mode of service. Data were stored in Microsoft Excel spread sheet. The data were edited, coded and transferred into intercool Stata (2009) version 7.0 (Stata Corporation, College Station, Texas, USA) for descriptive and analytical statistical univariate logistic regression analysis to look for identification of hypothesized risk factors in line with the result.

RESULTS

Overall prevalence

A total of 230 equines sera were examined by blocking ELISA technique. Out of which 54 equines were found to be seropositive which made the overall prevalence to be 23.47%.

Prevalence of AHS based on districts

An attempt was made to see the influence of location on the prevalence of AHS and accordingly, the prevalence of 52.72, 10.47 and 17.98% were found in Dale, Hula and Wonsho, respectively, in difference between Dale and other districts were found to be statistically significant (P<0.05) between the three locations (Table 1).

Prevalence of AHS based on agro ecology

AHS seropositivity was also assessed in relation to agro ecology and the prevalence of midland was 52.72% while it was 14.28% in the highland.

The difference between agro-ecology was statistically significant (P<0.05) (Table 2).

Prevalence of AHS based on species

The prevalence of AHS was 46.97, 13.66 and 33.33% in donkeys, horses and mules, respectively. There was statistically significant difference among donkeys, horses and mules (P<0.05) (Table 3).

Prevalence of AHS based on sex

The prevalence of AHS encountered in males were 28.66% while the correspondence value in female was 10.61% and this difference was seen to be significant statistically (P<0.05) (Table 4).

Prevalence of AHS based on mode of service

The prevalence of AHS infection among pack horses were 48.21%, while that of cart and race and pack were found to be 37.50% and that of cart and pack were 50% and statistically significant difference was observed between pack and combination of race and pack. Comparison of cart, and cart and pack need to be reserved as the number is not comparable (Table 5).

Table 2. Prevalence of AHS versus agro ecology.

Agro ecology	Number of equines examined	Number of equines seropositive	Prevalence (%) 95% CI
Midland	55	29	52.72 (39.01-66.35)
Highland	175	25	14.28 (9.05-19.52)
Total	230	54	23.47

Table 3. Prevalence of AHS in different species of equines.

Specie	Number tested	Number seropositive	Prevalence (%) 95%CI
Donkey	66	31	46.97 (34.61-59.33)
Horse	161	22	13.66 (8.30-1903)
Mule	3	1	33.33 (0.00-1.77)
Total	230	54	23.47

Table 3. Prevalence of AHS in different species of equines.

Specie	Number tested	Number seropositive	Prevalence (%) 95%CI
Donkey	66	31	46.97 (34.61-59.33)
Horse	161	22	13.66 (8.30-1903)
Mule	3	1	33.33 (0.00-1.77)
Total	230	54	23.47

Table 4. Prevalence of AHS in relation to sex.

Sex	Number tested	Number seropositive	Prevalence (%) 95%CI
Male	164	47	28.66 (21.67-35.65)
Female	66	7	10.61 (2.98-18.23)

Table 5. Prevalence of AHS based on mode of service.

Mode of service	Number tested	Number seropositive	Prevalence (%) 95%CI
Pack	56	27	48.21 (34.71-61.72)
Cart	8	3	37.5 (08.07)
Race and pack	163	22	13.5 (8.20-17.80)
Cart and pack	2	1	50% (0.00-685.3)
Total	230	53	23.47

DISCUSSION

This study revealed the overall prevalence of the three woredas' of Sidama zone, Hawassa, Ethiopia. The present overall prevalence report almost coincides with report of 25% prevalence in selected districts of Jimma zone (Molalegn et al., 2010) but it is not similar to the findings of Demissie (2013) in southern Ethiopia, who reported 33% prevalence. This might be attributed to geographical variation.

In this study, the prevalence difference observed between Dale and other districts (Wossho and Hula) were statistically significant ($P<0.05$). Similarly, the difference observed between midland and highland were also statistically significant ($P<0.05$). In this study, Dale was taken to be representative of midland, and Wonsho and Hula for highland. Therefore, the difference observed among districts is confounder, while agro-ecology (midland and highland) is an important factor. Ecology indicates the vector population is possibly manifested by prevalence. Hence, it is suggested that the prevalence in midland could be due to high density of vector population as the ecology favor its breeding (Ende et al., 2011; Tesfaye et al., 2013).

High prevalence was observed in donkeys as compared to horses and mules. The species comparison was made between donkeys and horses alone and the prevalence in donkeys was higher than in horses. The difference was statistically significant ($P<0.05$). This is contrary to the literature that donkeys and mules are resistant (Alemayehu and Benti, 2009). The deviation could be due to high exposure rate of donkeys which are usually in midland area of Dale.

It is also indicated that there was statistically significant difference ($P<0.05$) between sex and higher prevalence in male than in female. One of the probable reason was that most of the samples of midland were donkeys and of the male sex. This difference resulted from agro ecological variation rather than sex.

The study further revealed that there was lower prevalence in combined mode of service of race and pack than in pack. Horses are used in combined mode service of race and pack. Donkey is mainly used either as pack or cart. Most of the samples of horses were taken from highland and donkeys from midland land. The difference of the prevalence of AHS in the mode of service is not due to the mode of service they used, but the difference results from the distinct variation between the agro ecology from where the samples were taken. Comparison of cart, and cart and pack was not done because the numbers were not comparable.

The present finding showed that the hypothesized risk factors and agro-ecology is the predominant risk for the prevalence of African Horse sickness in the study area. Therefore, regular vaccination with potent vaccine in line with the disease epidemiology, awareness of the public on the disease epidemiology and further investigations should be done to identify the various risk factors.

ACKNOWLEDGEMENTS

The authors express their special thanks to the National Veterinary Institute (NVI) for allowing them to conduct this research and for their logistics support during the study. They are grateful to Mr. Getahun Abebe and Dr. Seid who unreservedly helped me in the work.

REFERENCES

Alemayehu L, Benti D (2009). Study on Reproductive Activity and Evaluation of Breeding Soundness of Jacks (*Equis asinus*) in and around Debre Zeit, Ethiopia. Livest. Res. Rur. Dev. 21:42-45.

Binepal VS, Wariru BN, Davies FG, Soi R, Olubayo R (2013). An attempt to define the host range for African Horse Sickness Virus (*Orbivirus*, Reoviridae) in East Africa, by a serological survey in some Equidae, Camelidae, Loxodontidae and Carnivore. Vet. Microbiol. 31:19-23.

Central Statistical Authority (2009). Federal Democratic Republic of Ethiopia. Central Statistical Authority (CSA), Agricultural sample survey 2008/2009 [2001E.C], Report on Livestock and Livestock characteristics (private peasant holding), Addis Ababa.

Cêtre-Sossah C, Mathieu B, Setier-Rio ML, Grillet C, Baldet T, Delécolle JC, Albina E (2008). Development and evaluation of a real-time quantitative PCR assay for Culicoides imicola, one of the main vectors of bluetongue (BT) and African horse sickness (AHS) in Africa and Europe. Res. Vet. Sci. 85(2):372-382.

Demissie GH (2013). Seroepidemiological Study of African Horse Sickness in Southern Ethiopia. Open Science Repository Veterinary Medicine 2013:e70081919.

Ende H, Tassew H, Gurmu EB, Amsalu K, Gizaw D (2011). Seroprevalence of African Horse Sickness at Central Highland of Ethiopia. Int. J. Agro Vet. Med. Sci. 9(4):139-148.

Ferhandey J, Ferhandey P, Rodriguey B, Sotelo E, Robles A, Arias M, Sanchey-vichiano J (2012). New advances in the molecular diagnosis of African Horse sickness (AHS). Proceedings of the 13th international symposium for the world association of veterinary laboratory Diagnosticians, 11-14 November, Melbourne, Australia.

Maclachlan NJ, Guthrie AJ (2010). Re-emergence of Bluetongue, African horse sickness and other Orbivirus diseases. Vet. Res. 41:35.

Molalegne B, Ashenafi A, Mihreteab B, Shiferaw J, Gelagay A and Esayas G (2010). Serological survey of African horse sickness in selected district of Jimma zone, southwestern Ethiopia. Trop. Anim. Health Prod. 43:1543-1547.

Mulualem T, Mekonnen A, Wudu T (2012). Seroprevalence and risk factors of African horse sickness in mules and donkeys in selected sites of West Amhara Region, Ethiopia African. J. Microbiol. Res. 6(19):4146-4151.

Office International Des Epizootics (OIE) (2004): Manual of Standards for Diagnostic Tests and Vaccines, African Horse sickness. pp. 73-80.

Office international epizootics (OIE) (2008). African horse sicknes, in manual of diagnostic tests and vaccine for terrestrial animals. 5th ed. New York, W.B. Saunders Company Ltd. pp. 582-583.

Rodriguez-Sanchez B, Fernandez-Pinero J, Sailleau C, Zientara S, Belak S, Arias M, Sanchez-Vizcaino JM (2008). Novel gel-based and real-time PCR assays for the improved detection of African Horse Sickness Virus. J. Virol. Method 151(1):87-94.

Sidama Zone of Agricultural and Rural Developments (SZARD), (2011). Personal Communication office data, Hawassa, Ethiopia.

Sidama Zone Planning and Economic Development Department (SZPEDD), (2004). Hawassa, Ethiopia.

STATA (2009). Stata Statistical Software, Release 7.0 Stata Corporation, College Station, Texas, USA.

Tesfaye T, Tadesse G, Tewodros F, Mersha C (2013). Seroprevalence and Associated Risk Factors of African Horse Sickness in Arsi and Bale Zones, Southeastern Ethiopia. Int. J. Anim. Vet. Adv. 4(5):326-332.

Thrusfield M (2005). Veterinary Epidemiology. 3rd ed., UK, Blackwell science Ltd, pp. 233-250.

Torrecuadrada M, Jorge L, Langeveld J, Venteo A, Sanz, A, Dalsgaard K, Hamilton W, Meloen R, Casal J (2011). Antigenic profile of African Horse Sickness virus serotype 4 VP5 and Identification of a Neutralizing Epitope shared with Blutongue virus and Epizootic Hemorrhagic Disease virus. Virology 257:449- 459.

Upadhyaya KA (2011). Text Book of Preventive Veterinary Medicine 1st ed. International Book Distributing Company, India. pp. 274-277.

9

Gastrointestinal nematodes of donkeys and horses in Gondar town northwest, Ethiopia

Anteneh Wondimu* and Getachew Sharew

College of Veterinary Medicine, Haramaya University P. O. Box 138 Dire Dawa, Ethiopia.

A study on the prevalence of gastrointestinal (GI) nematodes of equines was conducted from November 2011 to April 2012 in Gondar town to determine the prevalence and associated risk factors. A total of 103 horses and 281 donkeys were examined coprologicaly for the presence of GI nematode eggs using flotation techniques. Coprological result indicated horses and donkey harbor one or more nematodes infection in the total prevalence rate of 89.32% (92) and 98.22% (276) respectively. The two genera of parasite commonly encounter during the study period were strongyle type of egg (84.47 and 98.22%) and *Parascaris equorum* (43.69 and 23.35%) of horses and donkeys, respectively. Mixed infections were detected with prevalence of 76.9 and 40.8% in horses and donkeys, respectively. There was significant (P<0.05) difference in prevalence of strongyle type of eggs and *P. equorum* between species. Body condition is one factor which shows significant different in the numbers of nematodes eggs both in donkeys and horses as both the species with poor body condition harbor more parasitic egg than good body condition. Because of their importance and impact of disease on the use of equine a compressive study for strategic parasitic control measures should be implemented.

Key words: Gastrointestinal (GIT), nematodes, donkey, horse, Gondar, Ethiopia.

INTRODUCTION

Ethiopia has the largest livestock population of Africa country with estimated 35 million tropical livestock unit. This includes 2.03 million horses, and 7.43 million donkeys (CSA, 2015). According to CTA (1997) and Tegegne et al. (1999), 50% equine population of Africa is still found in Ethiopia. Equine play an important role in rural communities providing power and transport at low cost they can be used for various agricultural operations and also provide the much needed transport in rural areas for activities such as carrying water, building materials, agricultural products and people. Horses and mules are faster and more powerful animals for work but, on which is more costly to buy and maintain than a donkey (Pearson et al., 2003).

Despite its huge population size, equine remains marginal due to high prevalence of malnutrition, management constraints and disease like parasite. Parasitism represents a major obstacle to development of the livestock farming system in the country (Jobre et al., 1991) and characterized by high morbidity and mortality rates are to be mentioned.

Gastrointestinal nematodes are serious health hazards, contributing to poor body condition, reduced power output, poor productive performance and short life span

*Corresponding author. E-mail: anteneha7@gmail.com. Tel: +251 910172163.

(Pandey et al., 1994). Similarly, horses, donkeys and other equines is host for large numbers of internal parasites including blood protozoan parasites (Sumbria et al., 2014; Sumbria et al., 2015a, b; Sumbria et al., 2016). The vitality and other well-being of all ages are threaded by variety of internal parasites and the use of control measures ensures vigor and the best performance. The most common internal parasites are strongyles, *Parascaris*, pin worms (*Oxyuris equi*), and bots. Additionally, less important parasitic infection belongs to cestodes, lung worms, trematodes and intestinal thread worms (*Strongyloides*) (Powel and David, 1992; Hendrix and Charles, 2006). Despite the huge numbers and the increasing importance of equines in the Ethiopian economy, knowledge about the health problems affecting their welfare is limited for most parts of the country more over no previous study done on equine nematodes in and around Gondar town. Hence, it is necessary to examine the status and impact of these diseases and existing control measures (William and Masiga, 1998). Therefore, the objective of this study was to determine the prevalence of horses and donkeys gastrointestinal nematodes in the study area.

MATERIALS AND METHODS

Study area

The study was conducted in Gondar town and located 727 km North West of Addis Ababa. North Gondar zone located at an altitude ranging 1500 to 3500 m.a.s.l.. Numerous mountains, plateaus, hilly and sloppy areas, rivers, streams and lakes mark the topography of the zone. This zone is divided in to sub humid ("Wurch and Dega"), semi-arid ("Woynadega") and arid ("Kola"). The Gondar town is located at latitude of 12° 40'N and longitude of 27° 25'E with "Weyenadega" climate zone. The average minimum and maximum daily temperature of the area varies between 22, 30.7 and 12.3°C, respectively. The region receives a bimodal rain fall, the average annual precipitation rate being 1000mm. the short rains occur during the months of March, April and May while the long rains extend from June to September. The production system observed in the area combines mixed crop livestock production type. This zone had a livestock population of, 2.03 million cattle, 0.6 million sheep, 0.54 million goats, 0.25 million equine species and 1.9 million poultry (CSA, 2015).

Study population

The study animals were equines of two species (donkeys and horses) in Gondar town. All donkeys and horses were considered irrespective of age, sex and body condition score. These age classes were based on age of first work, productive age and the life span of Ethiopian donkeys (Svendsen, 1997). Donkeys were also grouped into different body condition score according to Svendsen (1997).

Study design

A cross-sectional study was carried out from November, 2011 to April, 2012 by collecting data on events associated with gastrointestinal nematodes of equines that are found in Gondar town.

Sample size determination

Simple random sampling strategy was followed to collect feces from individual animals. The sample size was decided based on the formula described by Thrusfield (2005) with 95% confidence interval at 5% desired absolute precision and by assuming the expected prevalence of 50%. The estimated sample size was calculated by the formula.:

$$N = \frac{1.96^2 \, Pexp\ (1\text{-}pexp)}{d^2} = 384$$

Where N = required sample size; Pexp = expected prevalence; d = desired absolute precision.

Methodology

Fecal sample was collected directly from the rectum of each animal using glove/freshly defecated feces with strict sanitation for each species, age and sex group and the sample placed in air and water tight vials and taken to the University of Gondar Veterinary Parasitology Laboratory. In the laboratory the sample was subjected to flotation technique and for identification of GIT nematodes egg of equines.

Parasitological examination

Saturated saline flotation technique

From collected sample, 3 g of fecal sample weighted and put into universal bottle and 42 ml of floatation fluid (NaCl) was added then mixed thoroughly. The presence of egg was appreciated using cover slip and test tube method (Urquhart et al., 1996).

Data management and analysis

The collected sample was entered into Microsoft excel and was analyzed using statistical software packages for social science (SPSS). Descriptive statics like percentage was used to determine the prevalence of GIT nematode and chi- square (χ^2) was used to look into the association of between prevalence of GIT nematodes and risk factors. In the analysis, confidence level was held at 95% and $p<0.05$ was set for significance.

RESULTS

The overall prevalence of GI nematodes was found as 368 (95.83%) as shown in Table 1. As indicated in Table 2 the prevalence of gastrointestinal nematodes on the basis of species shows 92(89.32%) and 276(98.22%) in horses and donkeys respectively. Out of the recorded eggs, 363(94.53%) was strongyle-type and 105(27.34%) of *P. equorum* eggs was recorded nematode eggs. The study also shows the prevalence rate of parasitic infection in different body condition of the animals. The result indicated the highest infection rate was recorded in poor body condition animals which was 99.07% but

Table 1. The overall prevalence of gastrointestinal nematode parasites.

No. of animals examined	No. % of positive animals	Prevalence
384	368	95.83%

Table 2. The prevalence of nematode parasites eggs on the basis of species and the type of nematode eggs.

Species	No. examined	No. of positive animals	Strongly type egg	*Parascaris equorum* egg
Horse	103	92(89.32%)	87(84.47%)	45(43.69%)
Donkey	281	276(98.22%)	276(98.22%)	60(21.35%)
Total	384	368(95.83%)	363(94.53%)	105(27.34%)

Pearson chi^2 (1) =14.9524; Pr=0.001.

Table 3. Prevalence of gastrointestinal nematode parasites on the basis of body condition.

Body condition score	No. of examined animas	No. of positive animals
Good	67	54(80.6%)
Medium	210	208(99.05%)
Poor	107	106(99.07%)
Total	384	368(95.83%)

Pearson chi^2(2) =47.1848; Pr=0.001.

medium and good body condition animals were relatively resistant for the nematode infection and the result was statically significant P>0.05 (Table 3)

The study indicate horses and donkeys were harboring one or mixed infection for strongyle and *P. equorum* parasite egg with the most frequently identified parasitic egg of strongyle type followed by *P. equorum* and there was significant difference in the prevalence rates of *P. equorum* and strongyle type of egg. Out of the total 103 donkey examined, 42(40.8%) were infected with strongyle type and *P. equorum* while out of the 281 horse examined, 216(76.9%) harbor both strongyle type and *P. equorum* egg type as described in Table 4.

DISCUSSION

Gastrointestinal nematode infection is the main disease condition affecting donkeys and horses in tropical and sub-tropical areas of the world (Svendsen, 1991). In the present study, microscopic fecal examination showed that the GI nematode parasite was an important health problem in the study area with over all prevalence rates of 95.83% which was 89.32 and 98.22%% in horse and donkey, respectively (Table 2). This is not much less than with the report by Tegegne et al. (1999) who indicated that no animal was found free out of 1340 examined from Adami Tulu, Ethiopia.

In the present study, the prevalence of strongyle species was 84.47 and 98.22% in horses and donkeys, respectively (Table 2) which was lower than those reported by Ayele et al. (2005) and Mulate (2005) who reported 100% prevalence in donkeys at Dugda Bora District and high land of Wollo provinces, respectively and Getachew et al. (2010) who reported 99% prevalence in working donkeys of Ethiopia. The prevalence was higher in the present study than the report of Saeed et al. (2010) and Seid (2011) who reported 65.51% on horses and 65.1% on both horses and donkeys, respectively. This difference may be due to ecological difference of those areas and deworming of animals when they went to the clinic for other bacterial diseases in the study areas.

In the present study, the prevalence of *P. equorum* was 43.69 and 21.35% in horses and donkeys respectively (Table 2). Similar report was generated by Ayele et al. (2005) at Dugda Bora District, Ethiopia. This is in agreement with the 34% prevalence reported by Tegegne et al. (1999) at Adami Tulu on donkey and also 32.5% prevalence reported by Ayele and Dinka. This might be due to the fact that horses were more frequently used in cart; also, they do not have enough time to graze on field only often in evening for one to two hours whereas donkeys have more time to graze on field. In this study age, and sex wise prevalence was not assessed because of the horses and donkeys were all adults and males that

Table 4. Prevalence of mix infection of GIT nematode based on egg type.

Species	No. of examined animals	No. of positive	Strongyle and *Parascaris equorum* mix found
Donkey	103	92(89.32%)	42 (40.8%)
Horse	281	276(98.22%)	216 (76.9%)

found in Gondar town working on cart and carrying of sand and stone besides the number of horses and donkeys are much vary because of few number of cart horses in the area.

CONCLUSION AND RECOMMENDATION

Besides the managerial problems from the owners there is also lack of knowledge on periodic deworming and treatment equines by taking to veterinary clinics when they get sick. Because of this reason almost all horse and donkey were positive for strongyles and moderately infected with *P. equorumin.* In line with above conclusion, the following recommendations are recommended:

1. Periodic deworming program shall be implemented for some animals by government for showing the importance until the community adapts.
2. Awareness should be created by teaching peoples in the meeting, by dramas on radio or television (mass media) about managerial systems and on the importance of GIT nematodes of equine.
3. Mixing of horses and donkey grazing should be avoided.

REFERENCES

Ayele G, Fesha G, Bojjia E, Getachew M, Alemayehu f, Tesfaye M, Amare B, Dereje N, Chala C, Asefa A, Anzunio G, Trawfod A (2005). Prevalence of Gastrointestinal Parasites of Donkeys in Dugda Bora districts, Ethiopia. pp. 14-21.

Central Statistical Agency (CSA) (2015). Federal Democratic Republic of Ethiopia; Agricultural Sample Survey 2014/15 Report On: Livestock and Livestock Characteristics: Statistical Bulletin, Volume II, P 22.

Getachew M, Trawford A, Feseha G, Reid SW (2010). Gastrointestinal parasites of working donkeys of Ethiopia. J. Trop. Anim. Health Prod. 42(1):27.

Hendrix G, Charles M (2006). Diagnostic Parasitology for Veterinary technician. 3rd edition, Linda, L, Duncan, Chaina.

Jobre Y, Gebreab F, Svendsen ED, Abdella M (1991). Health Problems of Working Donkeys in Debre Zeit and Menagesha of Ethiopia in Field. D and Pearson, R.A., (eds), Donkey, Mules and Horses in tropical agricultural development. Proceedings of colloquium held 3-6 September 1990.151-161.

Mulate B (2005). Preliminary study on helminthosis of Equines in South and North Wollo zones. Ethiopia Vet. J. 9(2):25-37.

Pandey VS, Khallaayoune K, Ouhelli H, Dakkak A (1994). Parasites of donkeys in Africa. Proceedings of the second colloquium on working equines (EDS. Bakkoury, M and Pretis, R.A.). Institutes of Agronomique et veterinary Hassan II. Rabat. Morocco. pp. 35-44.

Pearson RA, Simalenga TE, Krecek R (2003). Harnessing and hitching donkeys, horses and mules for work. Center for tropical veterinary medicine. University Of Edinburgh, UK and department of agriculture and rural engineering. University of venda for science and technology. South Africa. P 1.

Powel F, David G (1992). The health of horses. Great Britain.

Saeed K, Qadir Z, Ashraf K, Ahmad N (2010). Role Of Intrinsic And Extrinsic Epidemiological Factors on Strongylosis In Horses. J. Anim. plant Sci. 20(4):277-280.

Seid AA (2011). Prevalence of Equine strongylosis in and around Kombolcha, South Wollo Zone, Ethiopia. DVM thesis, Haramaya University, Haramaya Ethiopia.

Sumbria D, Moudgil AD, Singla LD (2014). Equine Piroplasmosis: Current status. *Veterinaria* 1(1):9-14.

Sumbria D, Singla LD, Kumar S, Sharma A, Dahiya RK, Setia R (2016). Spatial distribution, risk factors and haemato-biochemical alterationsassociated with Theileria equi infected equids of Punjab (India) diagnosed by indirect ELISA and nested PCR. Acta Trop. 155:104-112.

Sumbria D, Singla LD, Mandhotra A, Randhawa CS (2015b). Molecular Detection and Treatment of Equine Piroplasmosis. Philipp. J. Vet. Med. 52(2):131-136.

Sumbria D, Singla LD, Sharma A, Bal MS, Kumar S (2015a). Multiplex PCR for detection of *Trypanosoma evansi* and *Theileria equi* in equids of Punjab, India. Vet. Parasitol. 211:293-299.

Svendsen ED (1991). Donkeys; The international veterinary student 1(2):14-18.

Svendsen ED (1997).The professional Hand book of Donkey. Third edition. Whittet book LTD, W, 40 By, London.

Technical Center for Agricultural and Rural cooperation (CTA)(1997). Livestock development policies in Eastern and Southern Africa proceeding of seminar by CTA, OAU/ IBAR and the Ministry of Agriculture and cooperatives. Swaziland. pp. 216-220.

Tegegne T, Alemayehu A, Ayele GM (1999). Cross border livestock Trade and Food Security in the Southern and Southeastern Ethiopia Border lands. OSSREA. Developmental Report series. No.1 Commercial printing Enterprise. Addis Ababa, Ethiopia. pp. 1-6.

Thrusfield M (2005). Veterinary Epidemiology 2nd oxford. Blackwell science.

Urquhart G M, Armooky J, Duncan L, Dunn A and Mjenning F W (1996). Veterinary Parasitology, 2nd edition, Blackwell Science, Oxford, UK. P 307.

Williams A, Masiga W (1998). Viral diseases of animal in Africa. Nigeria, Lagos. Working Donkeys in Debre Zeit and Menagesha of Ethiopia in Field. D and Pearson, R.A., (eds), Donkey, Mules and Horses in tropical agricultural development. Proceedings of colloquium held 3-6 September 1990. pp. 151-161.

10

Bacterial pathogens of pigs with particular reference to *Escherichia coli*

Rukayya Hussain Abubakar[1], Evelyn Madoroba[2,3], Olubukola Adenubi[4], Darshana Morar-Leather[1] and Folorunso O. Fasina[1,5*]

[1]Department of Veterinary Tropical Diseases, Faculty of Veterinary Sciences, University of Pretoria, South Africa.
[2]Bacteriology Section, Agricultural Research Council–Onderstepoort Veterinary Research, South Africa.
[3]College of Agriculture and Environmental Sciences, University of South Africa, Florida Campus, South Africa.
[4]Department of Paraclinical Sciences, Faculty of Veterinary Sciences, University of Pretoria, South Africa .
[5]Emergency Centre for Transboundary Animal Diseases (ECTAD), Food and Agriculture Organization of the United Nations (FAO), UNON, Gigiri, Kenya.

Pigs are ungulate animals of the genus *Suis* and family Suidae. They are globally spread but restricted in certain countries due to religious and cultural beliefs. Pork serves as an important source of protein (38% of meat consumed in the world). While pig production remains a profitable enterprise, commercial and particularly the small-scale farmers face huge constraint in this husbandry practice, one of the most important being bacterial infections and its associated with morbidity and mortality. In this work, we reviewed the prevalence of bacterial infections in pigs with particular reference to *Escherichia coli*, a bacterium that is regularly isolated and can lead to multiple infections in pigs. Literatures were searched on selected veterinary and biological data bases in 2016 with focus on natural infections and isolates from natural infections with epidemiological details. Pathotypes, serotypes and serogroups of *E. coli*, the country of origin, source, growth stage, age of pigs infected, disease outbreak, the number of samples and type of samples, numbers and percentage of positive samples and isolates were used as filters. Pathotypes reported include enterotoxigenic *E. coli* (ETEC) 66.7%, enterotoxigenic *E. coli* and shiga toxigenic *E. coli* (ETEC and STEC) 14.3%, STEC only (7.9%), enterotoxigenic *E. coli*/enteropathogenic *E. coli*/enteroaggregative *E. coli* (ETEC/EPEC/EAE) 31.7%. Others were enterohaemorrhagic *E. coli* (EHEC), diffusely adherent *E. coli* (DAEC) (ETEC, EPEC, STEC) and extra-intestinal pathogenic *E. coli* (ExPEC). Twenty-nine countries with documented records of cases of *E. coli* were included with the USA reporting, the highest number followed by China. About 74% of the samples were taken from farms and others were from samples submitted to research laboratories and veterinary faculties for necropsy. Serogroups O141, O149, O139, O138, O8 and O9 were most common. Piglets were most affected (52.3%) followed by weaners (39.6%) and porkers (7.9%) with age ranging from 1 to 392 days old. A total of 24,854 isolates were considered, 10477 (42.2%) were positives and the following genes were carried: STa, STb, LT, stx1, stx2, Stx-2e, F4, F5, F6, F18, F41, AIDA, EAST1, eae, paa and hlyA. The diseases produced by *E. coli* were neonatal diarrhoea, colibacillosis, post-weaning diarrhoea and edema disease. The associated risk factors were poor housing, management and feed changes, extensive use of antibiotics as prophylaxis, overcrowding, and high humidity and temperature changes. India, USA, Japan, Slovakia, Denmark Sweden and Poland were countries with significant reports and high detection of virulence factors (72 to 100%).

Key words: *Escherichia coli,* diarrhea, serogroups, enterotoxigenic, colibacillosis.

INTRODUCTION

Pigs are ungulate animals of the genus *Suis* and family Suidae. Domesticated pigs originated from the European wild boar *Susscrofa* are indigenous to the Eurasian and African continents (Giuffra et al., 2000).The global pig population is estimated to be approximately one billion (Statista, 2016), and although this spread across the world, it may be restricted in certain countries due to religious and cultural beliefs. Pork serves as an important source of protein (38% of meat consumed in the world) and as a means of livelihood especially for women in developing countries (Madzimure et al., 2012). Pigs are also kept for leather, hair, as pets and use in human research (Gosh, 2014).

While pig production remains a profitable enterprise, commercial and particularly the small-scale farmers face huge constraints in this husbandry practice, one of the most important being bacterial infections and its associated with morbidity and mortality. We reviewed the prevalence of bacterial infections in pigs and paid particular attention to *Escherichia coli*, a bacterium that is regularly isolated and can lead to multiple infections in pigs.

The key words used to gather literature for review include; " *Escherichia coli* or *E.coli*", "pig, swine or porcine", "outbreak", "diarrhoea", "Oedema disease", "post weaning diarrhoea", "colibacillosis" and "prevalence". Literature searches were performed on selected veterinary and biological databases including the CAB Abstract, Medline, Pubmed, Science Direct and Google Scholar between January and November, 2016. Particular consideration was given to natural infections and isolates from natural infections with epidemiological details. Pathotypes, serotypes and serogroups of *E. coli*, the country of origin, source, growth stage, age of pigs infected, disease outbreak, the number of samples and type of samples, numbers and percentage of positive samples and isolates were used as filters. All literature considered were in English or where available then the English translations were used.

Extracted and compiled published manuscripts from peer reviewed journals were quality-checked and duplicate documents were removed. All remaining documents (n = 61) were filtered, harmonized and coded in a single Microsoft Excel® spreadsheet. The number of events, sample sizes and outcomes were calculated based on the available data. All data was analysed using the Fixed-effect model (precision-based estimates) in the Meta-analyses software on Excel (Neyellof et al., 2012). Comparison between individual studies was calculated in WinPepi v11.24 (Abramson, 2011) and presented in percentages with 95% confidence intervals. Cumulative events with measures of central tendencies were also produced in forest plots.

Bacterial pathogens of pigs

Based on our evaluation, the bacteria that affect pigs are diverse and vast but are not limited to the following, grouped by areas of primary lesions:

Cutaneous (skin) associated bacteria

Staphylococcus species

Infection in pigs is caused by *Staphylococcus hyicus* resulting in exudative epidermitis (Greasy pig disease) (Andresen, 1998). *Staphylococcus hyicus* is composed of both non-virulent and virulent strains which produces an exfoliative toxin, responsible for skin alteration in exudative epidermitis of pigs (Wegener et al., 1993; Andresen et al., 1997).

It is characterized by sudden onset of excess sebaceous secretion and exudation from the skin without pruritus leading to dehydration, growth depression and possibly death (Taylor, 2013). Other Staphylococcus species that could be isolated are *Staphylococcus chromogenes* and *Staphylococcus Sciuri* (Chen et al., 2007). *Staphylococcus aureus* is another important and common pathogen isolated from swollen ears, umbilical abscesses, subcutaneous abscesses and foot lesions, (Taylor, 2013; De Neeling et al., 2007).

Treponema species

Treponema species are associated with skin or mucous membrane diseases and cause skin ulcers in pigs regularly (Karlsson, 2014). Three major phylotypes are involved in infections which include: Treponema pedis (the most predominant), Treponema parvum and an undesignated phylotype (Karlsson, 2014).

Treponema pedis infection can occur as cutaneous spirochaetosis, ear necrosis and spirochaetal granuloma. They have been indicated as secondary bacterial infection in severe and chronic skin lesions of pigs (Taylor, 2013; Karlsson, 2014), such as ulcerative porcine stomatitis (Jensen et al., 2014) and periodic outbreaks of ear necrosis among weaners and gingival infections (Pringle et al., 2009; Karlsson et al., 2013).

*Corresponding author. E-mail: daydupe2003@yahoo.co.uk.

Reproductive system associated bacteria

Leptospira species

Leptospirosis, caused by *Leptospira* species is a disease that occurs worldwide in pigs and infection which is more common in animals kept outdoors (Ryley and Simmons, 1954). Route of infection is by ingestion, direct contact and through abrasions, trans-placental transmission or the veneral route (Taylor, 2013). *Leptospira* species are fine, spiral, aerobic, motile, gram negative bacteria (spirochete) of about 10 μm in length and 0.2 μm in diameter (Faine, 1994).

Approximately, 13 serovars of *Leptospira* are involved in infections in pigs and associated primarily with reproductive losses in breeding herds. The organisms persist in the kidneys and genital tracts of carrier pigs and are excreted in urine and genital fluids (Taylor, 2013). Routine vaccination may reduce the effect of the bacteria in a herd (Whyte et al., 1982), but elimination may be a difficult target because, pig is a reservoir host for leptospirosis.

Brucella species

Brucella suis infection in pigs, occurs mainly through the venereal or oral route (Xavier et al., 2010). Infection develops as bacteremia may persist for as long as 90 days which may lead to localisation in various tissues with resultant stillbirths, abortions, orchitis, lameness, posterior paralysis, spondylitis, occasional metritis and abscess formation. Infertility may occur in both sexes (Xavier et al., 2010; Deyoe, 1967).

Other pathogenic species in pigs are *B. abortus* and *B. mellitensis* (Godfroid, 2002). Diagnosis is mainly through the brucellosis card (Rose Bengal) test; but serum agglutination tests or complement fixation tests have also been used (Nicoletti, 2010). Brucellosis in pigs has a global distribution however its prevalence in domestic pigs is low in some countries and known to have been eradicated in USA (Godfroid, 2002).

Listeria species

Infection of pigs with *Listeria* species is common and previous study in Japan, Denmark and Yugoslavia suggested that approximately 10% of pigs at slaughter are infected (Taylor, 2013; Lungu et al., 2010). *Listeria monocytogenes* infection rarely causes disease, but sudden death in piglets, septicaemia and nervous signs have been recorded.

Most authors concurred that, porcine listeriosis occurs mainly as a septicaemia in piglets less than ten days old (Ladds et al., 1974; Long and Dukes, 1972; Busch et al., 1971) and multifocal hepatic necrosis is often the most notable necropsy finding in piglets (Lopez and Bildfell, 1989). Abortions, stillbirths and birth of weak piglets may also occur in sows (Taylor, 2013; Vannier, 1999). *Listeria* infection and carriage in domestic pigs or wild boar is a potential source of infection for man (Taylor, 2013; Borch et al., 1996).

Erysipelothrix species

Erysipelothrix rhusiopathiae is a small, facultative anaerobic, Gram positive (G+ve) rod that causes a condition known as swine erysipelas (Opriessnig et al., 2010; Wood and Steele, 1994). The disease outbreak may present as acute, sub-acute or chronic. It is characterized by sudden death or fever associated with characteristic diamond skin lesions (Opriessnig et al., 2010). Arthritis, vegetative endocarditis and abortion in pregnant sows may be observed (Schrauwen et al., 1993).

Necropsy lesions include enlarged and congested lymph nodes, oedematous and congested lungs, splenomegaly, hepatomegaly, petechial haemorrhages on the kidneys and heart. *E. rhusiopathiae* causes considerable economic losses and remains an animal hygiene problem in swine production areas of the world (Takeshi et al., 1999), and up to 50% of pigs in the world are estimated to harbour the organism in their tonsils and lymphoid organs (Opriessnig et al., 2010).

This status results in shedding of the organism in urine, faeces, saliva and nasal secretions (Opriessnig et al., 2004).

Respiratory system associated bacteria

Actinobacillus species

Actinobacillus suis and *Actinobacillus equuli* are two important species that may cause fatal septicaemia, endocarditis and arthritis in pigs of 1 to 6 weeks of age. In older animals, skin lesions and focal necrotising pneumonia, valvular endocarditis, abortion, metritis and polyarthritis may be seen (Radostits et al., 2000; Ramos-Vara et al., 2008). Clinical signs and post-mortem lesions are not specific but suggestive of the disease (Taylor, 2013).

Additionally, *Actinobacillus pleuropneumonia* may cause a respiratory infection of weaned, growing and finishing pigs in which there is fibrinous pleurisy and pneumonia with characteristic infarcts in the lungs. Infection which is highly contagious, often fatal and progressive weight loss in chronically affected pigs may be observed (Taylor, 2013; Frank et al., 1992).

Mycoplasma species

Mycoplasma organisms have been isolated from pigs but

only four species have repeatedly been associated with clinical disease namely (1) *Mycoplasma hyorhinis* which cause polyserositis and arthritis in young pigs of about 3 to 10 weeks; (2) *M. hyosynoviae* causes arthritis in growing pigs weighing between 35kg and 110kg live weight (Taylor, 2013); (3) *Mycoplasma hyopneumoniae* which is a primary pathogen of enzootic pneumonia, a chronic respiratory disease in pigs, highly prevalent in almost all pig producing areas. It is also considered to be one of the primary agents involved in the porcine respiratory disease complex (PRDC) (Thacker, 2006).

The organism is primarily found on the mucosal surface of the trachea, bronchi and bronchioles (Blanchard et al., 1992); and (4) *Mycoplasma suis* (formerly *Eperythrozoon suis*) infection which affects piglets 0 to 5 days of age, but weaners, growers and sowers may also be infected. Route of infection is by parenteral, transplacental or oral transmission and the clinical disease may manifests in 5 to 6 days.

The acute phase involves fever, anaemia, icterus, unthriftiness, jaundice and poor growth in weaned pigs, and is associated with low morbidity at high mortality rates (Messick, 2004). The chronic phase results in low reproductive efficiency, growth retardation, abortions, stillbirths and agalactia in sows (Messick, 2004; Heinritzi, 1989). In addition, a study revealed that *Mycoplasma arthritidis*, a rodent *Mycoplasma* has also been isolated from joints in an outbreak of conjunctivitis, severe polyarthritis and infertility in a boar stud (Binder et al., 1990).

Bordetella **species**

Bordetella bronchisepticais regarded as the aetiologic agent of atrophic rhinitis, colonises the ciliated epithelium of the upper and lower respiratory tract at about one week of age in piglets. It causes rhinitis characterised by sneezing, shortening or twisting of the snout, hypoplasia, mild nasal turbinate atrophy, persistent purulent bronchitis, haemorrhage, pneumonia and impaired growth (Giles, 1992; Duncan et al., 1966; Mazumder et al., 2012).

Bordetella bronchiseptica predisposes pigs to colonization and disease with other bacteria such as *Pasteurella multocida* and *Haemophilus parasuis* (Brockmeier, 2004; Brockmeier et al., 2001).

Pasteurella **species**

Pasteurella multocida is associated with pneumonia and atrophic rhinitis in pigs and can result in important economic losses on large pig farms worldwide (Davies et al., 2003; Dziva et al., 2008). Its strains are grouped into five capsular serogroups; A, B, D, E and F , however only serogroup A,B and D have been recovered from pigs (Davies et al., 2003; Townsend et al., 1998; Tang et al., 2009). Toxigenic *P. multocida* serogroups A and D together with *Bordetella bronchiseptica,* coexist to cause atrophic rhinitis (Davies et al., 2003; Backstrom et al., 1988).

Toxigenic *P. multocida* infection results in severe sneezing in non-immune piglets. This is later followed by atrophy of the turbinate bones and a distortion of the nasal septum, shortening and twisting of the upper jaw which may be accompanied by reduction in the rate of weight gain (Taylor, 2013). Similarly, pneumonic pasteurellosis is also a condition that results from the colonisation of existing lung lesions with *P. multocida* which may give rise to fever, respiratory distress and death in some cases and it is typically associated with sub-acute or chronic pleuritis. Common route of transmission is by nose-to-nose contact; however, both vertical and horizontal transfer may occur (Taylor, 2013; Davies et al., 2004).

Mannheimia (Pasteurella) haemolytica has been isolated in piglets from localised areas of fibrinous pleurisy or pleuropneumonia and from outbreaks of diarrhoea in pigs (Taylor, 2013).

Haemophilus **species**

Haemophilus parasuis is found in the upper respiratory tract of pigs as a commensal bacterium, but invades and cause severe systemic disease under favourable conditions (Oliveira et al., 2003). It causes Glassers disease and acute septicaemia (Peet et al., 1983; Riley et al., 1977). Glassers disease is an infectious, sometimes fatal polyserositis, polyarthritis and meningitis of young pigs (Amano et al., 1994). Bronchitis and other syndromes may occur in older animals in non-immune herds (Taylor, 2013).

Transmission is by direct contact and all age categories of pigs are susceptible to the infection (Oliveira and Pijoan, 2002).Post mortem lesions include serofibrinous or fibrino-purulent exudate on mucosal surfaces, usually in peritoneum, pericardium, pleura or joint surface. In the septicaemic form, petechial and ecchymotic haemorrhages are detected in liver, kidneys and brain (Amano et al., 1994).

Mycobacterium **species**

Several species of *Mycobacterium* such as *Mycobacterium porcinum, Mycobacterium avium* subsp. *hominisuis, Mycobacterium bovis, Mycobacterium intracellulare, Mycobacterium fortuitum* and *Mycobacterium tuberculosis* have been associated with tuberculosis in pigs. *Mycobacterium avium* subsp. *hominisuis* is an opportunistic pathogen, infecting mainly pigs and humans (Mijs et al., 2002; Inderlied et al., 1993; Thorel et al.,

2001).

A recent study demonstrated cross-reactions between avian and bovine tuberculin in pigs (Agdestein et al., 2011). *Mycobacteria bovis* is the main agent causing tuberculosis in cattle, while *M. tuberculosis* primarily causes tuberculosis in humans.

However, they both belong to the *M. tuberculosis* complex (MTC) and can lead to infections in pigs (Komijn et al., 1999; Biet et al., 2005). Tuberculosis is mostly observed in pigs at slaughter when gross lesions are detected primarily through the examination of the lymph nodes of the head and the visceral regions and partial or full carcasses condemnation usually follow, because it is a potential risk to human health.

Streptococcus **species**

Streptococcus suis is an encapsulated gram positive coccus and occurs singly in pairs, or occasionally in short chains. It is a normal flora in the upper respiratory tract of pigs, the genital and digestive tracts (Higgins and Gottschalk, 1999). *S. suis* causes septicaemia, arthritis and meningitis in suckling piglets and post-weaning pigs but less commonly in finishing pigs (Taylor, 2013; Gottschalk et al., 2007). The organism is an emerging zoonotic agent responsible for septicaemia which may sometimes be accompanied by septic shock and meningitis in humans (Goyette-Desjardins et al., 2014).

Streptococcus porcinus infection also occurs in pigs and is sometimes referred to as streptococcal lymphadenitis or streptococcal abcess. It causes abscess particularly in the cervical lymph nodes (Taylor, 2013). The Lancefield group C and β-haemolytic streptococci are other streptococci infections in pigs that are commonly isolated from the upper respiratory tract, pharynx, retropharyngeal lymph nodes and genital tract of carrier pigs. They are associated with vaginitis in sows and neonatal septicaemia in newborn piglets and may be isolated from arthritis and vegetative endocarditis in older animals and froms epticaemic and pneumonic lesions in older finishing pigs (Taylor, 2013). A presumptive diagnosis of infection in pigs is usually based on clinical signs and macroscopic lesions (Staats et al., 1997).

Digestive system associated bacteria

Clostridium **species**

Clostridial pathogens involved in pig infections include ***Clostridium*** *perfringens* (type A, C), *Clostridium defficiletyphocolitis, Clostridium tetani, Clostridium novyi, Clostridium botulinum, Clostridium septicum* and *Clostridium chauvoei* (Taylor, 2013; Baker et al., 2010). *Clostridium perfringens* type C is a large gram positive rod, which occasionally forms spores, bears attachment site and produces very potent toxins. The major toxin produced is protease/trypsin-sensitive β toxin which causes fatal necrotic and haemorrhagic enteritis in piglets less than seven days old and may cause chronic infection in older piglets. Clinical signs include profuse, bloody diarrhoea, loss of weight, palour and death within 12 to 24 h (Taylor, 2013; Songer and Meer, 1996).

C. perfringens Type A causes a similar syndrome but less severe with the major toxin produced being the α-toxin (Taylor, 2013; Songer and Uzal, 2005). *C. difficile* is toxigenic and produce two major toxins, A and B (Taylor, 2013; Diab et al., 2016). It is a recognized cause of antibiotic-associated diarrhoea and pseudomembranous colitis in humans, domestic and laboratory animals (Songer et al., 2000). Infection in pigs (neonatal enteritis) can be asymptomatic or result in diarrhoea and weight loss which may be chronic in suckling pigs (Taylor, 2013). Other clinical signs such as dyspnoea, mild abdominal distension, and scrotal oedema may be observed with characteristic ulcerative lesions present in the colon at post-mortem (Taylor, 2013).

C. tetani causes tetanus which presents as stiffness and abnormal gait leading to spasm and death. The condition occurs sporadically in young pigs and may be associated with umbilical infections, castration, or ovario hysterectomy (Taylor, 2013; Meseko and Oluwayelu, 2012). Additionally, *C. novyi* type B causes sudden death in large fattening pigs and sows. Incidence is worldwide and sporadic particularly in swill-fed pigs and older sows (Duran and Walton, 1997). Food-borne botulism is caused by *C. botulinum* through a preformed toxin of this organism in food resulting in a rare, sometimes fatal flaccid paralysis in pigs. The incidence is worldwide but rarely described (Taylor, 2013; Beiers and Simmons, 1967).

Salmonella **species**

Salmonellosis in pigs is caused by *Salmonella Enterica* serovar Choleraesuis var kunzendorf (Salmon and Smith, 1886; Stevens and Gray, 2013; Pedersen et al., 2015). It is a host specific, facultative, intracellular pathogen that causes paratyphoid (Gray et al., 1996).

The infection may result in enteric and fatal systemic disease, however, infected pigs may carry the organism in the tonsils, intestines and the gut-associated lymphoid tissue asymptomatically (Fedorka-Cray et al., 2000; Alban et al., 2012). Transmission is primarily through the faeco-oral route (Stevens and Gray, 2013), some studies have shown that the upper and lower respiratory tract may also serve as routes of infection (Fedorka-Cray et al., 1995).The infections may be present in different forms including (1) septicaemic form which is commonest in piglets with up to 100% mortality, (2) the acute enteric form in younger and weaned pigs,(3) the chronic enteric form and (4) the diarrheic form, which is usually due to the less invasive serotypes such as *Salmonella Typhimurium* (Taylor, 2013).

Brachyspira species

Brachyspira hyodysenteriae is a large anaerobic spirochaete that causes dysentery-infectious mucohaemorrhagic colitis of pigs (Wills, 2000). It affects pigs during the growth and finishing periods, and is characterized clinically by loss of condition with diarrhoea containing varying amounts of mucus, blood and necrotic material (Burrough, 2016).

The bacterium multiplies in the large intestine result in superficial mucosa degeneration, inflammation and multifocal points of bleeding along the mucosa. The organism does not infiltrate beyond the intestinal mucosa and results in decreased reabsorption of endogenous secretions from the unaffected small intestine leading to diarrhea (Kennedy et al., 1988). In instances, a proportion of untreated pigs may die while others may remain stunted (Taylor, 2013). Other *Brachyspira spirochaetes* that may also be involved in diarrhea are *Brachyspira innocens, Brachyspira murdochii, Brachyspira intermedia* and *Brachyspira pilosicoli* (Taylor, 2013).

Campylobacter species

Campylobacter is a gram negative, spiral, non-spore forming rod (Penner, 1988; Epps et al., 2013) and pigs are natural reservoirs with a prevalence rate of approximately 50 to 100% and excretion level of about 102 to 107 CFU/g (Jensen et al., 2006; Alter et al., 2005; Nielsen et al., 1997).*Campylobacter* infection causes a mucoid, creamy diarrhoea, which may contain blood in piglets 3 days-3weeks of age (Taylor, 2013). The species associated with disease in pigs include *Campylobacter coli* (the most common), *Campylobacter jejuni, Campylobacter hyointestinalis* and *Campylobacter sputorum* (Taylor, 2013; Alter et al., 2005).

Other *Campylobacter* species present in the porcine intestine, which may multiply and become associated with enteritis, are *C. hyointestinalis subsp. hyointestinalis, C. hyointestinalis subsp. lawsonii, Campylobacter mucosalis, Campylobacter hyoilei, Campylobacter lari* and *Campylobacter lanienae* (Taylor, 2013).

Helicobacter species

This infection in pigs is caused by *Helicobacter suis*, a gram negative, spiral-shaped bacterium that is commonly found in the gastric mucosa (Hellemans et al., 2007; Grasso et al., 1996; Park et al., 2004). Piglets and porkers have highest colonisation, found in the pyloric region, however, boars and sows, also have high colonization rates in the fundic region of the gastric mucosa (Hellemans et al., 2007).

The clinical infection by this organism is rare, and the main evidence for the pathogenicity of *H. suis* was from experimental studies that showed clear association between *H. suis* infection and the development of gastritis as well as a decrease in daily weight gain (De Bruyne et al., 2012).

Lawsonia species

This organism, *Lawsonia intracellularis* is an obligate, intracellular, gram negative, small, rod-shaped, intestinal, bacterium; it is the cause of proliferative enteropathyin pigs (Guedes and Gebhart, 2003), a frequent diarrhea disease of piglets and weaners characterised by hyperplasia and inflammation of the ileum and colon (Smith and McOrist, 1997).

Study has suggested that it infect mitotically the active epithelial cells of the intestinal crypts, which later multiply and spread in the cells as they divide (Boutrup et al., 2010). The condition is often mild and self-limiting but sometimes may result in necrotic enteritis, regional ileitis and proliferative haemorrhagic enteropathy. Affected pigs appear pale, may be stunted and may die suddenly with clotted blood in the lumen of the small intestine (Taylor, 2013; Guedes and Gebhart, 2003).

Yersinia species

Yersinia species are gram negative bacilli and the species associated with pig infection include (1) *Yersinia enterocolitica,* which easily colonise the gut of neonate piglets and subsequently become healthy carriers (Skjerve et al., 1998), it is capable of causing enteritis and typhilocolitis in weaned pigs and abortion in sows (Bhaduri et al., 2005); (2) *Yersinia pseudotuberculosis* which is also carried normally as gut resident (Taylor, 2013; Laukkanen, 2010).

Acute cases are characterized by enteritis, lymphadenitis and splenomegaly while chronic cases result in granulomatous nodules and localised abscesses affecting various organs, usually the liver and lungs (Brugmann et al., 2001). About 35 to 70% of herds and 4.5 to 100% of individual pigs carry *Yersinia* species asymptomatically (Bhaduri et al., 2005).

Enterococcus species

Enterococcus durans (Lancefield Group D) is a motile gram positive cocci that has been isolated from the intestines and faeces of 3 to 5 day old piglets, usually as commensals but may sometimes be associated with diarrhea (Taylor, 2013; Cheon and Chae, 1996).

Enterotoxins and mucosal damage have been identified with diarrhoea caused by *E. durans* however, decreased activity of digestive enzymes at the mucosal brush borders have suggested that the entire pathogenesis of diarrhoea due to *E. durans* has not been completely understood (Cheon and Chae, 1996; Tzipori et al., 1984).

***Bacillus* species**

Bacillus anthracis causes anthrax but are rare in pigs. Affected animals may die suddenly, pass bloody faeces or die after swelling of the neck. Route of entry is mainly by ingestion of contaminated feed (Taylor, 2013).

Other non-specific bacteria pathogens include

***Actinobaculum* species**

Actinomyces suis reclassified as *Actinobaculum suis* is associated with urinary tract infections in pigs (Lawson et al., 1997; Woldemeskel et al., 2002). It is linked with cystitis-pyelonephritis complex, a syndrome in which a small group of sows or gilts pass bloody purulent urine, often soon after service. They rapidly lose condition and sudden death may supervene (Taylor, 2013).

***Chlamydophila* species**

Chlamydophila pathogens in pigs are *Chlamydia suis, Chlamydophila pecorum, Chlamydophila psittaci* and *Chlamydophila abortus*. The infections from this organism may results in multiple lesions including conjunctivitis, enteritis, pneumonia, pleurisy, pericarditis, polyarthritis, orchitis, infertility, abortion and birth of weak piglets (Taylor, 2013; Szeredi et al., 1996; Jiang et al., 2013).

Miscellaneous bacteria pathogens isolated from pigs

(i) Since 1978, *Arcobacter* species have been associated with reproductive disorders, but excretion by clinically healthy pigs has been frequently reported as well. Information on *Arcobacter* colonization of the porcine gastrointestinal tract is lacking to date (De Smet et al., 2012).
(ii) *Aeromonas hydrophila* has been isolated from enteritis, urine infections and lymphnodes (Igbinosa et al., 2016; Gray and Stickler, 1989).
(iii) *Acinetobacter calcoaceticans, Trueperella (Arcanobacterium) pyogenes, Bacteroides fragilis*are found in the large intestine and have been isolated from diarrhoea in piglets both before and after weaning (Taylor, 2013; Hijazin et al., 2012; Myers and Shoop, 1987).
(iv) *Flavo bacterium*, a ciliated bacillus has been identified in the trachea of pigs. It has been recorded in cases of pneumonia and has been associated with lesions of active tracheitis (Nietfeld et al., 1995).
(v) *Corynebacterium pseudotuberculosis* has been recovered from the vagina and prepuce of healthy swine and from mandibular abscess of black Alentejano pigs (Kudo and Yanagawa, 1987; Oliveira et al., 2014) while *Corynebacterium ulcerance* was recovered from a case of caseous lymphadenitis in Germany (Contzen et al., 2011).
(vi) *Coxiella burneti* antibodies have been demonstrated in pigs (Taylor, 2013).
(vii) *Klebsiella* species sometimes are seen in chronic respiratory tract diseases, enteritis and mastitis (Došen et al., 2007; Ross et al., 1975; Wilcock, 1979).
(viii) *Legionella pneumophila* has been demonstrated in the sera of pneumonic pigs in the UK (Taylor, 2013).
(ix) *Burkholderia pseudomallei is* the cause of meliodosis in pigs in tropical and subtropical regions (Omar et al., 1962; Rampling, 1964).
(x) *Rhodococcus equi* usually present in granulomatous lesions in submandibular lymphnodes (Witkowski et al., 2016; Rzewuska et al., 2014).

Enteric bacteria in pigs

The pig gastrointestinal tract has a complex and dynamic microbial ecosystem, the composition of which differs between individuals, region of the gastrointestinal tract, as well as age of the animal (Konstantinov et al., 2004). This microbial flora has an important role as one of the major defence mechanisms of the animal mainly through competition for nutrients and attachment sites and stimulation of cross-reactive antibodies, which prepares the immune system in defence against pathogenic microbes (Tancrede, 1992).

The large intestine contains most of the microbial flora (over 400 species) (Sørum and Sunde, 2001) and consist of (a) strict Gram postive anaerobes and facultative anaerobes such as *Streptococci*, *Lactobacilli*, *Eubacteria*, *Bacteroides* species, *Fusobacterium* species, *Clostridium* species and *Peptostreptococcus* species; and (b) facultative anaerobes such as *E.coli, Klebsiella* species, *Enterobacter* species and *Enterococcus* species (Sørum and Sunde, 2001; Jensen, 2001). Factors which can cause microbial flora changes in the pig gastrointestinal tract include psychological and behavioural stressors, environment, weaning, age, feeding systems and the pigs genotype (Burrin and Stoll, 2003).

Global pig production is most frequently and economically affected by enteric bacterial infections (Moxley and Duhamel, 1999). Common clinical signs found include diarrhoea, reduced growth rate, weight loss and death (Moxley and Duhamel, 1999). Some changes found in the intestines of pigs with enteric bacterial infections include: attaching and effacing lesions, in enteropathogenic *E. coli* and *B.pilosicoli* infection, inflammation with *Salmonella enterica* and necrotizing and haemorrhagic lesions with certain *C. perfringens* (Moxley and Duhamel, 1999).

Lactobacilli family dominates the normal bacterial flora in pigs and produces lactic acid as an essential metabolic end-product. The concentration of lactic acid increases several-fold within the first few days post-weaning and results in decreased pH of the gut which eliminates other pathogenic enterobacteria (Janczyk et al., 2007; Pieper et al., 2008). This group of microorganisms is generally considered beneficial as their attachment to the mucosa may protect the animals from gut infection (Houdijk et al., 2002). Furthermore, cultivation-based studies have shown that lactic acid bacteria, *Enterobacteria* and *Streptococci* were the most important first colonisers of the pig intestine (Stewart, 1997). Similarly, 16S rRNA gene clone analysis indicated that ileal samples of two-day old piglets harboured a group of *E. coli, Shigella flexneri, Lactobacillus sobrius, Lactobacillus reuteri* and *Lactobacillus acidophilus* related sequences (Konstantinov et al., 2006).

E. coli

E. coli strains in pigs forms part of the normal faecal flora. However, when they acquire virulent genes they are able to cause disease (Taylor, 2013).These coliform bacteria are commonly used as representatives of the enterobacteria from faecal samples in culture based studies of the intestinal bacterial flora, as they are the major facultative anaerobic bacteria in the intestinal tract of most animal species (Dubreuil, 2012). *E. coli* are gram negative rods, flagellated with variable length and diameter of about 1μm.On culture colonies grow on solid media within 24 h after incubation and may be smooth, rough or mucoid (Fairbrother and Gyles, 2012). Major characteristics associated with pathogenic *E. coli* infections are proteins such as fimbriae and production of enterotoxins usually by the enterotoxigenic *E. coli* (ETEC) and Shiga toxin by Shigatoxigenic *E. coli* (STEC). Other toxins previously described are EAST1, cytotoxins, cytolethal distending toxin, hemolysin; outer membrane proteins (intimin) and adhesin involved in diffuse adherence (Taylor, 2013). In addition, study has shown that F18 was the main colonization factor for STEC and ETEC withF18ab and F18acas subgroups (Cheng et al., 2005).

E. coli strains have been identified as an important cause of several diseases in pigs worldwide including neonatal septicaemia, neonatal diarrhoea, post-weaning diarrhoea, oedema disease (bowel oedema or gut oedema), cystitis, septicaemia, polyserositis, coliform mastitis and urinary tract infections. They can also colonise existing lesions elsewhere in the body (Taylor, 2013; Fairbrother and Gyles, 2012). Post-weaning diarrhoea (post-weaning enteric colibacillosis) and oedema disease have a more significant impact in the porcine industry because they result in high economic losses due to high morbidity and mortality, decrease weight gain, the cost of treatments, vaccination and feed supplementation (Fairbrother and Gyles, 2012).The *E. coli* infections occur at different ages in the pigs. Coli septicaemia occurs in 0 to 4 days old piglets and may be associated with diarrhoea. Enteritis (enteric colibacillosis) which is also associated with diarrhoea, occurs at three main periods in the pigs life; neonatal diarrhoea occurs at 0 to 4 days of age, neonatal-weaning diarrhoea at 4 days to 3 to 4wks and post weaning diarrhoea usually associated with weaning, oedema disease occurs in recently weaned pigs while mastitis and cystitis occur in adult sows (Taylor, 2013).

Outbreaks of *E. coli* diarrhea have increased worldwide with post-weaning diarrhoea being the most common where F4 and F18 are usually associated with adhesion factors (Fairbrother and Gyles, 2006). This could be due to the emergence of more virulent *E. coli* clones, a benign commensal of the gut microflora which multiply rapidly and cause disease through colonisation of the intestinal mucosa or changes in the management of pigs (Fasina et al., 2015).

Furthermore, a potentially beneficial method of feeding behaviour and maintaining gastrointestinal health in pigs is through feeding weaners with liquid feed or fermented liquid feed, in contrast to dry feed, as it is considered a possible feeding strategy to maintain a high and regular feed and water intake of weaners (Canibe and Jensen, 2012). Avoiding a drastic decrease in feed and water intake after weaning is believed to ameliorate the post-weaning lag period in piglets which may predispose them to *E. coli* infections (Canibe and Jensen, 2012).

Classification of *E. coli*

The best approach to classify *E. coli* is by serotyping in association with virulent strains. However, only a small percentage of the organisms are typeable based on O, K, H and F antigens, and only about 175O, 80K, 56H and over 20F antigens have been officially recognized to date, based on proven or suspected pathogenicity of *E. coli* isolates (Fairbrother and Gyles, 2012).

Pathotype is the term used to classify *E. coli* by their virulence mechanisms. The broad classes identified include, Shiga toxin producing *E. coli* (STEC), enterohaemorrhagic *E. coli* (EHEC), enteropathogenic *E. coli* (EPEC) and extraintestinal pathogenic *E. coli* (ExPEC) (Fairbrother and Gyles, 2012) (Table 1).

Enteropathogenic *E. coli* (EPEC)

Enteropathogenic *E. coli* is a pathotype found in post weaning diarrhoea of pigs. This bacterium possesses a

Table 1. Important pathotypes of pathogenic *Escherichia coli* in pigs and associated virulent traits.

Pathotype	Adhesins	Toxins
ETEC	F5(K99), F6 (987P), F41	STa
	F4(K88)	STa, STb, LT, EAST-1, α-hemolysin
	F4(K88), AIDA,	STa, STb, LT, EAST-1, α-hemolysin
	F18, AIDA	STa, STb, LT, Stx (VT), EAST-1, α-hemolysin
EPEC	Eae (intimin)	
STEC (VTEC)	F18, AIDA	Stx2e,(VT2e), EAST-1, α-hemolysin
	Eae (intimin)	Stx1 and/or Stx2
ExPEC	P,S	CNF
	P,S	CNF

complex secretion system that injects over 20 effector proteins into the host enterocyte. This allows intimate adherence of the bacteria into the pigs intestinal epithelium to develop a characteristic "attaching and effacing" (AE) lesion. The EPEC together with other *E. coli* pathotypes that result in AE are collectively known as attaching and effacing *E. coli* (AEEC) (Zhu et al., 1994).

Shiga toxin producing *E. coli* (STEC)

Shiga toxin producing *E. coli,* produce a family of cytotoxins known as Shiga toxin (Stx) or verotoxin (VT). Many STEC are not pathogenic in the intestinal flora but when they possess additional virulence traits, they become highly pathogenic (Fairbrother and Gyles, 2012).

In pigs, the most pathogenic STEC are those that cause oedema disease known as oedema disease *E coli*, with apostrophes before and after as above (EDEC). EDEC produces stx2e and F18ab or F18 ac (DebRoy et al., 2009). Another subgroup of STEC is the enterohaemorrhagic *E. coli* (EHEC) which also possess eae and the same secretion system as EPEC (Fairbrother and Gyles, 2012). However, production of Shiga toxins alone may not be sufficient for *E. coli* O157:H7 pathogenicity (Mead and Griffin, 1998). Other virulence factors such as the intimin protein (involved in the attachment of the *E. coli* O157 to enterocytes), the presence of a plasmid encoded hemolysin, or both, are important in the pathophysiology of haemorrhagic disease (Mead and Griffin, 1998).

Extra intestinal pathogenic *E. coli* (ExPEC)

Extra intestinal pathogenic *E. coli* are a group of heterogeneous *E. coli* in the intestinal tract of pigs that can invade other systems to cause bacteraemia resulting in septicaemia or localised infections such as meningitis and arthritis (Fairbrother and Ngeleka, 1994). The ExPEC possess lipopolysaccharides which protect the bacteria from being killed by serum complement and phagocytes (Fairbrother and Gyles, 2012).

Enterotoxigenic *E. coli* (ETEC)

The ETEC pathotype is the most important among the pathogenic *E. coli* producing one or more enterotoxins that induce secretory diarrhoea in pigs (Fairbrother and Gyles, 2006).This pathotype produces two major enterotoxins; heat stable toxin (ST) and heat labile toxin (LT) which are both further subdivided into STa, STb, LTI and LTII, respectively (Evans et al., 1972; Czirók et al., 1992).The ETEC that causes neonatal diarrhoea produces only STa and possess one or more fimbriae F4 (K88), F5 (K99), F6 (987P) and F41 (Fairbrother and Gyles, 2012). Similarly, ETEC that causes post-weaning diarrhoea produces STa, STb, LT, and enteroaggregative heat stable enterotoxin (EAST-1) (Zhang et al., 2007) while ETEC isolates that produces STb or STb: EAST-1 from weaned pigs may also produce an adhesion involved in diffuse adherence (AIDA-I) (Mainil et al., 2002; Ngeleka et al., 2003; Niewerth et al., 2001).

Enterotoxigenic *E. coli* causes an estimated 840 million gastrointestinal infections and about 380,000 deaths worldwide each year in pigs (Gupta et al., 2008), leading to substantial economic losses for swine producers worldwide (Nagy and Fekete, 2005). The bacteria adhere to and colonize the intestinal mucosa of the small intestine (jejunum, ileum and to a lesser extent, the duodenum) (Arbuckle, 1970; Cox and Houvenaghel, 1993). They also adhere to enterocytes using surface fimbriae (pili) that adhere to specific receptors on enterocytes, without inducing morphological lesions but elaborate enterotoxins that act locally on enterocytes, leading to fluid secretion resulting in the exacerbation of the diarrhoeal illness in pigs (Verbrugghe et al., 2015). A very important illness induced by ETEC toxins is post-weaning diarrhoea in piglets (Verbrugghe et al., 2015).

E. coli post-weaning diarrhoea (PWD)

Post-weaning diarrhoea, also known as post-weaning enteric colibacillosis, is an important cause of death in weaned pigs worldwide. Infection usually occurs during the first weekpost weaning and often results in decreased weight gain (Taylor, 2013). Several factors, such as the stress of weaning, lack of antibodies originating from the sow's milk and dietary changes, contribute to the severity of the disease, manifesting as sudden death or severe diarrhea (Fairbrother, 1999; Amezcua et al., 2002; Maynard et al., 2003).

Most outbreaks have occurred in early-weaned piglets although traditional herds are being increasingly affected (Fairbrother, 1999; Amezcua et al., 2002; Maynard et al., 2003).

Virulence factors of *E. coli* associated with post-weaning diarrhea

Post-weaning diarrhea is caused primarily by ETEC, a pathotype that is characterized by the production of adhesins and alpha-hemolysin, which produce colonies with clear zones of haemolysis on blood agar. Several studies have shown that *E. coli* isolated from weaned pigs with diarrhoea were haemolytic (Frydendahl et al., 2003; Chen et al., 2004).

Alpha-hemolysin, an approximately 110 kDa pore-forming cytolysin, belongs to the RTX family of toxins. The hlyA gene that encodes the hemolysin is part of an operon that is found on plasmids in ETEC. It is a potent cytotoxin that can damage a variety of cells (Frydendahl, 2002). Serological typing has been expanded to include fimbrial antigens, which are virulence factors, as well as O and H antigens which are virulence markers (Chen et al., 2004). Some strains of ETEC that cause PWD possess additional genes that encode Shiga toxin 2e (Stx2e), allowing them to cause edema disease (ED). The ETEC strains that produce Stx (VT) are appropriately called ETEC/STEC or ETEC/VTEC (Nagy and Fekete, 1999).

Enteropathogenic *E. coli* have also been implicated in PWD (Zhu et al., 1994; Zhu et al., 2010; Janke et al., 1989; An et al., 2000). Identification of porcine EPEC (PEPEC) is challenging and veterinary diagnostic laboratories do not routinely seek to identify this pathotype of *E. coli* (Fairbrother, 1999). The eae (*E. coli* AE) gene is a marker for PEPEC, but some eae-positive porcine E. coli isolates may be non-pathogenic. O45 serogroup has been shown to possess genes of the locus of enterocyte effacement (LEE); a locus well established to confer ability for AE lesions (Zhu et al., 1994; An et al., 2000; Helie et al., 1991). Immunity to one strain of pathogenic *E. coli* does not essentially protect from others, while successive strains can pass through herds (Bertschinger, 1999).

Pathogenesis of post-weaning diarrhea

Post-weaning diarrhea is an enteric disease in pigs localised in the small intestine, where digesta flows quickly. The EPEC that causes this condition attaches to the enterocytes lining of the villi or to the mucus covering the villi with the fimbriae or pili, which prevents the bacteria from being flushed to the large intestine. Thereafter, the enterotoxigenic *E. coli* which have colonised the small intestine incites hypersecretory diarrhoea through the release of distinct enterotoxins such as the LT and ST. (Francis, 2002; Zhang et al., 2007).

The LT induces secretion of chloride ions, sodium ions, bicarbonate ions and water into the lumen by binding irreversibly to the mucosal cells and activating the adenylcyclase cyclic AMP system (Thiagarajah and Verkman, 2003; de Haan and Hirst, 2004, Fairbrother et al., 2005) while the ST (STa and STb) inhibits the absorption of sodium and chloride ions from the lumen into the epithelial cell via the guanylcyclase–cyclic GMP system, both resulting in fluid retention. Intestinal colonisation and diarrhoea typically last for about 4 to 14 days, with the organism being spread between animals by the faeco-oral route and aerosols (Bertschinger, 1999).

Pigs displaying PWD harbour massive numbers of haemolytic *E. coli* in the jejunum, whilst there is minimal change in numbers of other bacteria (Smith and Jones, 1963). It is common for EHEC to appear in the faeces of pigs in increased numbers, in the first week after weaning in both healthy and diarrhoeic pigs, although the numbers are higher in diarrhoeic pigs (Kenworthy and Crabb, 1963; Hampson et al., 1985) (Table 2).

The act of weaning is an essential precipitating factor for PWD, regardless of the age at weaning. All of the factors involved with weaning create an environment suitable for the proliferation of *E. coli* in the small intestine. Slower gut transit time and gut stasis immediately after weaning allow bacteria the opportunity to attach and time to multiply (Pluske et al., 2002). An inability of piglets to adequately thermoregulate, combined with sub-standard weaning accommodation, may result in cold stress. This alters intestinal motility and is thought to be a major factor in the pathogenesis of PWD (Wathes et al., 1989). Other factors include social stresses from mixing, fighting and crowding which trigger cortisol release, most likely increasing transit time and depressing the immune response to enhance bacterial infection; moving to a new pen increases the chance of exposure to microbes residing in fresh or dry matter in the environment; the presence of other pathogens such as rotavirus in the environment thereby increasing the likelihood and severity of disease (Lecce *et al.,* 1983). Poor hygiene will also increase the pathogenic *E. coli* load delivered to the small intestine because of faeco-oral cycling (Madec et al., 1998).

Table 2. *Escherichia coli* and its virulence profiles in pigs.

Country	Source	Sample	Pathotype	Serotype	Age(days)	Virulence factor	Summary of result	References
South Africa	Farm	Faeces and intestinal tissues	ETEC	-	35	EAST 1	*E. coli* associated endotoxaemia.	(Fasina et al.,2015)
China	lab samples	Bacterial isolates	ETEC and VTEC	-	-	F18+	F18+ is the main colonization factor for VTEC and ETEC.	(Cheng et al., 2005)
Norway	Abbatior	intestinal content	STEC	O157: H7		stx2, eae, *fliC*-H7	Prevalence of *E. coli* O157:H7 in pigs is low in Norway	(Johnsen et al., 2001)
US	Herd	Isolates	ETEC	-	14	K88, K99, 987P, ST, LT	ETEC produces k88,K99, 987P, LT and ST.	(Moon et al., 1980)
US	Slaughter facility	Colon(faeces)	STEC	O157: H7	-	stx1, stx2, eae, hly	Pigs in the US can habour *E. coli* O157:H7.	(Feder et al., 2003)
Denmark	Lab samples	intestinal content	PEC	O8, O45, O138, O139, O141, O147, O149 and O157	22	F4, F18, STa, STb, LT,ESAT1, VT2e	VTEC and ETEC in PWD and ED belong to limited serogroups and are haemolytic.	(Frydendahl, 2002)
US	Farm	faeces	STEC	-	140	stx1,stx2	The incidence of STEC in swine varies.	(Fratamico et al., 2004)
Canada	Farm	rectal swab	ETEC	O149	35	Sta, STb, LT, Vtx, F18 F4	PWECD is an economically important disease in pigs.	(Amezcua et al., 2002)
US	Farm	Faecal swabs, faeces or intestinal content	ETEC	-	35	K88, K99, STa, STb, LT, F18, F41, stx2e, EAST1, AIDA-1, paa, eae	Broad arrays of virulence genes are associated with PWD in pigs.	(Zhang et al., 2007)
China	Field isolates	Faecal swabs	-	O8, O9, O11, O20, O32, O91, O93, O101, O107, O115, O116 and O131	49	F4, F5, F6, F18, F41 STI, STII, stx2e	Pigs with PWD have *E. coli* enterotoxins and shiga toxin 2 variant.	(Chen et al., 2004)
Mexico	Farm	faeces swabs	-	-	11& 28	LT, STa, STb, Stx1, Stx2 and EAST 1, F4, F5, F6, F17, F18 and F41	There are a there wide variety of virulence genes associated with diarrhoea in piglets.	(Toledo et al., 2012)
Switzerland	Farm	intestinal content	ETEC and VTEC	O139, O141 and O149	56	F107 SLT-IIv, LTI, STIa, STII	F107 are a major colonisation factor in O139: K12 and O141: K85ab *E. coli* serogroups.	(Imberechts et al., 1994)
Japan	Necropsy specimen	intestinal content and rectal swab	ETEC	O149, O157, O141 and O8	26	Sta, LT, K88, K99, 987P, F41, 4F	There are clear differences in strains of ND and PWD in terms of ETEC strain, enterotoxin type and adhesins.	(Nakazawa et al., 1987)
Belgium	Farm	Serum	ETEC	-	392	F4	F4+ ETEC is highly prevalent and widely spread in non-vaccinated pig breeding farms in Belgium.	(Van den Broecket al.,1999)
India		Faeces	STEC and EPEC	O9, O20, O24, O59, O60, O85, O100, O103, O112, O113, O116, O118, O119, O123, O137 and O152	40	stx1, stx2, eaeA, hlyA	STEC and EPEC are associated with diarrhoea in piglets and infants.	(Begum et al., 2014)
Cuba	Farm	Fecal Isolates	EPEC	O141 and O157	30	STb, STa, VT2e, LT, F18, F6	ETEC and VTEC isolates from diarrhoic pigs belong to restricted number of serogroups and serotypes.	(Blanco et al., 2006)
India	Farm	Liver, Lung, Intestine (necropsy)	STEC	-	-	stx2, eae	eae and stx genes are the prime causes of oedema disease in pigs.	(Barman et al., 2008)
Germany	Field strains	Isolates -	STEC and ETEC	-	-	F18ac, F18ab	The F18 fimbrial subtypes are significantly associated with pathovars of *E. coli* strains.	(Barth et al., 2011)
Denmark	Institute	Faeces	ETEC	O149 and O138,	21	-	Diarrhoea occurrence is associated with faecal shedding of haemolytic *E. coli*.	(Carstensen et al., 2005)

Table 2. Contd.

Vietnam	Farm	Faeces, intestinal content	ETEC	O149 and O8	16	F4, F5, Sta,STb,LT	A large number of ETEC isolates belong to O8 serogroup, producing Sta, STb and LT but lacked fimbriae genes.	(Do et al., 2006)
Canada	Farm	Lab isolates	EPEC	O8, O116, O147, O138 and O45, O4 and O98	29	-	82% of *E. coli* isolates were enteropathogenic by the ligated intestine test in pigs.	(Gyles et al., 1971)
Uganda	Farm	Faeces	ETEC and VTEC	-	-	F18+, F4, LT, STa, STb and Stx2e	ETEC and VTEC infections are common in central uganda but clinical cases are masked by management practices.	(Okello et al., 2015)
China	Farm	Liver, spleen, kidney, heart, mesenteric lymph node		O107, O101, O9, O60 and O26.		-	O107, O101, O9, O26, and O60 are the dominant serotypes in southern china.	(Chen et al., 2013)
Korea	Farm	ileal contents	EAEC, ETEC	-	14	EAST 1, F4, F5, F6, F41, STa, STb, LT.	EAST1 is prevalent in *E. coli* and it is a virulence determinant in the pathogenesis of enteric colibacillosis of pre-weaned pigs.	(Choi et al., 2001b)
US	Research and diagnostic lab	Lab specimens	ETEC	O8, O9, O20, O101, O141, O149, O157, O138, and O139.		K88, LT, Stx2e; F18, STa, and STb	Loss of virulence genes is not uncommon in ETEC.	(Francis, 2002)
Spain	Farm	Isolates	ETEC	08, 09, 020, 0101, 0141 and 0149	15	F6 (987P), F5 (K99), F4 (K88) and F41	F6 fimbriae were found in higher rates than F5, F4, and F41 in younger and older piglets with ETEC strains.	(Garabal et al., 1997)
US	Farm	Isolates	STEC and ETEC	O138, O139, O141 and O147		f18, sta, stb, and stx2	Serogroup O147 may be a common serotype of oedema disease-causing *E. coli* in the United States.	(Helgerson et al., 2006)
England	Farm	Intestinal content	ETEC	O149	28	LT	Weaning at three weeks of age did not precipitate a profound change in the *E. coli* intestinal flora in the post-weaning period.	(Hinton et al., 1985)
Bulgeria	Farm	faeces and intestinal content	EHEC; VTEC	-	52	F18, F4	In the 2–3 post-weaning weeks, toxin producing *E. coli* that possesses the adhesion factor F4 is responsible for diarrhoea.	(Lyutskanov, 2011)
Zimbabwe	Farm	Faecal swabs	ETEC , VTEC	-	13	STa, STb, LT, Stx-2e F4, F18, F5 and F41, and F6	Vaccination or vaccine development based on F4, F5, F6, F18, and F41 antigens continues to be appropriate for ETEC infections.	(Madoroba et al., 2009)
Canada	Farm	Fecal swabs, faeces or intestinal content	ETEC and EPEC	O7, O157, O149, O26, O69, O139, O141, O103, O108, O109,O119, O20, O21 and O22	29	EAST1, AIDA-I, F4, F5, F6, F18, LT,STb,STa, EAE, Paa	AIDA-I/STb was dominant and EAST-I may not be an important marker for diarrhoea in pigs.	(Ngeleka et al., 2003)
Hungary	Farm	Intestine	-	O8, O138, O139, O141, O147, O149, and O157	49	K88, STa, STb, LT and VT	73% of K88 isolates had the capability to produce enterotoxins or VT which could contribute to post-weaning diarrhoea in pigs.	(Nagy et al., 1990)
Japan	Farm	Faece, cerebrum, liver, lung, heart blood, kidney, intestinal content, mesenteric lymph node	ETEC	O149: H-, O149: H10, O15:H9, O111:H- and OR: H6	19	STa, LT, K88,	Growth of ETEC was not active in healthy weaning pigs but infection with PRRS virus results in ETEC systemically with per acute death.	(Nakamine et al., 1998)
Germany	Farm			O138, O139, O139, O141, O141, O147 andO149	-	stx2e, fedA, orfA,orfB, AIDA	Porcine *E. coli* strains are a major reservoir for AIDA genes.	(Niewerth et al., 2001)
Canada	Animal health laboratory	Isolates	ETEC	O149		estA (STa), STb, LT, astA (EAST1), K88ac	Recent O149 ETEC associated with PWD in pigs in Ontario are different from the old O149 ETEC, and the new isolates has estAgene.	(Noamani et al., 2003)

Table 2. Contd.

Vietnam	Farm	small intestine, mesenteric lymph node, liver, lung, and spleen	-	O139, O141, O138, and O149	28	VT2e+, fedA(F18), AIDA, Sta, STb	0139:K82+/VT2e+/F18+/AIDA+ seropathotype was predominant and antibiotic resistances is widely distributed in *E. coli* causing ED in northern Vietnam.	(Oanh et al., 2010)
Poland	Farm	Faeces or rectal swabs	-	O139, O141 and O138	35	Stx2e, F18, STI, STII.	Molecular characterization of *E. coli* using the RAPD polymorphism analysis is a quick and convenient method to differentiate *E. coli* bacteria of the same and different serogroups.	(Osek, 2000)
China	Farm	rectal swab	ETEC	O80, O141, O139, O6, O9, O20, O101, O93, O138, O147, O157, O38 and O45.	26	K88, K99, F41, F18, 987P, STa, STb, LT, Stx2e	Novel serogroups O80, O6 and O38 of *E. coli* in pigs were identified in western China.	(Qi et al., 2012)
south Africa	Research council	rectal swab	ETEC, STEC, EAEC	-	73	STa, STb, LT, Stx2e, EAST-1, PAA, AIDA-I, EAE	PAA and AIDA-1 are important in South African pigs.	(Mohlatlole et al., 2013)
Korea	Farm	caecal and ileal contents	ETEC, STEC, DAEC	-	-	AIDA1, F18ab, Stx2e, Sta, STb, EAST1	AIDA gene is not restricted to DAEC strains.	(Ha et al., 2003)
Brazil	Farm	swabs		-	-	F4, F5, F6, F18, F41, STa, STb, LT and STx2e	*E. coli* strains isolated from pigs with diarrhoea possessed the genes for LT or/and ST enterotoxins.	(Vidotto et al., 2009)
Slovakia	Farm	Rectal swab and intestinal content	ETEC	O8, O54, O84, O101, O141, O141, O147, O149, O163, O2, O15, O84 andO157.	14	LT, Sta, STb, Stx1, Stx2, F4, F18, F6, F5, F41, F17, eae, EAST1	There is high prevalence of ETEC that possess LT and STb genes and the F4 colonization factor in piglets with diarrhoea in Slovakia.	(Vu-Khac et al., 2007)
China	Farm	Faeces	ETEC	-	-	EAST1, irp2, paa, STb, AIDA-I, LT-I, ler, hlyA, K88, eae, STa, sepA, F18, afaD, afaE, K99 and Stx2e	Relatively few isolates from the study express K88, K99, LT-I or STa, but EAST1, irp2, AIDA-I, paa and STb were frequent in *E. coli* strains in suckling pigs with diarrhoea in China.	(Liu et al., 2014)
Slovakia	Farm	Intestinal content	ETEC	-	21	F4, F5, F6, F18, F41, STa, STb, LT, STx2e, EAST1	There is a wide distribution of the astA gene among *E. coli* strains isolated from diarrhoeic piglets in Slovakia and a strong association of the astA gene with F4-positive strains.	(Vu-Khac et al., 2004)
Czech Republic	Farm	Rectal swab and intestinal content	ETEC and STEC	O149	-	LT+, STa+, K88, F18, EAST-1, paa.	There is a significantly higher prevalence of astA positive *E. coli* isolates among apparently healthy piglets in comparison with diarrheic piglets.	(Zajacova et al., 2012)
China	Farm	Rectal swab	ETEC and STEC	O141, O9, O32, O2, O116, O107, O147, O139, O91, O45 and O98.	49	AIDA-I, Sta, Stb, Lt, Stx2e, EAST1, F5, F6, F18, F41	AIDA-I represents an occasional virulence factor for PWD and ED in pigs and has the potential to transfer between porcine and human *E. coli*.	(Zhao et al., 2009)
Spain	Farm	Reactal swab	ETEC and VTEC	-	15	STa, LT, VT, CNF1, CNF2, α-hemolysin.	Majority of piglets in this study that produced verotoxin also produced STa enterotoxin but CNF1 was produced from only 1.5% of sick piglets.	(Garabal et al., 1995)
Korea	Pathology department	Ileal and cecal contents	ETEC, STEC	-	-	EAST1, STa, STb, LT, Stx2e, F4, F5, F6, F18, F41.	*E. coli* carries east1 gene in high prevalence in weaned pigs with diarrhoea and/or edema disease.	(Choi et al., 2001a)

Table 2. Contd.

Korea	Farm	Jejunal, ileal and caecal contents	ETEC, STEC	-	-	STa, STb, LT, Stx2e, F4, F5, F6, F18, F41	Genes for F18 and Stx2e are prevalent among *E coli* isolated from post-weaning pigs with diarrhoea or oedema disease.	(Kwon et al., 2002)
Denmark	national vet laboratory	Intestinal content and faeces	-	O149, O139, O138,O101 O8, O64, O147, O141 and O157	4,15,36 and 56	STa, STb, LT, VT, K88, 987P , F107, K99 and F41	Results correlation between genotypic and phenotypic methods was 97.7-100%. VT and F107 genes were more frequent in post-weaning than in neonatal *E.coli* strains.	(Ojeniyi et al., 1994)
Canada	vet medicine faculty	intestinal content	ETEC	O8,O9, O101, O9, O20,O64,O10, O157, O147,O149, O115, O138,O139,O141,O45,O26, O119,O15 and O108	31	F4, F5, F6, F41, STa, STb, LT and VT	The most important pathotypes among enterotoxigenic isolates in this study were F4:LT:STb, F5:STa, STb, F5:F41:STa, F4:STb, F6, STa, and LT.	(Harel et al., 1991)
Brazil	Farm	Faeces	ETEC, STEC	-	11	LT-I, STa, SLT-I, SLT-II, SLTIIv, F18ac.	eaeA gene and intimin production and/or Shiga-like toxins may be an important cause of diarrhoea among piglets.	(Martins et al., 2000)
Poland	Farm	Faeces or rectal swabs	-	-	35	LTI, STI, Stx2e, F4 F5 F6 F17 F18 and F41	Low prevalence of fimbria-positive *E. coli* strains isolated from pigs with PWD was found in this study.	(Osek, 1999)
Poland	Farm	Rectal swabs	ETEC	O1, O8, O9, O66, O138, O141, O147 and O149	35	EAST1-1, F4, LTI STI and STII	EAST1 gene is widely distributed among *E. coli* strains isolated from piglets with post-weaning diarrhoea.	(Osek, 2003)
Poland	Farm	Faecal swabs	ETEC	-	5& 42	Sta, LT, STb, K88, K99, 987P, F1	Enterotoxigenic (LT and STb) *E.coli* from suckling and weaned piglets with diarrhoea were 90.5% and 69.1% respectively and 18.5% of strains from healthy piglets were STa.	(Osek and Truszczyński, 1992)
Poland	Farm	Feaces	-	O157, O149, O66, O138, O139 and O141	-	F4, fedA, eltI, estI, estII, stx1, stx2e	*E. coli* from pigs with post-weaningdiarrhoea (13 out of 21 isolates) or from oedema disease (16 out of 19 strains) are able to produce F18 fimbriae.	(Osek et al., 1999)
Argentina	Farm	Rectal swabs spleen, kidney and liver	ETEC and VTEC	O8, O9, O64, O101, O138, O139, O149 and O162		STIa, STb, LTI, VT2e, VT1, VT2all	ETEC strains predominate in the group of animals with diarrhoea, STIa prevails in ETEC from pigs with diarrhoea, O64 prevails among ETEC and O138 prevails for ETEC/VTEC strains.	(Parma et al., 2000)
Sweden	Farm	faeces and intestinal content	ETEC	O149, O101, O9, O20, and O8,	25	LT, ST, K88, K99, 987P, F41	Frequency of O149 has been reduced, while that of O101 has increased to the same level as that of O149 in sweden.	(Soderlind et al., 1988)
Indonesia	Farm	Rectal swab		O20, O9 and O141	14	987P, ST, K88, K99.	Mixed infections with *E. coli* bearing different fimbrial antigens occur both within a group of piglets and in a single piglet.	(Hirst and Patten, 1991)
Slovakia	Farm	intestinal content and rectal swab	ETEC	-	15	F4, F5, F6 and F41	The frequency of occurrence of individual types of adherence antigens is related to geographical location.	(Vu-Khac et al., 2004)
Brazil	-	-	-	O139, O8, O9, O15, O20, O82, O101, O110 and O153	-	Stx2e, F18ab, STI, STII, LTI	Enterotoxin genes detected in high frequency are responsible for diarrhoea seen in pigs with oedema disease,	(da Silva et al., 2001)

Vaccination against pathogenic bacteria

Vaccination against pathogenic bacteria has become necessary as an alternative control measure due to the development of different serotypes of bacteria and bacterial resistance to a wide range of commonly used antibiotics (Fairbrother et al., 2005). Frequently used vaccines against bacterial diseases in swin

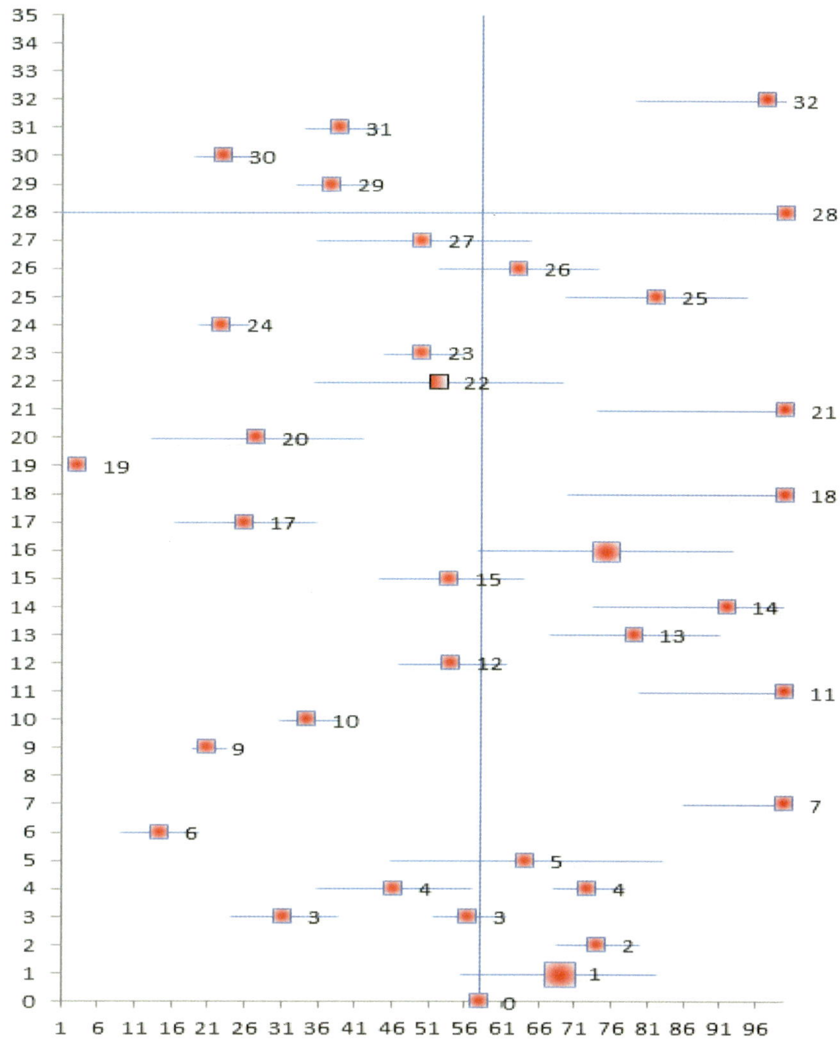

Figure 1. Forest plot of *prevalence of Escherichia coli* virulence factors

contain whole-cell killed micro-organisms, purified microbial components, or recombinant proteins (Haesebrouck et al., 2004). Vaccination against bacteria pathogens in pigs is directed towards either the extracellular bacteria or the exotoxin produced by the bacteria (Haesebrouck et al., 2004).

Exotoxins are produced within the bacterial cytoplasm. Some are excreted through the living cell wall, while others are released only by lysis of bacteria. In diseases caused by exotoxigenic bacteria, antibodies neutralizing that toxin play an important role in protection of the host against disease, provided they are able to prevent binding of the exotoxin to its receptor on the host cell. Vaccines containing the inactivated toxin (toxoid) or a non-toxic but antigenic recombinant protein derived from the exotoxin can be expected to provide protection against disease.

Antibodies generally mediate protection against the surface antigens and certain secreted antigens of extracellular bacteria. Cellular immunity may also play a role (Haesebrouck et al., 2004).

Oral immunization of piglets with live avirulent strains of bacteriais is a new vaccination strategy for bacterial diseases. An example is the administration of avirulent *E. coli* carrying the fimbrial adhesins or oral administration of purified F4 (K88) fimbriae.

Other approaches to control bacterial diseases include supplementation of the feed with egg yolk, antibodies from chickens immunized with F4 or F18 adhesins, breeding of F18 and F4 resistant animals, supplementation with zinc and/or spray-dried plasma, dietary acidification, phage therapy, or the use of probiotics. However, to date, no single strategy has proven to be totally effective (Fairbrother, 2005).

Results of meta-analysis

In the present review, 29 countries with documented records of cases of *E. coli* were included with the USA having the highest number of references followed by

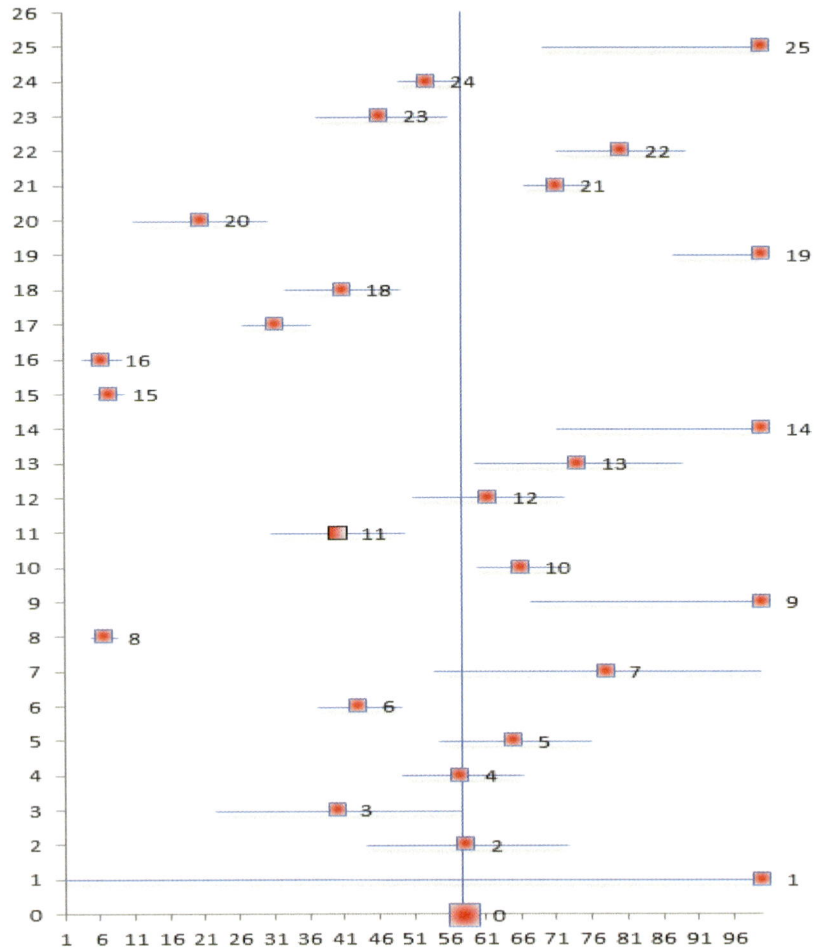

Figure 2. Forest plot for prevalence of *Escherichia coli* virulence factors in weaners.

China. About 74% of the samples were taken from farms and others were from samples submitted to research laboratories and veterinary faculties for necropsy.

In general 7 pathotypes were reported and 66.7% of the pathotypes identified were ETEC, 14.3% were ETEC and STEC, 7.9% were STEC, 31.7% were classified as ETEC/EPEC/EAEC, others were EHEC and DAEC (Table 2). Several serogroups were identified and the commonest were O141, O149, O139, O138, O8 and O9. 33.3% of samples collected were faecal swabs or faeces, 14.2% were intestinal segments, 17.4% were intestinal segments, feaces or rectal swabs and other organs, 6.3% were intestinal segments and other organs, 7.9% were lab isolates (Table 2). Piglets were 52.3%, 7.9% were porkers, 39.6% were weaners and all pigs were between 1 to 392 days old.

A total of 24,854 isolates were considered and 10477 were recorded as positives, the gene looked out for were STa, STb, LT, stx1, stx2, stx-2e F4, F5, F6, F18, F41, AIDA, EAST1, eae, paa, hlyA (Table 2). The diseases examined were diarrhoea in form of neonatal diarrhoea, colibacillosis, PWD and oedema disease. Some of the associated risk factors identified were poor housing, management and feed changes, extensive use of antibiotics as prophylaxis, overcrowding, high humidity and temperature changes (Table 2).

This study showed that India, USA, Japan, Slovakia and Denmark were the countries with the highest detection of virulence factors in piglets (100%; n = 3, 55, 42, 92 and 191 respectively), followed by Sweden (74%; n = 856) and Poland (72%; n =1125) (Table 3). For all the cases of virulence in piglets an overall prevalence of 57.93% (CI_{95}: 57.0 to 58.8) was estimated (n = 12970) (Table 3, Figure 1)

Similarly, South Africa, Cuba, Poland, Denmark, had the highest cases of virulence factor detection in *E. coli* in weaners (100%; n =2, 36, 46, and 240 respectively), followed by Canada (74.1% n = 135), the least detection was in found in China (6.5% n=324) (Table 4). The overall prevalence of virulence factor detection in weaners was 57.9% (CI_{95}: 56.99-58.83; n = 8058) (Table 4, Figure 2). Furthermore, in porkers the overall prevalence of *E. coli* virulence factor detection was36.45% (CI_{95}: 35.73- 37.57). The highest prevalence was found in the USA (70.5%; n = 687) and the lowest was in Norway (0.15% n= 1976) (Table 5, Figure 3).

Table 3. Prevalence of *Escherichia coli* virulence factors in piglets.

S/N	Study	Events	Sample Size	Outcome	SE	CI lower	CI upper	Forest Plot ID	Rate
1	US (herd)	108	111	0.972973	0.093624368	0.789469	1.156477	32	97.2973
2	Denmark (Diagnostic samples)	219	563	0.388988	0.026285344	0.337468	0.440507	31	38.89876
3	Mexico (Farm)	116	503	0.230616	0.021412186	0.188648	0.272584	30	23.06163
4	Japan (Necropsy samples)	214	567	0.377425	0.025800245	0.326857	0.427994	29	37.7425
5	India (Farm)	3	3	1	0.577350269	0.131607	2.131607	28	100
6	Denmark (Research institute)	45	90	0.5	0.074535599	0.35391	0.64609	27	50
7	Vietnam (Farm)	126	200	0.63	0.056124861	0.519995	0.740005	26	63
8	Canada (Farm)	164	200	0.82	0.064031242	0.694499	0.945501	25	82
9	Korea (Farm)	164	720	0.227778	0.017786456	0.192916	0.262639	24	22.77778
10	US (Research institute)	330	660	0.5	0.027524094	0.446053	0.553947	23	50
11	Spain (Farm)	36	69	0.521739	0.086956522	0.351304	0.692174	22	52.17391
12	US (Farm)	55	55	1	0.134839972	0.735714	1.264286	21	100
13	England (Farm)	14	51	0.27451	0.073365831	0.130713	0.418307	20	27.45098
14	Zimbabwe (Farm)	63	1984	0.031754	0.004000632	0.023913	0.039595	19	3.175403
15	Japan (Farm)	42	42	1	0.15430335	0.697565	1.302435	18	100
16	Germany (Farm)	27	104	0.259615	0.049963004	0.161688	0.357543	17	25.96154
17	Vietnam (Farm)	69	92	0.75	0.09028939	0.573033	0.926967	16	75
18	China (Farm)	112	208	0.538462	0.050879833	0.438737	0.638186	15	53.84615
19	Brazil (Farm)	92	100	0.92	0.09591663	0.732003	1.107997	14	92
20	Slovakia (Farm)	174	220	0.790909	0.059958663	0.67339	0.908428	13	79.09091
21	China (Farm)	206	381	0.540682	0.037671129	0.466847	0.614518	12	54.06824
22	Slovakia (Farm)	92	92	1	0.104257207	0.795656	1.204344	11	100
23	Czech Republic (Farm)	277	800	0.34625	0.020804146	0.305474	0.387026	10	34.625
24	Spain (Farm)	280	1334	0.209895	0.012543629	0.18531	0.234481	9	20.98951
25	Denmark (Research Laboratory)	191	191	1	0.072357461	0.858179	1.141821	7	100
26	Denmark (Research Laboratory)	28	194	0.14433	0.027275787	0.090869	0.19779	6	14.43299
27	Brazil (Farm)	45	70	0.642857	0.095831485	0.455027	0.830687	5	64.28571
28	Poland (Farm)	819	1125	0.728	0.025438379	0.678141	0.777859	4	72.8
29	Argentina (Farm)	70	223	0.313901	0.037518387	0.240365	0.387437	3	31.39013
30	Sweden (Farm)	634	856	0.740654	0.029415136	0.683001	0.798308	2	74.06542
31	Indonesia (Farm)	484	858	0.564103	0.025641026	0.513846	0.614359	3	56.41026
32	Slovakia (Farm)	74	160	0.4625	0.053764533	0.357122	0.567878	4	46.25
33	Brazil (Farm)	99	144	0.6875	0.06909635	0.552071	0.822929	1	68.75
-	-	-	-	0.579256	0.0047	0.570044	0.588468	Central Tendency	57.92558

Table 4. Prevalence of *Escherichia coli* virulence factors in weaners.

Serial number	Study	Events	Sample Size	Outcome	SE	CI lower	CI upper	Forest plot ID	Rate
1	south Africa (Farm)	2	2	1	0.707106781	-0.38593	2.385929	1	100
2	China (Lab samples)	63	108	0.583333	0.073493092	0.439287	0.72738	2	58.33333
3	Canada (Farm)	20	50	0.4	0.089442719	0.224692	0.575308	3	40
4	US (Farm)	175	304	0.575658	0.043515647	0.490367	0.660949	4	57.56579
5	China (Field isolates)	140	215	0.651163	0.0550333	0.543298	0.759028	5	65.11628
6	Mexico (Farm)	194	450	0.431111	0.030951974	0.370445	0.491777	6	43.11111
7	Switzerland (Farm)	39	50	0.78	0.12489996	0.535196	1.024804	7	78
8	India	48	720	0.066667	0.009622504	0.047807	0.085527	8	6.666667
9	Cuba (Farm)	36	36	1	0.166666667	0.673333	1.326667	9	100
10	Bulgeria (Farm)	409	619	0.660743	0.032671645	0.596707	0.72478	10	66.07431
11	Canada (Farm)	68	170	0.4	0.048507125	0.304926	0.495074	11	40

Table 4. Contd.

12	Hungary (Farm)	126	205	0.614634	0.054755962	0.507312	0.721956	12	61.46341
13	Canada (Animal health Lab)	100	135	0.740741	0.074074074	0.595556	0.885926	13	74.07407
14	Poland (Farm)	46	46	1	0.147441956	0.711014	1.288986	14	100
15	Korea (Farm)	45	604	0.074503	0.011106298	0.052735	0.096272	15	7.450331
16	China (Farm)	21	324	0.064815	0.014143752	0.037093	0.092537	16	6.481481
17	Korea (Pathology Department)	149	476	0.313025	0.025644024	0.262763	0.363287	17	31.30252
18	Korea (Farm)	94	230	0.408696	0.042153738	0.326074	0.491317	18	40.86957
19	Denmark (National Vet Lab)	240	240	1	0.064549722	0.873483	1.126517	19	100
20	Denmark (National Vet Lab)	17	83	0.204819	0.049675971	0.107454	0.302184	20	20.48193
21	Canada (Vet Medicine Faculty)	872	1226	0.711256	0.024086171	0.664047	0.758465	21	71.12561
22	Poland (Farm)	298	372	0.801075	0.046405044	0.710121	0.892029	22	80.10753
23	Poland (Farm)	96	207	0.463768	0.047333135	0.370995	0.556541	23	46.37681
24	Poland (Farm)	608	1146	0.530541	0.021516279	0.488369	0.572713	24	53.0541
25	Poland (Farm)	40	40	1	0.158113883	0.690097	1.309903	25	100
-	-	-	-	0.579062	0.0047	0.56985	0.588274	Central Tendency	57.90619

Table 5. Prevalence of *Escherichia coli* virulence factors in porkers.

S/No	Study	Events	Sample Size	Outcome	SE	CI lower	CI upper	Forest plot ID	Rate
1	Norway	3	1976	0.001518219	0.000876544	-0.0002	0.003236	1	0.151822
2	US	6	305	0.019672131	0.008031114	0.003931	0.035413	2	1.967213
3	US	484	687	0.704512373	0.03202329	0.641747	0.767278	3	70.45124
4	Belgium	95	135	0.703703704	0.072198477	0.562195	0.845213	4	70.37037
5	south Africa	106	263	0.403041825	0.039146883	0.326314	0.47977	5	40.30418
-	-	-	-	0.36648965	0.0047	0.357278	0.375702	Central Tendency	36.64897

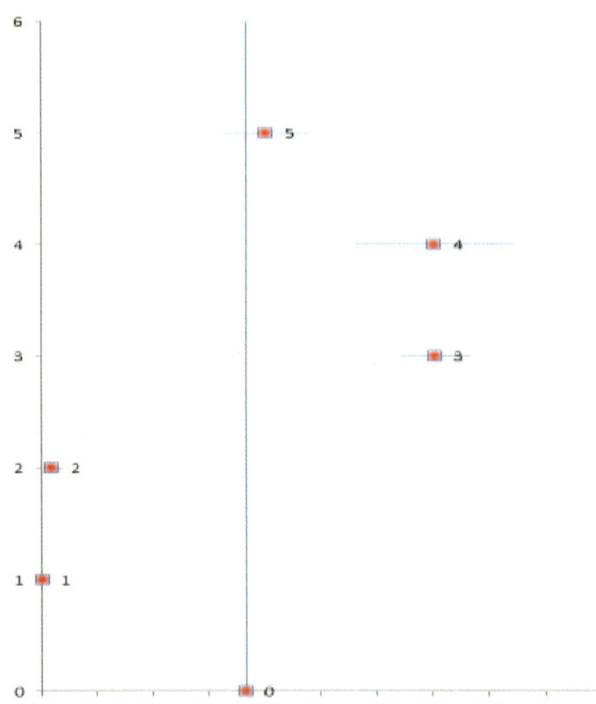

Figure 3. Forest plot for prevalence of *Escherichia coli* virulence factors in porkers.

REFERENCES

Abramson JH (2011). WINPEPI updated: computer programs for epidemiologists, and their teaching potential. Epidemiol. Perspect. Innov. 8:1.

Agdestein A, Johansen TB, Polaček V, Lium B, Holstad G, Vidanović D, Aleksić-Kovačević S, Jørgensen A, Žultauskas J, Nilsen SF (2011). Investigation of an outbreak of mycobacteriosis in pigs. BMC Vet. Res. 7(1):10.118.

Alban L, Baptista F, Møgelmose V, Sørensen L, Christensen H, Aabo S, Dahl J (2012). *Salmonella* surveillance and control for finisher pigs and pork in Denmark: a case study. Food Res. Int. 45(2):656-665.

Alter T, Gaull F, Kasimir S, Gürtler M, Mielke H, Linnebur M, Fehlhaber K (2005). Prevalences and transmission routes of Campylobacter spp. strains within multiple pig farms Vet. Microbiol.108(3):251-261.

Amano H, Shibata M, Kajio N, Morozumi T (1994). Pathologic observations of pigs intranasally inoculated with serovar 1, 4 and 5 of *Haemophilus parasuis* using immunoperoxidase method. J. Vet. Med. Sci. 56(4):639-644.

Amezcua R, Friendship RM, Dewey CE, Gyles C, Fairbrother JM (2002). Presentation of postweaning *Escherichia coli* diarrhoea in southern Ontario, prevalence of hemolytic *E. coli* serogroups involved and their antimicrobial resistance patterns. Can. J. Vet. Res. 66(2):73-78.

An H, Fairbrother JM, Désautels C, Mabrouk T, Dugourd D, Dezfulian H, Harel J (2000). Presence of the LEE (locus of enterocyte effacement) in pig attaching and effacing *Escherichia coli* and characterization of eae, espA, espB and espD genes of PEPEC (pig EPEC) strain 1390. Microb. Pathog.28(5):291-300.

Andresen LO (1998). Differentiation and distribution of three types of exfoliative toxin produced by *Staphylococcus hyicus* from pigs with exudative epidermitis.FEMS Immunol. Med. Microbiol.20(4):301-310.

Andresen LO, Bille-Hansen V, Wegener HC (1997). Staphylococcus hyicusexfoliative toxin: purification and demonstration of antigenic diversity among toxins from virulent strains. Microb. Pathog. 22(2):113-122.

Arbuckle J (1970). The location of *Escherichia coli* in the pig intestine. J. Med. Microbiol.3(2):333-340.

Backstrom LR, Brim TA, Collins MT (1988). Development of turbinate lesions and nasal colonization by *Bordetella bronchiseptica* and *Pasteurella multocida* during long-term exposure of healthy pigs to pigs affected by atrophic rhinitis. Can. J. Vet. Res. 52(1):23-29.

Baker AA, Davis E, Rehberger T, Rosener D (2010). Prevalence and diversity of toxigenic *Clostridium perfringens*and *Clostridium difficile* among swine herds in the midwest. Appl. Environ. Microbiol. 76(9):2961-2967.

Barman N, Deb R, Ramamurthy T, Sharma R, Borah P, Wani S, Kalita D (2008). Molecular characterization of shiga like toxin-producing *Escherichia coli* (STEC) isolates from pigs oedema. Indian J. MedRes.127(6): 602-606.

Barth S, Schwanitz A, Bauerfeind R (2011). Polymerase chain reaction-based method for the typing of F18 fimbriae and distribution of F18 fimbrial subtypes among porcine Shiga toxin-encoding *Escherichia coli* in Germany. J. Vet. Diagn. Invest. 23(3):454-464.

Begum J, Dutta T, Chandra R, Choudhary PR, Varte Z, Bitew M (2014). Molecular and phenotypic characterization of shigatoxigenic *Escherichia coli* (STEC) and enteropathogenic *E. coli* (EPEC) from piglets and infants associated with diarrhoea in Mizoram, India Afr .J. Biotechnol. 13(12):1452-1461.

Beiers P, Simmons G (1967). Botulism in pigs. Aust.Vet. J. 43(7):270-271.

Bertschinger H (1999). Postweaning *Escherichia coli* diarrhea and edema disease. Diseases of swine 8:441-454

Bhaduri S, Wesley IV, Bush EJ (2005). Prevalence of pathogenic *Yersinia enterocolitica* strains in pigs in the United States. Appl. Environ. Microbiol. 71(11):7117-7121.

Biet F, Boschiroli ML, Thorel MF, Guilloteau LA (2005). Zoonotic aspects of *Mycobacterium bovis* and *Mycobacterium avium-intracellulare* complex (MAC). Vet. Res. 36(3):411-436.

Binder A, Aumüller R, Likitdecharote B, Kirchhoff H (1990). Isolation of *Mycoplasma arthritidis* from the joint fluid of boars. J. Vet. Med. Series B. 37(1-10):611-614.

Blanchard B, Vena MM, Cavalier A, Le Lannic J, Gouranton J, Kobisch M (1992). Electron microscopic observation of the respiratory tract of SPF piglets inoculated with *Mycoplasma hyopneumoniae*. Vet. Microbiol. 30(4):329-341.

Blanco M, Lazo L, Blanco JE, Dahbi G, Mora A, López C, González EA, Blanco J (2006). Serotypes, virulence genes, and PFGE patterns of enteropathogenic *Escherichia coli* isolated from Cuban pigs with diarrhea.Int. Microbiol. 9(1):53-60.

Borch E, Nesbakken T Christensen H (1996). Hazard identification in swine slaughter with respect to foodborne bacteria. Int. J. Food Microbiol. 30(1): 9-25.

Boutrup TS, Boesen H, Boye M, Agerholm JS, Jensen TK (2010). Early pathogenesis in porcine proliferative enteropathy caused by *Lawsonia intracellularis*. J. Comp. Pathol. 143(2):101-109.

Brockmeier SL (2004). Prior infection with *Bordetella bronchiseptica* increases nasal colonization by*Haemophilus parasuis* in swine. Vet. Microbiol. 99(1):75-78.

Brockmeier SL, Palmer MV, Bolin SR, Rimler RB (2001). Effects of intranasal inoculation with *Bordetella bronchiseptica*, porcine reproductive and respiratory syndrome virus, or a combination of both organisms on subsequent infection with *Pasteurella multocida* in pigs. Am. J. Vet. Res. 62(4):521-525.

Brugmann M, Peters M, Mumme J (2001). Case report: *Yersinia enterocolitica* septicemia in an American minipig. Dtsch. Tierarztl. Wochenschr 108(6):257-260.

Burrin D, Stoll B (2003). 12 Intestinal nutrient requirements in weanling pigs.Weaning the pig: concepts and consequences. P 301.

Busch R, Barnes D, Sautter J (1971). Pathogenesis and pathologic changes of experimentally induced listeriosis in newborn pigs. Amer. J. Vet. Res. Available at: http://agris.fao.org/agris-search/search.do?recordID=US201302348493

Canibe N, Jensen BB (2012). Fermented liquid feed-Microbial and nutritional aspects and impact on enteric diseases in pigs. Anim. Feed Sci.Technol. 173(1):17-40.

Carstensen L, Ersbøll AK, Jensen KH, Nielsen JP (2005). *Escherichia coli* post-weaning diarrhoea occurrence in piglets with monitored exposure to creep feed. Vet. Microbiol. 110(1):113-123.

Chen R, Li B, Zhang X, Liu H, He D (2013). Diversity of *Escherichia coli* Isolated from Southern China. J. Anim. Vet. Adv. 12(14):1233-1236.

Chen S, Wang Y, Chen F, Yang H, Gan M, Zheng SJ (2007). A highly pathogenic strain of *Staphylococcus sciuri* caused fatal exudative epidermitis in piglets. PLoS One 2(1):e147.

Chen X, Gao S, Jiao X, Liu XF (2004). Prevalence of serogroups and virulence factors of *Escherichia coli* strains isolated from pigs with post-weaning diarrhoea in eastern China. Vet. Microbiol. 103(1):13-20.

Cheng D, Sun H, Xu J Gao S (2005). Prevalence of fimbial colonization factors F18ab and F18ac in *Escherichia coli* isolates from weaned piglets with oedema and/or diarrhoea in China. Vet. Microbiol. 110(1):35-39.

Cheon DS, Chae C (1996). Outbreak of diarrhoea associated with *Enterococcus durans* in piglets. J. Vet. Diagn. Invest. 8(1):123-124.

Choi C, Cho W, Chung H, Jung T, Kim J, Chae C (2001a). Prevalence of the enteroaggregative *Escherichia coli* heat-stable enterotoxin 1 (EAST1) gene in isolates in weaned pigs with diarrhea and/or edema disease. Vet. Microbiol. 81 (1): 65-71.

Choi C, Kwon D, Chae C (2001b). Prevalence of the enteroaggregative *Escherichia coli* heat-stable enterotoxin 1 gene and its relationship with fimbrial and enterotoxin genes in *E. coli* isolated from diarrheic piglets. J. Vet. diagn. Invest. 13(1): 26-29.

Contzen M, Sting R, Blazey B, Rau J (2011). *Corynebacterium ulcerans* from diseased wild boars. Zoonoses Public Health 58(7):479-488.

Cox E, Houvenaghel A (1993). Comparison of the in vitro adhesion of K88, K99, F41 and P987 positive *Escherichia coli* to intestinal villi of 4-to 5-week-old pigs.Vet. Microbiol. 34(1):7-18.

Czirók É, Semjen G, Steinrück H, Herpay M, Milch H, Nyomärkay I,

Stverteczky Z, Szeness A (1992). Comparison of rapid methods for detection of heat-labile (LT) and heat-stable (ST) enterotoxin in *Escherichia coli*. J. Med. Microbiol. 36(6):398-402.

da Silva AS, Valadares GF, Penatti MPA, Brito BG, da Silva Leite D (2001). *Escherichia coli* strains from oedema disease: O serogroups, and genes for Shiga toxin, enterotoxins, and F18 fimbriae. Vet. Microbiol. 80(3): 227-233.

Davies RL, MacCorquodale R, Baillie S, Caffrey B (2003). Characterization and comparison of *Pasteurella multocida* strains associated with porcine pneumonia and atrophic rhinitis. J. Med. Microbiol. 52(1):59-67.

Davies RL, MacCorquodale R, Reilly S (2004). Characterisation of bovine strains of Pasteurella multocida and comparison with isolates of avian, ovine and porcine origin. Vet. Microbiol. 99(2):145-158.

De Bruyne E, Flahou B, Chiers K, Meyns T, Kumar S, Vermoote M, Pasmans F, Millet S, Dewulf J, Haesebrouck F (2012). An experimental Helicobacter suis infection causes gastritis and reduced daily weight gain in pigs.Vet. Microbiol. 160(3):449-454.

de Haan L, Hirst TR (2004). Cholera toxin: a paradigm for multi-functional engagement of cellular mechanisms. Molec. Membrane Biol. 21:77-92.

De Neeling A, Van den Broek M, Spalburg E, Van Santen-Verheuvel M, Dam-Deisz W, Boshuizen H, Van De Giessen A, Van Duijkeren E, Huijsdens X (2007). High prevalence of methicillin resistant *Staphylococcus aureus* in pigs.Vet. Microbiol.122(3): 366-372.

De Smet S, De Zutter L, Houf K (2012). Spatial distribution of the emerging foodborne pathogen *arcobacter* in the gastrointestinal tract of pigs. Foodborne pathog. Dis. 9(12):1097-1103.

DebRoy C, Roberts E, Scheuchenzuber W, Kariyawasam S, Jayarao BM (2009). Comparison of genotypes of *Escherichia coli* strains carrying F18ab and F18ac fimbriae from pigs. J. Vet. Diagn Invest. 21(3):359-364.

Deyoe B (1967) Pathogenesis of three strains of Brucella suis in swine.Am J. Vet. Res. 28:951-957.

Diab SS, Uzal FA, Songer JG, Prescott JF, Popoff MR (2016). Diseases produced by *Clostridium difficile*.Clostridial Diseases of Animals, Wiley-Blackwell. pp. 177-195.

Do TN, Cu PH, Nguyen HX, Au TX, Vu QN, Driesen SJ, Townsend KM, Chin JJ, Trott DJ (2006). Pathotypes and serogroups of enterotoxigenic *Escherichia coli* isolated from pre-weaning pigs in north Vietnam.J. Med. Microbiol. 55(1): 93-99.

Došen R, Prodanov J, Milanov D, Stojanov I, Pušić I (2007). The bacterial infections of respiratory tract of swine. Biotechnol. Anim. Husbandry. 23(5-6-2):237-243.

Dubreuil JD (2012). The whole Shebang: the gastrointestinal tract, *Escherichia coli* enterotoxins and secretion. Curr. Issues Mol. Biol. 14(2):71-82.

Duncan JR, Ross RF, Switzer WP, Ramsey FK (1966). Pathology of experimental *Bordetella bronchiseptica* infection in swine: atrophic rhinitis. Am. J. Vet. Res. 27(117):457-466.

Duran C, Walton J (1997). *Clostridium novyi* sudden death in sows: toxaemia or post mortem invader. Pig J. 39:37-53

Dziva F, Muhairwa AP, Bisgaard M, Christensen H (2008). Diagnostic and typing options for investigating diseases associated with *Pasteurella multocida*. Vet. Microbiol. 128(1):1-22.

Epps SV, Harvey RB, Hume ME, Phillips TD, Anderson RC, Nisbet DJ (2013). Foodborne *Campylobacter*: infections, metabolism, pathogenesis and reservoirs.Int. J. Environ. Res Public Health 10(12):6292-6304.

Evans DJ, Chen LC, Curlin GT, Evans DG (1972). Stimulation of adenyl cyclase by *Escherichia coli* enterotoxin. Nature 236(66):137-138.

Faine S (1994). *Leptospira* and leptospirosis.CRC Press Inc. Boca Raton.

Fairbrother J (1999) Identification, nomenclature, and diagnosis of pathogenic *Escherichia coli*.In: Proceedings of the Annual Meeting of the Western Canadian Association of Swine Practitioners, Saskatoon, Canada, pp. 21-31.

Fairbrother J, Gyles C (2006).Post-weaning *Escherichia coli* diarrhoea and oedema disease: Diseases of Swine. Blackwell Publishing. (9):649-662.

Fairbrother J, Gyles C (2012). Colibacillosis: Diseases of swine. Blackwell Publishing.10:723-749.

Fairbrother J, Ngeleka M (1994). Extraintestinal *Escherichia coli* infections in pigs: In *Escherichia coli* in domestic animals and humans. CAB international, Wallingford, United Kingdom. pp. 221-236.

Fairbrother JM, Nadeau E, Gyles CL (2005). Escherichia coli in post-weaning diarrhea in pigs: an update on bacterial types, pathogenesis, and prevention strategies. Anim. Health Re. Rev. 6(01):17-39.

Fasina FO, Bwala DG, Madoroba E (2015). Investigation of multidrug-resistant fatal colisepticaemia in weanling pigs.Onderstepoort J. Vet. Res. 82(1):1-6.

Feder I, Wallace FM, Gray JT, Fratamico P, Fedorka-Cray PJ, Pearce RA, Call JE, Perrine R, Luchansky JB (2003). Isolation of *Escherichia coli* O157: H7 from intact colon faecal samples of swine. Emerg Infect Dis. 9(3):380-383.

Fedorka-Cray PJ, Gray JT, Wray C (2000). *Salmonella* infections in pigs:*Salmonella* in domestic animals.CABI publishing, Oxon, Great Britain pp. 191-207.

Fedorka-Cray PJ, Kelley LC, Stabel TJ, Gray JT, Laufer JA (1995). Alternate routes of invasion may affect pathogenesis of *Salmonella typhimurium* in swine. Infect. Immun. 63(7):2658-2664.

Francis DH (2002). Enterotoxigenic *Escherichia coli* infection in pigs and its diagnosis. J. Swine Health Prod. 10(4):171-175.

Frank RK, Chengappa MM, Oberst RD, Hennessy KJ, Henry SC, Fenwick B (1992). Pleuropneumonia caused by *Actinobacillus pleuropneumoniae* biotype 2 in growing and finishing pigs. J. Vet. Diagn. Invest. 4(3):270-278.

Fratamico PM, Bagi LK, Bush EJ, Solow BT (2004). Prevalence and characterization of shiga toxin-producing *Escherichia coli* in swine feces recovered in the National Animal Health Monitoring System's Swine 2000 study. Appl. Environ. Microbiol. 70(12):7173-7178.

Frydendahl K (2002). Prevalence of serogroups and virulence genes in *Escherichia coli* associated with post-weaning diarrhoea and oedema disease in pigs and a comparison of diagnostic approaches. Vet. Microbiol. 85(2):169-182.

Frydendahl K, Jensen TK, Andersen JS, Fredholm M, Evans G (2003).Association between the porcine *Escherichia coli* F18 receptor genotype and phenotype and susceptibility to colonisation and post-weaning diarrhoea caused by *E. coli* O138: F18. Vet. Microbiol. 93(1).39-51.

Garabal J, González E, Vazquez F, Blanco J, Blanco M (1995). Toxigenic *Escherichia coli* in Spanish piggeries from 1986 to 1991. Vet. Microbiol. 47(1):17-25.

Garabal J, Vázquez F, Blanco J, Blanco M, González E (1997). Colonization antigens of enterotoxigenic *Escherichia coli* strains isolated from piglets in Spain.Vet. Microbiol. 54(3):321-328.

Giles C (1992). Bordetellosis: Diseases of swine.Iowa State University Press, Ames. pp. 436-445.

Giuffra E, Kijas JM, Amarger V, Carlborg O, Jeon JT, Andersson L (2000). The origin of the domestic pig: independent domestication and subsequent introgression. Genetics 154(4):1785-1791.

Godfroid J (2002). Brucellosis in wildlife. Rev. Sci. Technol. 21(1):277-286.

Gosh L (2014). Why pigs are so valuable for medical.Available at: https://a-z-animals.com/animals/pig/

Gottschalk M, Segura M, Xu J (2007).*Streptococcus suis* infections in humans: the Chinese experience and the situation in North America. Anim. Health Res. Rev. 8(01):29-45.

Goyette-Desjardins G, Auger J, Xu J, Segura M, Gottschalk M (2014). *Streptococcus suis*, an important pig pathogen and emerging zoonotic agent-an update on the worldwide distribution based on serotyping and sequence typing. Emerg. Microbes Infect. 3(6):e45.

Grasso G, Ripabelli G, Sammarco M, Ruberto A, Iannitto G (1996). Prevalence of *Helicobacter*-like organisms in porcine gastric mucosa: a study of swine slaughtered in Italy.Comp. Immun. Microbiol. Infect. Dis. 19(3):213-217.

Gray JT, Fedorka-Cray PJ, Stabel TJ, Kramer TT (1996).Natural transmission of *Salmonella choleraesuis* in swine. Appl. Environ. Microbiol. 62(1):141-146.

Gray S, Stickler D (1989). Some observations on the faecal carriage of mesophilic *Aeromonas* species in cows and pigs. Epidemiol. Infect. 103(03):523-537.

Guedes RM, Gebhart CJ (2003). Comparison of intestinal mucosa homogenate and pure culture of the homologous *Lawsonia intracellularis* isolate in reproducing proliferative enteropathy in swine. Vet Microbiol. 93(2):159-166.

Gupta S, Keck J, Ram P, Crump J, Miller M, Mintz E (2008). Part III. Analysis of data gaps pertaining to enterotoxigenic *Escherichia coli* infections in low and medium human development index countries, 1984-2005.Epidemiol. Infect. 136(06):721-738.

Gyles CL, Stevens JB, Craven JA (1971). A study of *Escherichia coli* strains isolated from pigs with gastro-intestinal disease. Can. J. Comp. Med. 35(3):258-266.

Ha SK, Choi C, Chae C (2003). Prevalence of a gene encoding adhesin involved in diffuse adherence among *Escherichia coli* isolates in pigs with post-weaning diarrhoea or oedema disease.J. Vet. Diagn. Invest. 15(4):378-381.

Chiers K, Maes D, Ducatelle R, Decostere A (2004). Efficacy of vaccines against bacterial diseases in swine: what can we expect. Vet. Microbiol. 100(3):255-268.

Hampson D, Hinton M, Kidder D (1985). Coliform numbers in the stomach and small intestine of healthy pigs following weaning at three weeks of age. J. Comp. Pathol. 95(3):353-362.

Harel J, Lapointe H, Fallara A, Lortie LA, Bigras-Poulin M, Lariviere S, Fairbrother JM (1991). Detection of genes for fimbrial antigens and enterotoxins associated with *Escherichia coli* serogroups isolated from pigs with diarrhoea.J. Clin. Microbiol. 29(4):745-752.

Heinritzi K (1989). *Eperythrozoon* infection in swine as a disease factor. Berl. Munch. Tierarztl. Wochenschr. 102(10):337-342.

Helgerson AF, Sharma V, Dow AM, Schroeder R, Post K, Cornick NA (2006). Edema disease caused by a clone of *Escherichia coli* O147. J. Clin. Microbiol. 44(9):3074-3077.

Helie P, Morin M, Jacques M, Fairbrother JM (1991). Experimental infection of newborn pigs with an attaching and effacing *Escherichia coli* O45:K"E65" strain. Infect. Immun. 59(3):814-821.

Hellemans A, ChiersK, Maes D, De Bock M, Decostere A, Haesebrouck F, Ducatelle R (2007). Prevalence of '*CandidatusHelicobacter suis*' in pigs of different ages. Vet. Rec. 161(6):189-192

Higgins R, Gottschalk M (1999). *Streptococcal* diseases. Diseases of swine, 8th ed. Iowa State University Press, Ames. pp. 563-578.

Hijazin M, Metzner M, Erhard M, Nagib S, Alber J, Lämmler C, Hassan A, Prenger-Berninghoff E, Zschöck M (2012). First description of *Trueperella* (*Arcanobacterium*) bernardiae of animal origin. Vet. Microbiol. 159(3):515-518.

Hinton M, Hampson D, Hampson E, Linton A (1985). A comparison of the ecology of *Escherichia coli* in the intestine of healthy unweaned pigs and pigs after weaning. J. Appl. Bacteriol. 58(5):471-477

Hirst R, Patten B (1991). The importance of enterotoxigenic *Escherichia coli* containing the 987P antigen in causing neonatal colibacillosis in piglets in Indonesia.Vet. Microbiol. 26(4):393-400.

Houdijk J, Hartemink R, Verstegen M, Bosch M (2002). Effects of dietary non-digestible oligosaccharides on microbial characteristics of ileal chyme and faeces in weaner pigs. Arch. Anim. Nutr. 56(4):297-307.

Igbinosa IH, Igbinosa EO, Okoh AI (2016). Antibiogram characterization and putative virulence genes in *Aeromonas* species isolated from pig faecal samples. Environ. Sci. Pollut Res. 23:1-7.

Imberechts H, Bertschinger H, Stamm M, Sydler T, Pohl P, De Greve H, Hernalsteens J, Van Montagu M, Lintermans P (1994). Prevalence of F107 fimbriae on *Escherichia coli* isolated from pigs with oedema disease or postweaning diarrhoea.Vet Microbiol. 40(3-4):219-230.

Inderlied CB, Kemper CA, Bermudez LE (1993). The *Mycobacterium avium* complex.Clin. Microbiol. Rev. 6(3):266-310

Janczyk P, Pieper R, Smidt H, Souffrant WB (2007). Changes in the diversity of pig ileal *lactobacilli* around weaning determined by means of 16S rRNA gene amplification and denaturing gradient gel electrophoresis. FEMS Microbiol. Ecol. 61(1):132-140.

Janke BH, Francis DH, Collins JE, Libal MC, Zeman DH, Johnson DD (1989). Attaching and effacing *Escherichia coli* infections in calves, pigs, lambs, and dogs. J. Vet. Diagn. Invest. 1(1):6-11.

Jensen AN, Dalsgaard A, Baggesen DL, Nielsen E (2006). The occurrence and characterization of *Campylobacter jejuni* and *C. coli* in organic pigs and their outdoor environment. Vet. Microbiol. 116(1):96-105.

Jensen BB (2001). Possible ways of modifying type and amount of products from microbial fermentation in the gut: Manipulation of the gut environment in pigs. Nottingham University Press pp. 12-14.

Jensen TK, Strijkstra G Gruys E, Baumgärtner W, Schou KK, Boye M (2014). Detection of polytreponemal infection in three cases of porcine ulcerative stomatitis by Fluorescent in situ hybridization.Cutting Edge Pathology.Available at: http://orbit.dtu.dk/fedora/objects/orbit:133307/datastreams/file_0da61419-92b4-43a7-b63e-6c2156d8e594/content

Jiang H, Huang S, Zhang W, Zhao L, Xu C, Deng S, Zhu X (2013). Seroprevalence of *Chlamydia* infection in pigs in Jiangxi province, south-eastern China. J. Microbiol. 62(12):1864-1867.

Johnsen G, Wasteson Y, Heir E, Berget OI, Herikstad H (2001). *Escherichia coli* O157: H7 in faeces from cattle, sheep and pigs in the southwest part of Norway during 1998 and 1999. Int. J. Food Microbiol. 65(3): 193-200.

Karlsson F (2014).*Treponema* spp. in porcine skin ulcers. Phd. Thesis, Swedish University of Agricultural Sciences, Uppsala.

Karlsson F, Svartström O, Belák K, Fellström C, Pringle M (2013). Occurrence of Treponema spp. in porcine skin ulcers and gingiva. Vet. Microbiol. 65(3):402-409.

Kennedy M, Rosnick D, Ulrich R, Yancey J R (1988). Association of *Treponema hyodysenteriae* with porcine intestinal mucosa. Microbiology 134(6):1565-1576.

Kenworthy R, Crabb W (1963). The intestinal flora of young pigs, with reference to early weaning, *Escherichia coli* and scours. J. Comp. Pathol. Ther. 73: 215-228.

Komijn RE, de Haas PE, Schneider MM, Eger T, Nieuwenhuijs JH, van den Hoek RJ, Bakker D, van Zijd Erveld FG, van Soolingen D (1999). Prevalence of *Mycobacterium avium* in slaughter pigs in The Netherlands and comparison of IS1245 restriction fragment length polymorphism patterns of porcine and human isolates. J. Clin. Microbiol. 37(5):1254-1259.

Konstantinov SR, Awati AA, Williams BA, Miller BG, Jones P, Stokes CR, Akkermans AD, Smidt H, De Vos WM (2006). Post-natal development of the porcine microbiota composition and activities. Environ. Microbiol. 8(7): 1191-1199.

Konstantinov SR, Favier CF, Zhu WY, Williams BA, Klüß J, Souffrant W, de Vos WM, Akkermans AD, Smidt H (2004). Microbial diversity studies of the porcine gastrointestinal ecosystem during weaning transition. Anim. Res. 53(4):317-324.

Kudo Y, Yanagawa R (1987). Isolation and numerical taxonomic study of urease-positive aerobic *corynebacteria* from lower urinary tract of healthy swine. Jpn. J. Vet. Res. 35(3):181-193.

Kwon D, Choi C, Jung T, Chung HK, Kim JP, Bae SS, Cho WS, Kim J, Chae C (2002). Genotypic prevalence of the fimbrial adhesins (F4, F5, F6, F41 and F18) and toxins (LT, STa, STb and STx2e) in *Escherichia coli* isolated from post-weaning pigs with diarrhoea or oedema disease in Korea.Vet. Rec. 150(2):35-37.

Ladd P, Dennis S, Njoku C (1974). Pathology of listeric infection in domestic animals. Vet. Bull. 44(2): 67-74.

Laukkanen R (2010). Enteropathogenic *Yersinia* in pork production. Academic dessertation, Department of Food Hygiene and Environmental Health Faculty of Veterinary Medicine University of Helsinki Helsinki, Finland.

Lawson PA, Falsen E, Åkervall E, Vandamme P, Collins MD (1997). Characterization of some *Actinomyces*-like isolates from human clinical specimens: reclassification of *Actinomyces suis* (Soltys and Spratling) as *Actinobaculum suis* comb. nov. and description of *Actinobaculum schaalii* sp. nov.Int. J. Syst. Evol. Microbiol. 47(3):899-903.

Lecce JG, Clare DA, Balsbaugh RK, Collier DN (1983). Effect of dietary regimen on rotavirus-*Escherichia coli* weanling diarrhoea of piglets. J. Clin. Microbiol. 17(4):689-695.

Liu W, Yuan C, Meng X, Du Y, Gao R, Tang J, Shi D (2014). Frequency of virulence factors in *Escherichia coli* isolated from suckling pigs with diarrhoea in China. Vet. J. 199(2):286-289.

Long JR, Dukes TW (1972). Listeriosis in newborn swine. Can. Vet. J. 13(2):49-52.

Lopez A, Bildfell R (1989). Neonatal porcine listeriosis. Can. Vet. J. 30(10):828-829.

Lungu B, Ricke SC, Johnson MG (2010). Occurrence of Listeria

monocytogenes in Raw and Ready-to-Eat Foods and Food-Processing Environments and Intervention Strategies for Control. Perspectives on Food-Safety Issues of Animal-Derived Foods. P 129.
Lyutskanov M (2011). Epidemiological characteristics of post-weaning diarrhoea associated with toxin-producing *Escherichia coli* in large intensive pig farms. Trakia J. Sci. 9(3):68-73.
Madec F, Bridoux N, Bounaix S, Jestin A (1998). Measurement of digestive disorders in the piglet at weaning and related risk factors. Prev. Vet. Med. 35(1):53-72.
Madoroba E, Van Driessche E, De Greve H, Mast J, Ncube I, Read J, Beeckmans S (2009). Prevalence of enterotoxigenic *Escherichia coli* virulence genes from scouring piglets in Zimbabwe.Trop. Anim. Health Prod. 41(7):1539-1547.
Madzimure J, Chimonyo M, Zander KK Dzama K (2012). Potential for using indigenous pigs in subsistence-oriented and market-oriented small-scale farming systems of Southern Africa. Trop. Anim. Health Prod. 45(1):135-142.
Mainil JG, Jacquemin E, Pohl P, Kaeckenbeeck A, Benz I (2002). DNA sequences coding for the F18 fimbriae and AIDA adhesin are localised on the same plasmid in Escherichia coliisolates from piglets. Vet. Microbiol. 86(4):303-311.
Martins MF, Martinez-Rossi NM, Ferreira A, Brocchi M, Yano T, Castro AFP, Silveira, WD (2000). Pathogenic characteristics of *Escherichia coli* strains isolated from newborn piglets with diarrhea in Brazil. Vet Microbiol. 76(1):51-59.
Maynard C, Fairbrother JM, Bekal S, Sanschagrin F, Levesque RC, Brousseau R, Masson L, Lariviere S, Harel (2003). Antimicrobial resistance genes in enterotoxigenic *Escherichia coli* O149:K91 isolates obtained over a 23-year period from pigs. Antimicrob. Agents Chemother. 47(10):3214-3221.
Mazumder Y, Das A, Kar D, Shome B, Dutta B, Rahman H (2012). Isolation of *Bordetella bronchiseptica* from pigs in North East India. J. Anim. Sci. Adv. 2(4):396-406.
Mead PS, Griffin PM (1998). *Escherichia coli* O157: H7. Lancet. 352(9135):1207-1212.
Meseko C, Oluwayelu D (2012). Clinical Tetanus in Pigs in a Pig Farming Complex, Lagos, Nigeria. Nig. Vet. J. 33(4):666-669
Messick JB (2004). *Hemotrophic mycoplasmas* (hemoplasmas): a review and new insights into pathogenic potential. Vet. Clin. Pathol. 33(1):2-13.
Mijs W, de Haas P, Rossau R, Van Der Laan T, Rigouts L, Portaels F, van Soolingen D (2002). Molecular evidence to support a proposal to reserve the designation *Mycobacterium avium* subsp. *avium* for bird-type isolates and'*M. avium* subsp. *hominissuis*' for the human/porcine type of *M. avium*. Int. J. Syst. Evol. Microbiol. 52(5):1505-1518.
Mohlatlole RP, Madoroba E, Muchadeyi FC, Chimonyo M, Kanengoni AT, Dzomba EF (2013). Virulence profiles of enterotoxigenic, shiga toxin and enteroaggregative *Escherichia coli* in South African pigs. Trop. Anim. Health Prod. 45(6):1399-1405.
Moon HW, Kohler EM, Schneider RA, Whipp SC (1980). Prevalence of pilus antigens, enterotoxin types, and enteropathogenicity among K88-negative enterotoxigenic *Escherichia coli* from neonatal pigs. Infect. Immun. 27(1):222-230.
Moxley RA, Duhamel GE (1999). Comparative pathology of bacterial enteric diseases of swine: Mechanisms in the Pathogenesis of Enteric Diseases 2. Springer 83-101.
Myers LL, Shoop DS (1987). Association of enterotoxigenic *Bacteroides fragilis* with diarrheal disease in young pigs. Am. J. Vet. Res. 48(5):774-775.
Nagy B, Casey TA. Moon HW (1990). Phenotype and genotype of *Escherichia coli* isolated from pigs with post-weaning diarrhoea in Hungary. J. Clin. Microbiol. 28(4): 651-653.
Nagy B, Fekete PZ (1999). Enterotoxigenic *Escherichia coli* (ETEC) in farm animals.Vet. Res. 30(2-3):259-284.
Nagy B, Fekete PZ (2005). Enterotoxigenic *Escherichia coli* in veterinary medicine. Int. J. Med. Microbiol. 295(6):443-454.
Nakamine M, Kono Y, Abe S, Hoshino C, Shirai J, Ezaki T (1998). Dual infection with enterotoxigenic *Escherichia coli* and porcine reproductive and respiratory syndrome virus observed in weaning pigs that died suddenly. J. Vet. Med. Sci. 60(5):555-561.
Nakazawa M, Sugimoto C, Isayama Y, Kashiwazaki M (1987). Virulence factors in *Escherichia coli* isolated from piglets with neonatal and post-weaning diarrhea in Japan. Vet. Microbiol. 13(4):291-300.
Neyelloff JL, Fuchs SC, Moreira LB (2012). Meta-analyses and forest plots using a Microsoftexcel spreadsheet: step-by-step guide focusing on descriptive data analysis. BMC Res. Notes. 5 (52) 0500-5-52.
Ngeleka M, Pritchard J, Appleyard G, Middleton DM, Fairbrother JM (2003). Isolation and association of *Escherichia coli* AIDA-I/STb, rather than EAST1 pathotype, with diarrhea in piglets and antibiotic sensitivity of isolates. J. Vet. Diagn. Invest. 15(3):242-252.
Nicoletti P (2010). Brucellosis: past, present and future. Contributions of Macedonian Academy of Sciences & Arts. (1):21-32.
Nielsen EM, Engberg J, Madsen M (1997). Distribution of serotypes of Campylobacter jejuni and C. coli from Danish patients, poultry, cattle and swine.FEMS Immun. Med. Microbiol.19(1): 47-56.
Nietfeld JC, Franklin CL, Riley LK, Zeman DH, Groff BT (1995). Colonization of the tracheal epithelium of pigs by filamentous bacteria resembling cilia-associated respiratory bacillus. J. Vet. Diagn. Invest. 7(3): 338-342.
Niewerth U, Frey A, Voss T, Le Bouguenec C, Baljer G, Franke S, Schmidt MA (2001). The AIDA autotransporter system is associated with F18 and stx2e in Escherichia coli isolates from pigs diagnosed with edema disease and postweaning diarrhea. Clin. Diagn. Lab. Immun. 8(1):143-149.
Noamani BN, Fairbrother JM, Gyles CL (2003). Virulence genes of O149 enterotoxigenic *Escherichia coli* from outbreaks of postweaning diarrhea in pigs.Vet. Microbiol. 97(1):87-101.
Oanh TKN, Nguyen VK, Do TN, Goddeeris BM, De Greve H (2010). *Escherichia coli* strains causing oedema disease in northern Vietnam share an identical verotoxin 2e.Trop. Anim. Health Prod. 42(8):797-1804.
Ojeniyi B, Ahrens P, Meyling A (1994). Detection of fimbrial and toxin genes in *Escherichia coli* and their prevalence in piglets with diarrhoea. The application of colony hybridization assay, polymerase chain reaction and phenotypic assays. J. Vet. Med. 41(1-10):49-59.
Okello E, Moonens K, Erume J, De Greve H (2015). Enterotoxigenic *Escherichia coli* strains are highly prevalent in Ugandan piggeries but disease outbreaks are masked by antibiotic prophylaxis.Trop. Anim. Health Prod.47(1): 117-122.
Oliveira M, Barroco C, Mottola C, Santos R, Lemsaddek A, Tavares L, Semedo-Lemsaddek T (2014). First report of *Corynebacterium pseudotuberculosis* from caseous lymphadenitis lesions in Black Alentejano pig (*Sus scrofa domesticus*). BMC Vet. Res.10:218
Oliveira S, Blackall P, Pijoan C (2003). Characterization of the diversity of *Haemophilus parasuis* field isolates by use of serotyping and genotyping. Am. J. Vet. Res. 64(4):435-442.
Oliveira S, Pijoan C (2002). Diagnosis of *Haemophilus parasuis* in affected herds and use of epidemiological data to control disease. J. Swine Health Prod.10(5):221-225.
Omar A, Kheong CK, Mahendranathen T (1962). Observations on porcine melioidosis in Malaya. Br. Vet. J.118:421-429.
Opriessnig T, Bender JS, Halbur PG (2010). Development and validation of an immunohistochemical method for rapid diagnosis of swine erysipelas in formalin-fixed, paraffin-embedded tissue samples. J. Vet. Diagn. Invest.. 22(1):86-90.
Opriessnig T, Hoffman LJ, Harris DL, Gaul SB, Halbur PG (2004). *Erysipelothrix rhusiopathiae*: genetic characterization of midwest US isolates and live commercial vaccines using pulsed-field gel electrophoresis. J. Vet. Diagn. Invest. 16(2):101-107.
Osek J (1999). Prevalence of virulence factors of *Escherichia coli* strains isolated from diarrhoeic and healthy piglets after weaning. Vet. Microbiol. 68(3):209-217.
Osek J (2000). Virulence factors and genetic relatedness of *Escherichia coli* strains isolated from pigs with post-weaning diarrhea.Vet. Microbiol. 71(3):211-222.
Osek J (2003). Detection of the enteroaggregative *Escherichia coli* heat-stable enterotoxin 1 (EAST1) gene and its relationship with fimbrial and enterotoxin markers in *E. coli* isolates from pigs with diarrhoea.Vet. Microbiol. 91(1):65-72.
Osek J, Gallien P, Truszczyński M, Protz D (1999). The use of polymerase chain reaction for determination of virulence factors of *Escherichia coli* strains isolated from pigs in Poland.Comp. Immun. Microbiol. Infect. Dis. 22(3):163-174.

Osek J, Truszczyński M (1992). Occurrence of fimbriae and enterotoxins in *Escherichia coli* strains isolated from piglets in Poland.Comp. Immun. Microbiol. Infect. Dis. 15(4):285-292.
Park J, Seok S, Cho S, Baek M, Lee H, Kim D, Park J (2004) .The high prevalence of *Helicobacter* sp. in porcine pyloric mucosa and its histopathological and molecular characteristics. Vet. Microbiol. 104(3):219-225.
Parma A, Sanz M, Vinas M, Cicuta M, Blanco J, Boehringer S, Vena M, Roibon W, Benitez M, Blanco J (2000). Toxigenic *Escherichia coli* isolated from pigs in Argentina.Vet. Microbiol. 72(3):269-276.
Pedersen K, Sørensen G, Löfström C, Leekitcharoenphon P, Nielsen B, Wingstrand A, Aarestrup FM, Hendriksen RS, Baggesen DL (2015).Reappearance of *Salmonella serovar Choleraesuis var. Kunzendorf*in Danish pig herds. Vet. Microbiol. 176(3):282-291.
Peet R, Fry J, Lloyd J, Henderson J, Curran J, Moir D (1983). *Parasuis* septicaemia in pigs. Aust. Vet. J. 60(6):187-187.
Penner JL (1988). The genus Campylobacter: a decade of progress. Clin. Microbiol. Rev. 1(2):157-172.
Pieper R, Janczyk P, Zeyner A, Smidt H, Guiard V Souffrant WB (2008). Ecophysiology of the developing total bacterial and *Lactobacillus* communities in the terminal small intestine of weaning piglets. Microb. Ecol. 56(3):474-483.
Pluske JR, Pethick DW, Hopwood DE, Hampson DJ (2002). Nutritional influences on some major enteric bacterial diseases of pig. Nutr. Res. Rev 15(02):333-371.
Pringle M, Backhans A, Otman F, Sjölund M, Fellström C (2009). Isolation of spirochetes of genus *Treponema* from pigs with ear necrosis. Vet. Microbiol. 139(3):279-283.
Qi X, Huang N, Zhao B, Wang C. Zhao X (2012). Prevalence of serogroups and genotypes for fimbriae and enterotoxins in *Escherichia coli* isolated from diarrheic piglets in western China. J. Swine Health Prod. 20(6):290-293.
Radostits O, Gay C, Blood D, Hinchcliff K (2000). Actinobacillosis in pigs. Veterinary Medicine. A Text book of the disease of cattle, horses, sheep, pigs and goats. Bailler, Tindal, London. P 942.
Ramos-Vara JA, Wu CC, Mitsui I, Lin TL, Miller MA (2008). Metritis, valvular endocarditis, and septicemia by *Actinobacillus equuli*in a gilt in the United States. Vet. Pathol. 45(4):495-499.
Rampling A (1964). Porcine melioidosis in the territory of Papua and New Guinea. Aust. Vet. J. 40(6):241-241.
Riley MG, Russell EG, Callinan RB (1977). *Haemophilus parasuis* infection in swine. J. Am. Vet. Med. Assoc. 171(7): 649-651.
Ross RF, Zimmerman BJ, Wagner WC, Cox DF (1975). A field study of coliform mastitis in sows. J. Am. Vet. Med. Assoc. 167(3):231-235.
Ryley J, Simmons G (1954). Leptospirosis of pigs. Aust. Vet. J. 30(7):203-208.
Rzewuska M, Witkowski L, Cisek AA, Stefańska I, Chrobak D, Stefaniuk E, Kizerwetter-Świda M ,Takai S (2014). Characterization of *Rhodococcus equi* isolates from submaxillary lymph nodes of wild boars (*Sus scrofa*), red deer (*Cervus elaphus*) and roe deer (*Capreolus capreolus*). Vet. Microbiol.172(1):272-278.
Salmon D, Smith T (1886).The bacterium of swine plague. Am. Month Microbiol. J. 7:204.
Schrauwen E, Devriese L, Hoorens J, Takahashi T (1993). *Erysipelothrix-tonsillarum* endocarditis in a dog-a case-report.Vlaams Diergen. Tijds 62(5):160-161.
Skjerve E, Lium B, Nielsen B, Nesbakken T (1998). Control of *Yersinia enterocolitica* in pigs at herd level. Int. J. Food Microbiol. 45(3):195-203.
Smith HW, Jones J (1963). Observations on the alimentary tract and its bacterial flora in healthy and diseased pigs. J. Pathol. Bacteriol. 86(2):387-412.
Smith S, McOrist S (1997). Development of persistent intestinal infection and excretion of *Lawsonia intracellularis* by piglets.Res. Vet. Sci. 62(1):6-10.
Soderlind O, Thafvelin B, Mollby R (1988). Virulence factors in *Escherichia coli* strains isolated from Swedish piglets with diarrhea. J. Clin. Microbiol. 26(5): 879-884.
Songer JG, Meer RR (1996). Genotyping of*Clostridium perfringens*by Polymerase Chain Reaction is a Useful Adjunct to Diagnosis of Clostridial Enteric Disease in Animals. Anaerobe 2(4):197-203.
Songer JG, Post KW, Larson DJ, Jost BH, Glock RD (2000). Diagnostic Notes: Infection of neonatal swine with *Clostridium difficile*. Swine Health Prod. 8:185-190.
Songer JG, Uzal FA (2005). Clostridial enteric infections in pigs. J. Vet. Diagn. Invest. 17(6):528-536.
Sørum H, Sunde M (2001). Resistance to antibiotics in the normal flora of animals.Vet. Res. 32(3-4):227-241.
Staats J, Feder I, Okwumabua O, Chengappa M (1997). *Streptococcus suis*: past and present. Vet. Res. Commun. 21(6):381-407.
Statista (2016). Number of pigs worldwide from 1990 to 2013.Available at: *http://www.statista.com/statistics/263963/number-of-pigs-worldwide-since-1990/*
Stevens MP, Gray JT (2013). 13 Salmonella Infections in Pigs: *Salmonella* in Domestic Animals. P 263.
Stewart CS (1997). Microorganisms in hindgut fermentors: Gastrointestinal microbiology. Chapman and Hall, New York. 2:142-186.
Szeredi L, Schiller I, Sydler T, Guscetti F, Heinen E, Corboz L, Eggenberger E, Jones GE, Pospischil A (1996). Intestinal Chlamydia in finishing pigs. Vet. Pathol. 33(4):369-374.
Takeshi K, Makino S, Ikeda T, Takada N, Nakashiro A, Nakanishi K, Oguma K, Katoh Y, Sunagawa H, Ohyama T (1999). Direct and rapid detection by PCR of *Erysipelothrix* sp. DNAs prepared from bacterial strains and animal tissues. J. Clin. Microbiol. 37(12):4093-4098.
Tancrede C (1992). Role of human microflora in health and disease. Eur. J. Clin. Microbiol. Infect. Dis. 11(11):1012-1015.
Tang X, Zhao Z, Hu J, Wu B, Cai X, He Q, Chen H (2009). Isolation, antimicrobial resistance, and virulence genes of *Pasteurella multocida* strains from swine in China. J. Clin. Microbiol. 47(4):951-958.
Taylor DJ (2013). Pig diseases 9th ed, North Birbiston Road, Lennoxtown.
Thacker EL (2006). Mycoplasmal diseases. Dis. swine 9:701-717.
Thiagarajah JR,Verkman AS (2003). CFTR pharmacology and its role in intestinal fluid secretion. Curr. Opin. Pharmacol. 3:594-599.
Thorel MF, Huchzermeyer HF, Michel AL (2001). *Mycobacterium avium* and *Mycobacterium intracellulare* infection in mammals. Rev. Sci. Technol. 20(1):204-218.
Toledo A, Gomez D, Cruz C, Carreon R; Lopez J, Giono S.Castro AM (2012). Prevalence of virulence genes in *Escherichia coli* strains isolated from piglets in the suckling and weaning period in Mexico. J. Med. Microbiol. 61(1):148-156.
Townsend KM, O'Boyle D, Phan TT, Hanh TX, Wijewardana TG, Wilkie I, Trung NT, Frost AJ (1998). Acute septicaemic pasteurellosis in Vietnamese pigs.Vet. Microbiol. 63(2):205-215
Tzipori S, Hayes J, Sims L, Withers M (1984). *Streptococcus durans*: an unexpected enteropathogen of foals. J. Infect. Dis. 150(4):589-593.
Van den Broeck W, Cox E, Goddeeris BM (1999). Seroprevalence of F4 enterotoxigenic *Escherichia coli* in regions with different pig farm densities.Vet. Microbiol. 69(3):207-216.
Vannier P (1999). Infectious causes of abortion in swine.Reprod. Domest. Anim. 34(3-4):367-376.
Verbrugghe E, Van Parys A, Leyman B, Boyen F, Arnouts S, Lundberg U, Ducatelle R, Van den Broeck W, Yekta MA, Cox E (2015). Heat-labile enterotoxin of *Escherichia coli* promotes intestinal colonization of *Salmonella enterica*.Comp. Immun. Microbiol. Infect. Dis.43:1-7.
Vidotto MC, Lima N, Fritzen JT, Freitas JCD, Venâncio EJ, Ono MA (2009). Frequency of virulence genes in *Escherichia coli* strains isolated from piglets with diarrhoea in the North Parana State, Brazil. Braz. J. Microbiol. 40(1):199-204.
Vu-Khac H, Holoda E, Majerčiak M, Gašpar G, Pilipčinec E (2004). Genotyping of fimbrial adhesins in*Escherichia coli* strains isolated from Slovak piglets suffering from diarrhoea. Folia Microbiol. 49(1):59-63.
Vu-Khac H, Holoda E, Pilipcinec E, Blanco M, Blanco J, Dahbi G, Mora A, López C, González E, Blanco J (2007). Serotypes, virulence genes, intimin types and PFGE profiles of *Escherichia coli* isolated from piglets with diarrhoea in Slovakia. Vet. J. 174(1):176-187.
Wathes C, Miller B, Bourne F (1989). Cold stress and post-weaning diarrhoea in piglets inoculated orally or by aerosol. Anim Prod. 49(03):483-496.
Wegener HC, Andresen LO, Bille-Hansen V (1993). *Staphylococcus hyicus* virulence in relation to exudative epidermitis in pigs. Can. J.

Vet. Res. 57(2):119-125.
Whyte P, Dobson K, Ratcliff R, Cargill C (1982). Protection of pregnant swine by vaccination against Leptospira infection. Aust. Vet. J. 59(2):41-45.
Wilcock BP (1979). Experimental *Klebsiella* and *Salmonella* infection in neonatal swine.Can. J .Comp. Med. 43(2):200-206.
Wills RW (2000). Diarrhea in growing-finishing swine. Vet. Clin. North Am. Food Anim. Pract. 16(1):135-161.
Witkowski L, Rzewuska M, Takai S, Kizerwetter-Świda M, Kita J (2016). Molecular epidemiology of *Rhodococcus equi* in slaughtered swine, cattle and horses in Poland. BMC Microbiol. 16(1):10.1186.
Woldemeskel M, Drommer W, Wendt M (2002). Microscopic and ultrastructural lesions of the ureter and renal pelvis in sows with regard to *Actinobaculum suis* infection. J. Vet. Med. Series A. 49(7):348-352.
Wood RL, Steele JH (1994). *Erysipelothrix* infections: Handbook of Zoonoses. pp. 83-91.
Xavier NM, Paixao AT, den Hartigh BA, TsolisMR, SantosLR (2010). Pathogenesis of *Brucella spp*. Open Vet. Sci. J. 4(1):109-118.
Zajacova ZS, Konstantinova L, Alexa P (2012). Detection of virulence factors of *Escherichia coli* focused on prevalence of EAST1 toxin in stool of diarrhoeic and non-diarrhoeic piglets and presence of adhesion involving virulence factors in astA positive strains. Vet. Microbiol. 154(3):369-375.
Zhang W, Zhao M, Ruesch L, Omot A, Francis D (2007). Prevalence of virulence genes in *Escherichia coli* strains recently isolated from young pigs with diarrhea in the US. Vet. Microbiol. 123(1):145-152.
Zhao L, Chen X, Xu X, Song G, Liu X (2009). Analysis of the AIDA-I gene sequence and prevalence in *Escherichia coli* isolates from pigs with post-weaning diarrhoea and oedema disease.Vet. J. 180(1):124-129.
Zhu C, Harel J, Jacques M, Desautels C, Donnenberg MS, Beaudry M, Fairbrother JM (1994). Virulence properties and attaching-effacing activity of *Escherichia coli* O45 from swine postweaning diarrhea. Infect. Immun. 62(10):4153-4159.
Zhu W, Lomsadze A, Borodovsky M (2010). Ab initio gene identification in metagenomic sequences. Nucleic acids Res. 38(12):e132.

Supplementary Table 1. *Escherichia coli* virulence factors in piglets based on published information from different countries.

Location of study	Events	Sample Size	Outcome (es)	SE	Var	w	w*es	w*(es²)	w²	w_v	w_v*es	w_v*(es²)	w_v^2
US (herd)	108	111	0.9730	0.0936	0.0088	114.083333	111	108	13015.0069	114.08333	111.00000	108.00000	13015.00694
Denmark (Diagnostic samples)	219	563	0.3890	0.0263	0.0007	1447.34703	563	219	2094813.43	1447.34703	563.00000	219.00000	2094813.431
Mexico (Farm)	116	503	0.2306	0.0214	0.0005	2181.11207	503	116	4757249.86	2181.11207	503.00000	116.00000	4757249.857
Japan (Necropsy samples)	214	567	0.3774	0.0258	0.0007	1502.28505	567	214	2256860.36	1502.28505	567.00000	214.00000	2256860.362
India (Farm)	3	3	1.0000	0.5774	0.3333	3	3	3	9	3.00000	3.00000	3.00000	9
Denmark (Research institute)	45	90	0.5000	0.0745	0.0056	180	90	45	32400	180.00000	90.00000	45.00000	32400
Vietnam (Farm)	126	200	0.6300	0.0561	0.0032	317.460317	200	126	100781.053	317.46032	200.00000	126.00000	100781.0532
Canada (Farm)	164	200	0.8200	0.0640	0.0041	243.902439	200	164	59488.3998	243.90244	200.00000	164.00000	59488.39976
Korea (Farm)	164	720	0.2278	0.0178	0.0003	3160.97561	720	164	9991766.81	3160.97561	720.00000	164.00000	9991766.805
US (Research institute)	330	660	0.5000	0.0275	0.0008	1320	660	330	1742400	1320.00000	660.00000	330.00000	1742400
Spain (Farm)	36	69	0.5217	0.0870	0.0076	132.25	69	36	17490.0625	132.25000	69.00000	36.00000	17490.0625
US (Farm)	55	55	1.0000	0.1348	0.0182	55	55	55	3025	55.00000	55.00000	55.00000	3025
England (Farm)	14	51	0.2745	0.0734	0.0054	185.785714	51	14	34516.3316	185.78571	51.00000	14.00000	34516.33163
Zimbabwe (Farm)	63	1984	0.0318	0.0040	0.0000	62480.254	1984	63	3903782136	62480.25397	1984.0000	63.00000	3903782136
Japan (Farm)	42	42	1.0000	0.1543	0.0238	42	42	42	1764	42.00000	42.00000	42.00000	1764
Germany (Farm)	27	104	0.2596	0.0500	0.0025	400.592593	104	27	160474.425	400.59259	104.00000	27.00000	160474.4252
Vietnam (Farm)	69	92	0.7500	0.0903	0.0082	122.666667	92	69	15047.1111	122.66667	92.00000	69.00000	15047.11111
China (Farm)	112	208	0.5385	0.0509	0.0026	386.285714	208	112	149216.653	386.28571	208.00000	112.00000	149216.6531
Brazil (Farm)	92	100	0.9200	0.0959	0.0092	108.695652	100	92	11814.7448	108.69565	100.00000	92.00000	11814.7448
Slovakia (Farm)	174	220	0.7909	0.0600	0.0036	278.16092	220	174	77373.4972	278.16092	220.00000	174.00000	77373.49716
China (Farm)	206	381	0.5407	0.0377	0.0014	704.665049	381	206	496552.831	704.66505	381.00000	206.00000	496552.8306
Slovakia (Farm)	92	92	1.0000	0.1043	0.0109	92	92	92	8464	92.00000	92.00000	92.00000	8464
Czech Republic (Farm)	277	800	0.3463	0.0208	0.0004	2310.46931	800	277	5338268.45	2310.46931	800.00000	277.00000	5338268.451
Spain (Farm)	280	1334	0.2099	0.0125	0.0002	6355.55714	1334	280	40393106.6	6355.55714	1334.0000	280.00000	40393106.6
Denmark (Research Laboratory)	191	191	1.0000	0.0724	0.0052	191	191	191	36481	191.00000	191.00000	191.00000	36481
Denmark (Research Laboratory)	28	194	0.1443	0.0273	0.0007	1344.14286	194	28	1806720.02	1344.14286	194.00000	28.00000	1806720.02
Brazil (Farm)	45	70	0.6429	0.0958	0.0092	108.888889	70	45	11856.7901	108.88889	70.00000	45.00000	11856.79012
Poland (Farm)	819	1125	0.7280	0.0254	0.0006	1545.32967	1125	819	2388043.79	1545.32967	1125.0000	819.00000	2388043.79
Argentina (Farm)	70	223	0.3139	0.0375	0.0014	710.414286	223	70	504688.457	710.41429	223.00000	70.00000	504688.4573
Sweden (Farm)	634	856	0.7407	0.0294	0.0009	1155.73502	856	634	1335723.43	1155.73502	856.00000	634.00000	1335723.427
Indonesia (Farm)	484	858	0.5641	0.0256	0.0007	1521	858	484	2313441	1521.00000	858.00000	484.00000	2313441
Slovakia (Farm)	74	160	0.4625	0.0538	0.0029	345.945946	160	74	119678.598	345.94595	160.00000	74.00000	119678.5975
Brazil (Farm)	99	144	0.6875	0.0691	0.0048	209.454545	144	99	43871.2066	209.45455	144.00000	99.00000	43871.20661
-	-	-	-	-	-	-	-	-	-	-	-	-	-
-	-	-	-	-	-	-	-	-	-	-	-	-	-
K	16	-	-	-	Sums:	91256.4598	12970	5472	3980098538	91256.45979	12970	5472	3980098538
Df	15	-	-	-	-	-	-	-	-	-	-	-	-

Supplementary Table 1. Contd.

-		-	-	-	-	-	-	-	-	v	0.0758493	-	-
Q	3628.61	-	-	Q_v	3628.6138	-	-	-	-	-	-	-	-
I^2	99.5866	-	-	I^2_v	99.586619	-	-	-	-	-	-	-	-
-		-	-	-	-	-	-	-	-	-	-	-	-
es (fixed)	0.14213	-	-	es (random)	0.1421269	-	-	-	-	-	-	-	-
SEes (fixed)	0.00331	-	-	SEes (random)	0.0033103	-	-	-	-	-	-	-	-
CI (fixed)	0.13564	0.1486151	-	CI (random)	0.1356387	0.14861513	-	-	-	-	-	-	-

Supplementary Table 2. *Escherichia coli* virulence factors in weaners based on published information from different countries.

Location of study	Events	Sample Size	Outcome (es)	SE	Var	w	w*es	w*(es²)	w²	w_v	w_v*es	w_v*(es²)	w_v^2
south Africa (Farm)	2	2	1.0000	0.7071	0.5000	2	2	2	4	2.00000	2.00000	2.00000	4
China (Lab samples)	63	108	0.5833	0.0735	0.0054	185.14286	108	63	34277.878	185.14286	108.00000	63.00000	34277.878
Canada (Farm)	20	50	0.4000	0.0894	0.0080	125	50	20	15625	125.00000	50.00000	20.00000	15625
US (Farm)	175	304	0.5757	0.0435	0.0019	528.09143	304	175	278880.56	528.09143	304.00000	175.00000	278880.56
China (Field isolates)	140	215	0.6512	0.0550	0.0030	330.17857	215	140	109017.89	330.17857	215.00000	140.00000	109017.89
Mexico (Farm)	194	450	0.4311	0.0310	0.0010	1043.8144	450	194	1089548.6	1043.81443	450.00000	194.00000	1089548.6
Switzerland (Farm)	39	50	0.7800	0.1249	0.0156	64.102564	50	39	4109.1387	64.10256	50.00000	39.00000	4109.1387
India	48	720	0.0667	0.0096	0.0001	10800	720	48	116640000	10800.00000	720.00000	48.00000	116640000
Cuba (Farm)	36	36	1.0000	0.1667	0.0278	36	36	36	1296	36.00000	36.00000	36.00000	1296
Bulgeria (Farm)	409	619	0.6607	0.0327	0.0011	936.82396	619	409	877639.13	936.82396	619.00000	409.00000	877639.13
Canada (Farm)	68	170	0.4000	0.0485	0.0024	425	170	68	180625	425.00000	170.00000	68.00000	180625
Hungary (Farm)	126	205	0.6146	0.0548	0.0030	333.53175	205	126	111243.43	333.53175	205.00000	126.00000	111243.43
Canada (Animal health Lab)	100	135	0.7407	0.0741	0.0055	182.25	135	100	33215.063	182.25000	135.00000	100.00000	33215.063
Poland (Farm)	46	46	1.0000	0.1474	0.0217	46	46	46	2116	46.00000	46.00000	46.00000	2116
Korea (Farm)	45	604	0.0745	0.0111	0.0001	8107.0222	604	45	65723809	8107.02222	604.00000	45.00000	65723809
China (Farm)	21	324	0.0648	0.0141	0.0002	4998.8571	324	21	24988573	4998.85714	324.00000	21.00000	24988573
Korea (Pathology Department)	149	476	0.3130	0.0256	0.0007	1520.6443	476	149	2312359.1	1520.64430	476.00000	149.00000	2312359.1
Korea (Farm)	94	230	0.4087	0.0422	0.0018	562.76596	230	94	316705.52	562.76596	230.00000	94.00000	316705.52
Denmark (National Vet Lab)	240	240	1.0000	0.0645	0.0042	240	240	240	57600	240.00000	240.00000	240.00000	57600
Denmark (National Vet Lab)	17	83	0.2048	0.0497	0.0025	405.23529	83	17	164215.64	405.23529	83.00000	17.00000	164215.64
Canada (Vet Medicine Faculty)	872	1226	0.7113	0.0241	0.0006	1723.711	1226	872	2971179.6	1723.71101	1226.00000	872.00000	2971179.6
Poland (Farm)	298	372	0.8011	0.0464	0.0022	464.37584	372	298	215644.92	464.37584	372.00000	298.00000	215644.92
Poland (Farm)	96	207	0.4638	0.0473	0.0022	446.34375	207	96	199222.74	446.34375	207.00000	96.00000	199222.74
Poland (Farm)	608	1146	0.5305	0.0215	0.0005	2160.0592	1146	608	4665855.8	2160.05921	1146.00000	608.00000	4665855.8

Supplementary Table 2. Contd.

Poland (Farm)	40	40	1.0000	0.1581	0.0250	40	40	40	1600	40.00000	40.00000	40.00000	1600
K	16	-	-	-	Sums:	35706.95	8058	3946	220994363	35706.95028	8058	3946	220994363
Df	15	-	-	-	-	-	-	-	-	-	-	-	-
-	-	-	-	-	-	-	-	-	-	v	0.0715685	-	-
Q	2127.5483	-	-	Q_v	2127.548312	-	-	-	-	-	-	-	-
I^2	99.294963	-	-	I^2_v	99.29496313	-	-	-	-	-	-	-	-
es (fixed)	0.2256704	-	-	es (random)	0.225670351	-	-	-	-	-	-	-	-
SEes (fixed)	0.005292	-	-	SEes (random)	0.005292046	-	-	-	-	-	-	-	-
CI (fixed)	0.2152979	0.23604	-	CI (random)	0.215297941	0.2360428	-	-	-	-	-	-	-

Supplementary Table 3. *Escherichia coli* virulence factors in porkers based on published information from different countries.

Location of study	Events	Sample Size	Outcome (es)	SE	Var	w	w*es	w*(es^2)	w^2	w_v	w_v*es	w_v*(es^2)	w_v^2
Norway	3	1976	0.0015	0.0009	0.0000	1301525.3	1976	3	1.694E+12	51.06604	0.07753	0.00012	2607.7405
US	6	305	0.0197	0.0080	0.0001	15504.167	305	6	240379184	50.90039	1.00132	0.01970	2590.8494
US	484	687	0.7045	0.0320	0.0010	975.14256	687	484	950903.02	48.52671	34.18767	24.08563	2354.8415
Belgium	95	135	0.7037	0.0722	0.0052	191.84211	135	95	36803.393	40.33179	28.38163	19.97226	1626.6533
south Africa	106	263	0.4030	0.0391	0.0015	652.53774	263	106	425805.5	47.36150	19.08867	7.69353	2243.1118
-	-	3366	0.3664897	-	-	-	-	-	-	-	-	-	-
K	16	-	-	-	Sums:	1318849	3366	694	1.694E+12	238.18643	82.736812	51.771239	11423.197
Df	15	-	-	-	-	-	-	-	-	-	-	-	-
-	-	-	-	-	-	-	-	-	-	v	0.0195817	-	-
Q	685.40921	-	-	Q_v	23.031651	-	-	-	-	-	-	-	-
I^2	97.811526	-	-	I^2_v	34.872232	-	-	-	-	-	-	-	-
es (fixed)	0.0025522	-	-	es (random)	0.3473616	-	-	-	-	-	-	-	-
SEes (fixed)	0.0008708	-	-	SEes (random)	0.064795	-	-	-	-	-	-	-	-
CI (fixed)	0.0008455	0.0042589	-	CI (random)	0.2203634	0.4743598	-	-	-	-	-	-	-

11

Clinical survey on major ruminant diseases in Kola Tembein and Tanqua Abergelle Districts, Central Zone of Tigray, Northern Ethiopia

Guash Abay[1*], Mulalem Zenebe[2], Daniel Desta[2], Hailai Hagos[1], Minister Berhanie[1] and Tsegay Teame[1]

[1]Abergelle Agricultural Research Center, Abyi-Adi, Ethiopia.
[2]Shire-Mytsebri Agricultural Research Center, Shire, Ethiopia.

Diseases are the major detriment in ruminant production and productivity in the study districts. A cross sectional study was conducted to assess the major animal health constraints of ruminants. 461 species of sick ruminants were examined and diagnosed tentatively. Similarly, samples were collected and identified in the laboratory for confirmation of the cases. Of the clinically identified ruminant diseases, sheep and goat pox (11.93%), abortion (8.24%), pasteurellosis (8.46%), lice infestation (9.98%), tick infestation (5.86%), and flea infestation (5.21%) accounted for higher values. The proportion of infectious, non-infectious, ectoparasitic infestation, and reproductive diseases among clinically sick ruminants was 51.63, 9.97, 26.25, and 12.15%, respectively. The higher ectoparasitic infestation in the study district was lice infestation (38.02%) followed by tick (22.31%), flea (19.83%), mange mite (11.57%), and leech infestation (8.26%). The reproductive problems encountered were abortion (67.86%), retained placenta (25%), and dystocia (7.14%). The most prevalent infectious diseases encountered were sheep and goat pox (23.11), pastuerellosis (16.39), gastrointestinal tract parasitism (13.03), and anthrax (6.30). The most encountered non-infectious diseases were abscess (28.26) and bloat (17.39). In conclusion, infectious diseases and external parasites cause serious economic loss in the study districts. So, regular surveillance of animal disease coupled with vaccination of animals with available vaccines, regular spraying of acaricides and more importantly, public awareness in prevention and control of major livestock diseases in the districts is recommended.

Key words: Clinical survey, Kola Tembien, ruminants, Tanqua Abergelle.

INTRODUCTION

Ethiopia has the largest livestock population in Africa which is estimated to be 54 million cattle, 29.33 million sheep, 24.06 million goats, 1.78 million horses, 5.57 million donkeys, 380 thousand mules, 1 million camels,

*Corresponding author. E-mail: guashaba81@gmail.com.

39.6 million chicken, and 4.7 million beehives (Central Statistical Agency (CSA), 2015). The majority of the livestock populations are local breeds, which are found in rural areas under subsistence type of farming system and the remaining are hybrid and exotic breeds (CSA, 2015). The livestock subsector has an enormous contribution to Ethiopian national economy and livelihoods of many Ethiopians. It contributes about 16.5% of national gross domestic product (GDP) and 35.6% of the agricultural GDP. It also contributes 15% export earnings and 30% of agricultural employment (Leta and Mesele, 2014). Despite huge livestock population and existing favorable environmental conditions, the current livestock output of the country is little. This is associated with a number of factors. Of these factors, disease is a major challenge in the livestock production and productivity (Negassa et al., 2011). In Ethiopia, the aggregate annual economic losses from animal diseases through direct mortality and reduced productive and reproductive performance were estimated at US$150 million (Berhanu, 2002).

The study district favors the development and propagation of infectious agents which makes it difficult to resist the annoying effect of these parasites on the host and makes the control of disease difficult (Singla 1995; Singh et al., 2000). However, as the major predisposing factors and enormous economic losses caused by disease, detailed studies on their prevalence and distribution is required. So far limited efforts have been made to investigate an overall situation of ruminant disease in Aberegele Research Center mandate areas. Therefore, the objective of this study was to have baseline information on ruminant disease and to determine the prevalence of major ruminant diseases.

MATERIALS AND METHODS

Description of the study areas

The study was conducted in Kola Tembien and Tanqua Abergele districts for disease investigation and sample collection.

The study districts were categorized as hot to warm sub-moist lowlands (SM1-4) sub-agro ecological zone of the region with an altitude of 1300 to 1500 m above sea level and the mean annual rainfall ranging from 400 to 600 mm which is characterized by low, erratic, and variable rainfall. The annual temperature ranges from 28 to 42°C (Bureau of Agricultural and Rural Development of Woreda Tanqua Abergelle and Woreda Kola Tembien, 2015) (Figure 1).

Clinical disease survey

Throughout the research period, any ruminant disease either in a form of outbreak or individual cases was vigorously investigated so as to arrive at tentative disease diagnosis.

Study design and animals

A cross-sectional study design was conducted from July 2012 to June 2013 on the survey of major ruminant disease on 461 heads of ruminants consisting of different age groups, sex, breed, body condition scoring, and production systems. The animals include those coming to veterinary open air clinics, animals belonging to small holder dairy farms, and animals in the field. Tentative diagnosis was made based on history of illness and clinical examination. Samples were also taken to Abergelle Agricultural Research Center Laboratory and were examined immediately. For this study, a total of 461 clinical cases coming to veterinary clinics were thoroughly and purposively investigated for cause of abnormalities or dysfunction.

Data analysis

All data recorded were entered into Microsoft Excel and subsequently analyzed using Stata version 11 computer program. Descriptive statistics was used to know the frequency of the disease in the study area.

RESULTS

Various age group, breed and species of animals were brought to clinics seeking for veterinary service. Thirty ruminant diseases were identified in districts of Tanqua Abergelle and Kola Tembien from 461 clinical sick animals which were presented to Yechila and Abi Adi veterinary open air clinics. All these clinical cases were examined based on the history of the patient and general and systemic clinical examination, and laboratory examination protocols so as to arrive at tentative diagnosis. Table 1 shows the percentile and relative frequencies of these diseases.

Of the 30 clinically identified ruminant diseases, sheep and goat pox, abortion, pasturellosis, lice infestation, tick infestation and flea infestation accounted for the higher values in both districts with relative percentile of 11.93, 8.24, 8.46, 9.98, 5.86, and 5.21%, respectively.

Proportion of disease categories in Tanqua Abergele and Kola Tembien

Based on the nature and cause of illness, the diseases were categorized as infectious, non-infectious, ectoparasitic infestation, and reproductive diseases. Diseases such as anthrax, black leg, sheep and goat pox, contagious ecthyma (Orf), actinobacillosis, actinomycosis, colibacillosis, mastitis, pasturelosis, parasitic bronchitis, gastrointestinal tract parasitism, Peste desPetitis Ruminants, foot root, and kerato conjuctivitis were grouped as infectious. Tick infestation, lice infestation, flea infestation, mange mite infestation and leech infestation were grouped as ectoparasitic infestation. Bloat, milk fever, trauma of eye, fracture of limbs and horn, wart, abscess and incisional hernia were grouped under disease category of non-infectious whereas abortion, retained placenta and dystocia were also grouped under reproductive problems category.

The proportion of infectious, non-infectious,

Table 1. The prevalence of major ruminant diseases in Tanqua Abergelle and Kola Tembien districts.

Tentative diagnosis	Frequency	Percent
GIT Parasitism	31	6.72
PPR	5	1.08
Abortion	38	8.24
Abscess	13	2.82
Actinobacillosis	8	1.74
Actinomycosis	9	1.95
Anthrax	15	3.25
Black leg	8	1.74
Bloat	8	1.74
Colibacillosis	7	1.52
Dystocia	4	0.87
Flea infestation	24	5.21
Foot rot	3	0.65
Fracture of horn	1	0.22
Fracture of limb	4	0.87
Incisional hernia	4	0.87
Keratoconjunctivitis	15	3.25
Leech infestation	10	2.17
Lice infestation	46	9.98
Mange mite infection	14	3.04
Mastitis	11	2.39
Milk fever	3	0.65
Orf	17	3.69
Parasitic bronchitis	15	3.25
Pastuerellosis	39	8.46
Sheep and goat pox	55	11.93
Retained placenta	14	3.04
Tick infestation	27	5.86
Trauma of eye	7	1.52
Wart	6	1.30

ectoparasitic infestation and reproductive diseases in both district were 51.63, 9.97, 26.25, and 12.15%, respectively. Of these, infectious and ectoparasitic infestation accounted for higher proportion as compared to reproductive and non-infectious diseases.

The status of external parasite infestation in the study districts

The overall prevalence of ectoparasite infestation in the study districts was 26.25% (121/461). The ectoparasite infestation disease category includes lice, tick, flea, mange mite, and leech infestation and their prevalence is shown in Table 2.

Higher infestation was found in lice (38.02%) and followed by tick (22.31%), flea (19.83%), mange mite (11.57%) and leech infestation (8.26%) in the study districts.

The status of reproductive problems in the study districts

The overall prevalence of reproductive problem categories in districts of Tanqua Abergelle and Kola Tembien was 12.15%. The reproductive problem category comprises of abortion, retained placenta and dystocia with their prevalence of 67.86, 25, and 7.14%, respectively. The higher proportions of reproductive diseases were abortion (Table 3).

The prevalence of infectious diseases in the study districts

The overall prevalence of infectious disease categories in

Table 2. The status of external parasite infestation in the districts of Tanqua Abergele and Kola Tembein.

Type of parasite	Frequency	Percent
Lice infestation	46	38.02
Tick infestation	27	22.31
Flea infestation	24	19.83
Mange mite infestation	14	11.57
Leech infestation	10	8.26

Table 3. The prevalence of reproductive disease in the study area.

Disease category	Tanqua Abergelle (%)	Kola Tembien (%)	Total (%)
Retained placenta	17.86	7.14	25
Abortion	66.07	1.79	67.86
Dystocia	5.36	1.79	7.14
Total	89.29	10.71	100

Table 4. The status of prevalènce of infectious disease in districts of Tanqua Abergele and Kola Tembien.

Infectious disease	Frequency	Percent
Anthrax	15	6.30
Black leg	8	3.36
Actinomycosis	9	3.78
Actinobacilosis	8	3.36
Mastitis	11	4.62
GIT parasitism	31	13.03
Sheep and goat pox	55	23.11
Orf	17	7.14
Colibacillosis	7	2.94
Kerato conjunctivitis	15	6.30
Foot rot	3	1.26
PPR	5	2.10
Pasturellosis	39	16.39
Parasitic bronchitis	15	6.30
Total	238	100.00

the study districts were 51.63% which is the leading among the disease category and exerts major effect on the livestock industry. Pasturellosis, gastrointestinal parasitism, parasitic bronchitis and sheep and goat pox was the leading prevailing infectious disease among the infectious disease category in the study districts (Table 4).

The prevalence of non-infectious disease in the study districts

The overall prevalence of non-infectious disease in both districts is 9.97% which is the least among disease category. Of all the non-infectious disease in the study districts, bloat has higher percentage followed by trauma of eye due to whip lash (Table 5).

DISCUSSION

The study reveals that sheep and goat pox, abortion, pasteurellosis, lice infestation, tick infestation and flea infestation were the major animal health constraints of ruminants in the study districts. This study agrees with the finding of Haftu et al. (2014) in which pasteurellosis and ectoparasite infestation were the major health constraints in Ganta Afeshum district.

Table 5. The status of non-infectious diseases in the study districts.

List of abnormalities	Frequency	Percent
Bloat	8	17.39
Trauma of eye	7	15.22
Fracture of horn	1	2.17
Incisional hernia	4	8.70
Wart	6	13.04
Milk fever	3	6.52
Abscess	13	28.26
Fracture of limbs	4	8.70
Total	46	100

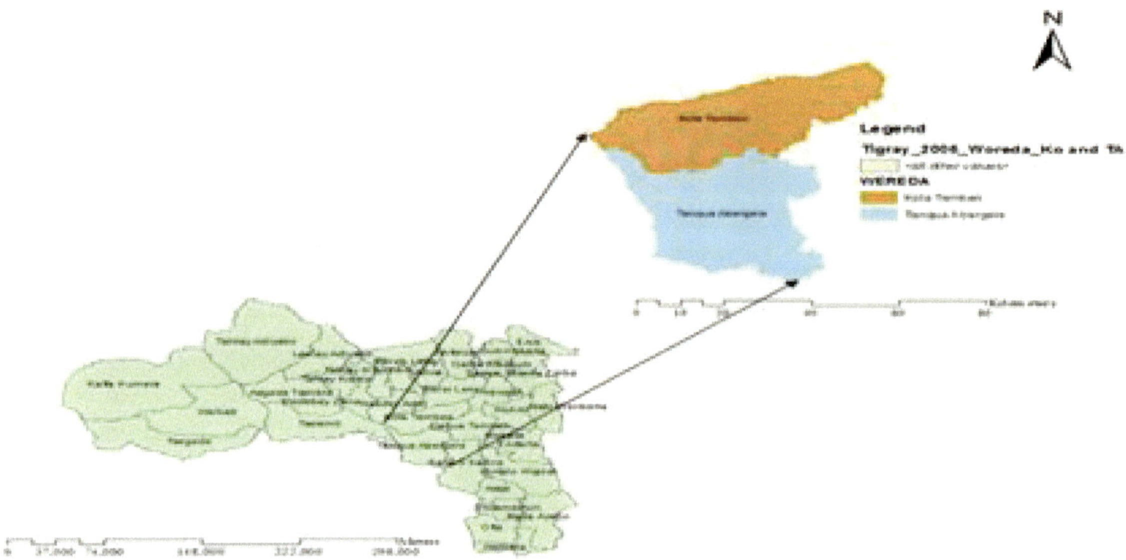

Figure 1. Topographic map of Tanqua Abergele and Kola Tembien.

The overall prevalence of ectoparasites in the study districts was 26.25%. However, it is higher than the study conducted in Ganta Afeshum district (15.4%) reported by Haftu et al. (2014) and it is lower than the study conducted in Gondar (78.38%) reported by Fentahun et al. (2012). These variations might be due to different management practice of the animals, agro ecology, and ectoparasite control practices in the different study districts.

The major infectious diseases of small ruminants identified in this study were pastuerellosis, gastrointestinal tract parasitism, parasitic bronchitis and sheep and goat pox. These diseases were also identified in different areas of the country like Urgessa et al. (2012) who reported the existence of these diseases in Ilu Abba Bora Zone of Oromia Regional State, in Ganta Afeshum district of Eastern Zone of Tigray (Haftu et al., 2014).

The major reproductive problems identified in these study districts were abortion (67.8%), retained placenta (25%), and dystocia (7.14%). The present findings revealed the existence of small ruminant abortion and retained placenta at a high prevalence. The present finding with regards to abortion was higher than the report in Dire Dawa (51.02%) by Negash et al. (2012). This report was also higher than the report by Fentahun and Fresebehat, (2012) in Gonder areas (15%). The present finding also revealed higher prevalence of retained placenta and dystocia. This report also disagrees with those of Feleke (2008) who reported higher prevalence (25%) of retained fetal membrane and very low prevalence of dystocia (0.3%) was reported in Bure districts. In the present study, the higher prevalence of abortion, retained placenta and dystocia might be associated with infectious and non-infectious causes. Similarly, this may also be due to different management factors and agro ecology (Juyal et al., 2011). Most researches on reproductive problems especially abortion put as a serious constraint small ruminant production, because this causes high mortality amongst kids and lambs and it has a high zoonotic potential (Gizaw et al., 1995; Gojam et al., 1995; Solomon and Gemeda, 2000; Tibbo, 2006).

The overall investigated infectious diseases in ruminants in the study districts were anthrax (6.3%), blackleg (3.36%), actinomycosis (3.78%), actinobacillosis (3.36%), mastitis (4.62%), gastrointestinal tract parasitism (13.03%), sheep and goat pox (23.11%), Orf (7.14%), colibacillosis (2.94%), keratoconjunctivitis (6.3%), foot rot (11.26%), and pastuerellosis (16.39%). Different reports were described about infectious diseases of ruminants in different parts of Ethiopia; in Ganta Afeshum reported by Haftu et al. (2014) for anthrax (6.8%), blackleg (5.8%), pastuerellosis (15.9%), and gastrointestinal tract parasitism (16.1%). Amsalu (2007), Mekonnen (2007), Yohannes (2007) and Abraha (2007) also reported the importance of anthrax and blackleg.

The present study showed that pasteurellosis was the most serious economically important bacterial infectious disease of ruminants in the study districts. This result is in agreement with the findings of Haftu et al. (2014) who reported the prevalence in Ganta Afeshum to be 15.9%. Pasteurellosis being commensally of the upper respiratory tract selectively proliferate and colonize the lower part of the respiratory tract. This occurs during the times of ill-defined factors of which inclement weather is one example (Radostits et al., 2006). Similarly, the high occurrence of the diseases in the study districts may be due to stress factors.

Sheep/goat poxviruses in the present study were found to be frequently occurring viral infectious diseases in the districts. Factors predisposing for poxvirus infection include climate, housing, and shortage of feed during the long dry season. Similar, study was reported by Haffize (2001) in Central Ethiopia. This finding is also in agreement with the finding of Feleke (2008) who studied major animal health problems of market oriented livestock development in Bure district and reported the prevalence of sheep and goat pox in Bure woreda to be 18.35 and 31.25%, respectively.

In the study districts, different non infectious diseases were investigated. Among these non-infectious diseases, bloat was at higher prevalence rate (17.39%). The present finding was different from the report of Haftu et al. (2014) who reported that the prevalence was 4.7%; this may be due to agro ecology and management difference. In addition to this, Feleke (2008) also reported that eye trauma was investigated; although it was in a low prevalence (0.3%).

CONCLUSIONS AND RECOMMENDATION

In the study districts, health problems such as sheep and goat pox, abortion, pasturellosis, lice infestation, tick infestation and flea infestation were the major identified health problem of ruminants. Other diseases of economic importance included black leg, mastitis; peste des petits ruminants (PPR) and anthrax were also identified. Based on these findings, the following recommendations are made:

(1) Provision of adequate budget for procurement of drugs and veterinary equipment may be made.
(2) Identification of strains of different diseases in the district is needed.
(3) Provision of regular in-service training to animal health workers in the district is required.
(4) Training farmers and extension agents in prevention and control of major livestock diseases in the district may be stressed.
(5) Provision of regular vaccinations and treatment of major livestock diseases in the district is recommended.

ACKNOWLEDGEMENT

The authors would like to thank Tigray Agricultural Research Institute who supported financially.

REFERENCES

Abraha GG (2007). Major animal health problems of market oriented livestock development in Atsbi Womberta woreda, Tigray Regional State (Doctoral dissertation, Addis Ababa University).
Amsalu K (2007). Major animal health problems of market oriented livestock development in Fogera woreda (Doctoral dissertation, Addis Ababa University) Ethiopia.
Berhanu A (2002, June). Welcome address: Animal health and poverty reduction strategies. In Proceedings of the 16th Annual Conference of the Ethiopian Veterinary Association (EVA), held. 56:117-137.
Central Statistical Agency (CSA) (2015). Central statistics for livestock population in Ethiopia, Addis Ababa, Ethiopia.
Feleke A (2008).Major animal health problems of market oriented livestock development in Bure woreda (Doctoral dissertation, Haramaya University).
Fentahun T, Fresebehat A (2012). Listeriosis in Small Ruminants: A Review. Adv. Biol. Res. 6(6):202-209.
Fentahun T, Woldemariam F, Chanie M, Berhan M (2012). Prevalence of ectoparasites on small ruminants in and around Gondar Town. American-Eurasian J. Sci. Res. 7(3):106-111.
Gizaw S, Abegaz S, Gojam Y (1995). Factors affecting preweaning survival of Horro lambs at Bako Research Center. In 3. National Conference of the Ethiopian Society of Animal Production, Addis Abeba (Ethiopia), 27-29 Apr 1995. ESAP.
Gojam Y, Gizaw S, Thwaites CJ, Awgichew K (1995). Influence of birth weight and postpartum age on lamb mortality in Ethiopian Horro sheep. In 3. National Conference of the Ethiopian Society of Animal Production, Addis Abeba (Ethiopia), 27-29 Apr 1995. ESAP.
Haffize M (2001). Study on skin diseases of small ruminants in central Ethiopia. DVM Thesis, Faculty of Veterinary Medicine, Addis Ababa University, DebrezeZeit, Ethiopia.
Haftu B, Asresie A, Haylom M (2014). Assessment on Major Health

Constraints of Livestock Development in Eastern Zone of Tigray: The Case of “Gantaafeshum Woreda” Northern Ethiopia. J. Vet. Sci. Technol. 5:174.

Juyal PD, Bal MS, Singla LD (2011) Economic impact, diagnostic investigations and management of protozoal abortions in farm animals. In: All India SMVS’ Dairy Business Directory 11:39-46.

Leta S, Mesele F (2014). Spatial analysis of cattle and shoat population in Ethiopia: growth trend, distribution and market access. Springer plus. 3(1): 310.

Mekonnen K (2007). Major animal health problems of market oriented livestock development in Alaba woreda, Southern Nations Nationalities and Peoples Region (Doctoral dissertation, Addis Ababa University), Ethiopia.

Negash E, Shimelis, Desta B (2012). Seroprevalence of small ruminant brucellosis and its public health awareness in selected sites of Dire Dawa region, Eastern Ethiopia. J. Vet. Med. Anim. Health 4(4):61-66.

Negassa A, Rashid S, Gebremedhin B (2011). Livestock Production and Marketing. ESSP II Working Paper 26. International Food Policy Research Institute/ Ethiopia Strategy Support Program II, Addis Ababa, Ethiopia.

Radostits OM, Gay CC, Hinchcliff KW, Constable PD (Eds.) (2006). Veterinary Medicine E-Book: A textbook of the diseases of cattle, horses, sheep, pigs and goats. Elsevier Health Sciences.

Singh AP, Singla LD, Singh A (2000) A study on the effects of macroclimatic factors on the seasonal population dynamics of *Boophilus micropus* (Canes, 1888) infesting the cross-bred cattle of Ludhiana district. Int. J. Anim. Sci. 15(1):29-31.

Singla LD (1995) A note on sub-clinical gastro-intestinal parasitism in sheep and goats in Ludhiana and Faridkot districts of Punjab. Indian Vet. Med. J. 19:61-62.

Solomon A, Gemeda D (2000). Genetic and phenotypic parameters of growth, reproductive and survival performance of Horro sheep at Bako Research Center. Research fellowship report. International Livestock Research Institute (ILRI), Addis Ababa, Ethiopia.

Tibbo M (2006). Productivity and health of indigenous sheep breeds and crossbreds in the central Ethiopian highlands. P 51.

Urgessa D, Duguma B, Demeka S, Tolamariam T (2012). A survey of sheep and goat diseases in Ilu Abba Bora Zone of Oromia Regional State, Southwestern Ethiopia. Glob. Vet. 9 (5):552-556.

Yohannes T (2007). Major animal health problems of market oriented livestock development in Alamata Woreda. DVM thesis, Faculty of Veterinary Medicine, Addis Ababa Universty, Debre Zeit, Ethiopia.

12

Public health risk and transmission route of Middle East respiratory syndrome (MERS): MERS coronavirus in dromedary camel

Andualem Yimer* and Sisay Fanta

School of Veterinary Medicine, Wollo University, Dessie, Ethiopia.

Middle East respiratory syndrome corona virus (MERS-CoV) is a novel enzootic beta origin corona virus which was described in September 2012 for the first time. According to the reports of different researchers, the prevalence of MERS-CoV antibodies, during serological examination, is very high in dromedary camels of Eastern Africa and the Arabian Peninsula. However, the infection in camel is mostly asymptomatic. In contrast to the camel case, the clinical signs and symptoms of MERS-CoV infection in humans ranges from an asymptomatic or mild respiratory illness to severe pneumonia and multi-organ failure with an overall mortality rate of about 35%. Therefore, the objective of this paper was to review the public health risk, transmission routes of Middle East respiratory syndrome and to recommend the disease for further research. The identification of MERS-CoV RNA and viable virus from dromedary camels, including samples with respiratory symptoms by different studies have been detected especially in isolation of identical strains of MERS-CoV from epidemiologically linked humans and camels are the suggestive evidence for inter-transmission of the virus, primarily from camels to humans and its public health risks. Though inter-human spread within health care settings is responsible for the majority of reported MERS-CoV human cases, the virus is currently incapable of causing sustained human-to-human transmission (pandemic occurrence). Phylogenetic studies and viral sequencing results strongly suggest that MERS-CoV originated from bat ancestors after evolutionary recombination process, primarily in dromedary camels in Africa, before its exportation to the Arabian Peninsula through the camel trading routes. Currently, there is no specific drug or vaccine available for treatment and prevention of infections due to MERS-CoV in patients. The important measures to control MERS-CoV spread are strict regulation of camel movement, regular herd screening and isolation of infected camels, use of personal protective equipment by camel handlers and awareness creation on the public, especially in African pastoralists where consumption of unpasteurized camel milk is common. Therefore, urgent global epidemiological studies are required, especially in the poor camel rearing African countries to understand the transmission patterns and the human cases of MERS-CoV and also for the proper implementation of the above mentioned control measures.

Key words: Dromedary camel, epidemiology, MERS-CoV, public health, respiratory syndrome.

INTRODUCTION

Middle East respiratory syndrome coronavirus (MERS-CoV) is a novel lineage C beta corona virus derived from bats which can cause acute viral respiratory disease in humans (WHO, 2014a) and in camels (also known as camel flu) (Richard, 2015). Dromedary camels in the Middle East have high sero prevalence for MERS-CoV and MERS-CoV RNA has been consistently detected in these animals, especially in settings such as camel abattoirs, where camels from multiple origins are assembled, but the exact source of infection in camels has not been identified. More than 60% of the global population of dromedary camels is distributed in African countries and some of these countries are important camel exporters to the Arabian Peninsula (Faye and Bonnet, 2012). MERS-CoV antibodies were also found with high prevalence in dromedary camels in these African countries with positive rates higher than 80% for the animals in Egypt, Ethiopia, Nigeria and Sudan, and 30 to 54% in Tunisia (Reusken et al., 2014).

According to WHO (2015c), there were 1,618 laboratory-confirmed cases of MERS reported with 579 human deaths and camels are believed to be involved in its spread to humans but its way of transmission is unclear (Zumla et al., 2015). This disease in human is zoonotic in origin, although clusters of human-to-human transmission have been reported, especially in health care or family settings (WHO, 2015a). However, this human zoonotic disease has so far been reported only from countries in the Middle-East, the reason for the absence of zoonotic disease report from Africa is unclear (Chu et al., 2014) and it should be of great concern to researchers.

In humans, the virus is graver and opportunistic pathogen associated with the death rate of 40% from infection cases report. It is yet to be established whether infections thought to have been acquired from an animal origin produce a more severe outcome than those spread between humans (WHO, 2013a). Therefore, the objective of this paper was to review the public health risk, transmission routes of Middle East respiratory syndrome and to recommend the disease for further research.

PUBLIC HEALTH RISK AND DESCRIPTIONS OF MERS CORONA VIRUS

History and origin

The first zoonotic introduction of a corona virus into the human population occurred by the severe acute respiratory syndrome corona virus (SARS-CoV) in 2002. According to WHO (2003), SARS-CoV causes a world pandemic, outbreak with 8,400 recorded infection cases and 800 deaths, similarly MERS-CoV marks the second known zoonotic introduction of a highly pathogenic of evidence currently support this theory: the very close phylogenetic similarity with the bat *Beta corona viruses* such as, BtCoV-HKU4 and BtCoV-HKU5 (van-Boheemen et al., 2012); closely related corona virus sequences have been recovered from bats in Africa, Asia, the Americas and Eurasia. Therefore, MERS-CoV uses the evolutionary conserved dipeptidyl peptidase-4 (DPP4) protein in *Pipistrellus pipistrellus* bats for cell entry (Raj et al., 2013).

Middle East respiratory syndrome in human was first identified in 2012, in Saudi Arabia and more than 1000 infection cases of the disease have been reported in May, 2015 and about 40% of those who were infected died due to the disease (Zaki et al., 2012), accordingly, most cases have occurred in the Arabian Peninsula (Zumla et al., 2015). HCoV-EMC/2012 is a strain of MERS-CoV that is detected in the first infected person in London in 2012, which was found to have a 100% identical viral sequencing to the strain identified in Egypt from tomb bats (Zaki et al., 2012); this result is suggestive that bats are the primary origin of MERS-CoV.

Etiology

Middle East respiratory syndrome is caused by the newly identified MERS corona virus (MERS-CoV), with single-stranded RNA belonging to the genus beta corona virus which is distinct from SARS corona virus and the common-cold corona virus (Saey, 2013). According to Eckerle et al. (2014), MERS-CoV uses the DPP4 (CD26) receptor to gain entry and effectively replicate in camel cell lines and neutralizing antibodies for MERS-CoV have been detected in dromedary camels from Africa and Middle East (Milne- Price et al., 2014).

Different studies suggested that the mean incubation period of the virus is 5 to 6 days, it will take 13 to 14 days to show clinical illness in infected person and to subsequently spread to another person. In progressively diseased patients, death can occur within 11 to 13 days, sometimes it will range from 5 to 27 days (Chan et al., 2014; Ki, 2015).

Pathogenesis and clinical sign

The disease in human initially showed simple respiratory problem with mild fever, chills, muscle ache and respiratory stress (shortness of breath). Then it leads to severe pneumonia within 2 to 3 days after infection progressively after some period of time it will develop into severe acute respiratory syndrome (SARS) or acute corona virus, probably originating from bats. Three lines

*Corresponding author. E-mail: anduyimer007@gmail.com.

respiratory distress syndrome (ARDS). In later cases, MERS-CoV causes clinical symptoms of upper and lower respiratory tract infections specific signs and symptoms including high-grade fever, non-productive cough, dyspnea, headache, myalgia, nausea, vomiting, and diarrhea that may precede the respiratory symptoms (Guery et al., 2013). Finally, death may occur in almost half of the cases, especially in unmanaged patients, more death rate will occur (Abdullah et al., 2013).

Laboratory result on admission of patients indicates leukopenia, lymphopenia, thrombocytopenia, and elevated lactate dehydrogenase levels (Assiri et al., 2013). MERS-CoV can also cause severe pneumonia with acute respiratory distress syndrome (ARDS), requiring mechanical ventilation and intensive care admission (Drosten et al., 2013). Incontrast to the human cases, camel showed minor clinical signs of the disease, including of rhinorrhea and a mild increase in body temperature but no other clinical signs were observed (Ahsa, 2013) and the nasal discharge drained from both nostrils varied in character from serous to purulent (Daniella et al., 2014)

Diagnosis

The definitive diagnosis of cases of coronavirus infection basically rely on advanced diagnostic perceptions like the detection of unique sequences of viral RNA by real-time reverse-transcriptase polymerase chain reaction (RTPCR) and immunofluorescence because the disease has no pathognomonic clinical manifestation both in human and in camel (WHO, 2013b). However, antibodies against beta coronaviruses are identified to cross-react within the other species of the genus due to their characteristic antigenic similarity. Therefore, immunofluorescence antibody tests effectively limit their use to confirmatory diagnosis of the disease (Memish et al., 2014).

Throat swabs, urine, faeces and serum samples were collected from wild bats in Saudi Arabia including the area where the first MERS-CoV patient had reported and worked, this study result indicate that, 227of the samples was found positive for nucleotide fragment of the RNA-dependent RNA polymerase region of MERS-CoV genome from the examined different 1003 samples; this result suggest that bats are the evolutionary origin of the virus for camel and human infections (Memish et al., 2013).

EPIDEMIOLOGY OF THE DISEASE

Distribution

According to WHO (2014b) official report, 707 infected patients were identified in 21 countries from three continents of the world. From those detected human cases, 252 patients have died due to MERS-CoV, indicating the case fatality rate of the disease to be about 35% (Drosten et al., 2013). The infection so far has been acquired either directly through a probable zoonotic source, or as a result of human to human transmission through close contacts (Hijawi et al., 2012). An unexplained observation has shown the seasonal variation in the number of reported cases, with a peak occurrence from April to June of each year. The number of cases reported during April, 2014 alone was alarming, because it was greater than the cumulative number of cases reported since the outbreak began (http://coronamap.com, 2014). The possible justification for the seasonal variation of camel case reports may be that it coincides with camel breeding season, and younger camels seem to be more often infected than older camels in the herds (Holmes et al., 2014). Human cases have also been reported in Kuwait, Yemen, Oman, Iran, Lebanon, Tunisia, Algeria, Bangladesh, Malaysia, even in non-camel rearing countries like France, Italy, Germany, the Netherlands, United Kingdom, Greece, Italy and United States (WHO, 2014c), which is suggestive of the presence of other probable intermediate hosts in addition to camel. Furthermore, sero positive camels for MERS-CoV antibodies were identified in Egypt, Kenya, Nigeria, Tunisia and Ethiopia (Figure 1), suggesting that there may be MERS-CoV human cases that are undetected in Africa (Reusken et al., 2014).

Species affected, reservoirs and route of transmission

The disease due to MERS-Cov is thought to be zoonotic because of its close genetic similarity to bat corona viruses (Karesh et al., 2012). Identical strains with human MERS-Cov have been isolated from camels in Egypt, Qatar and Saudi Arabia and MERS-CoV antibodies have also been detected in camels of Africa and the Middle East (Memish et al., 2014). According to Reusken et al. (2013), camels are thought to be a source of human infection, this is because genetic sequence similarities have been determined between human and camel corona viruses (Memish et al., 2014). Transmission from dromedary camels to humans has been shown with RT-PCR and viral genome sequence analysis, molecular detection and phylogenetic analysis have been also performed to investigate transmission (Azhar et al., 2014). Other animals, such as goats, cows, sheep, buffalo, pigs and wild birds have been tested for MERS-CoV antibodies, but no positive findings have been reported, these investigation results provide evidence that camels are a primary probable source of the MERS-CoV zoonotic infection for humans (Reusken et al., 2013). Bats are known natural reservoirs for several

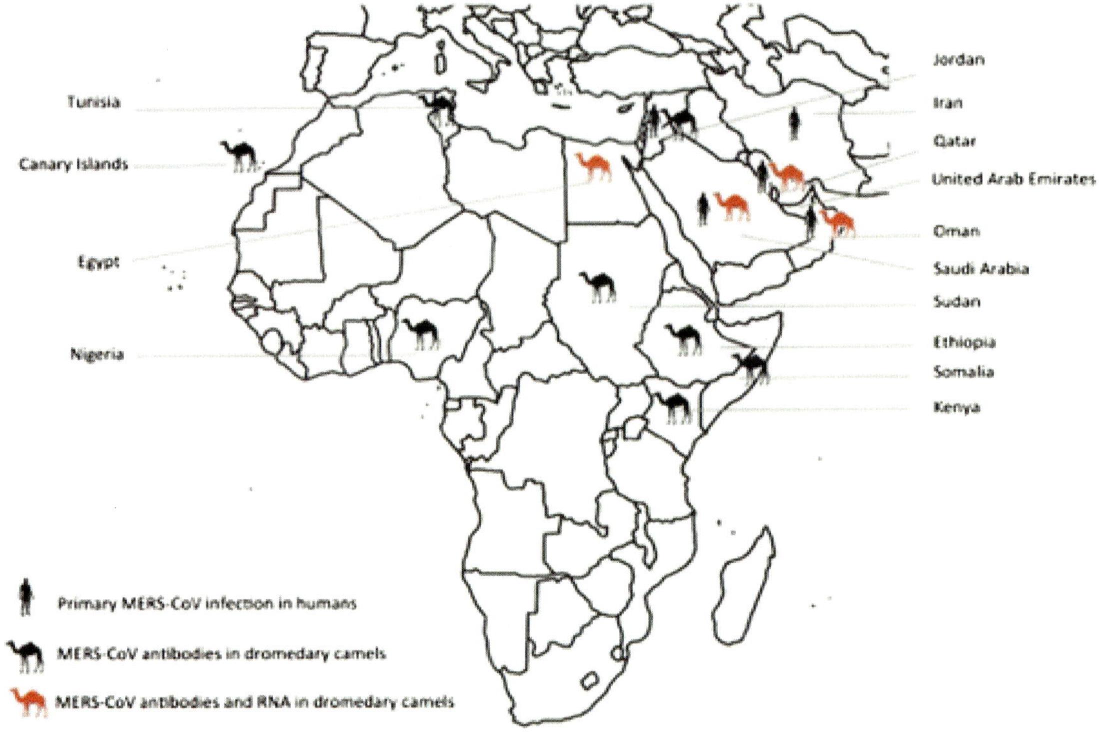

Figure 1. Distribution of human MERS-CoV cases and prevalence of MERS-CoV based on serological and RNA detection in dromedary camels (Source: Taylor and Francis, 2016).

emerging viral infections in humans including rabies, Nipah virus, Hendra virus and Ebola virus (Han et al., 2015). Due to their extremely diverse species with a long evolutionary history, bats have co-evolved with a variety of viruses and due to their lack of B-cell-mediated immune responses which allows them to carry viruses without showing overt clinical signs of viral infections (Dobson, 2005; Karesh et al., 2012). As a result of their low metabolic rate and suppressed immune response during bats' hibernation time, there is delayed viral clearance, which make them the potential reservoirs for different viruses (George et al., 2011). Generally, species affected by Middle East respiratory syndrome and used as source of infection are *Homo sapiens* (human), camels and bats (Augustina et al., 2013).

MERS-CoV is a zoonotic virus that is transmitted from animals to humans (WHO, 2015b). The route of transmission from animal to human is not fully understood(Zumla and Memish, 2014), but researchers hypothesize that camels are a likely reservoir host for MERS-CoV (Figure 2) and most likely, camels are the animal which is source of infection for humans (Saad and Said, 2011).

In some areas of the Arabian Peninsula, the consumption of unpasteurized milk is common and, in some cultural practices of the region, camel milk and urine are consumed for their believed medicinal effects (Saad and Said, 2011). Researchers have proved that MERS-CoV in milk can survive for prolonged periods (van-Doremalen et al., 2014). Contact with a MERS-CoV-infected animal, such as a dromedary, or its bodily fluids may be responsible for zoonotic transmission to humans, but investigations continue to better clarify this question (Aburizaiza et al., 2014).

Transmission of MERS-CoV from human-to-human occurs similarly to other corona viruses. It is believed that it is transmitted by contact with the respiratory secretions of an infected individual that are aerosolized by coughing or sneezing (WHO, 2015a). Many of those infected with MERS-CoV were associated with healthcare settings such as hospitals, but the virus does not have a chance to pass easily from human to human if there is not direct close contact with the infected individual (Oboho et al., 2014).

Group at risk

Studies on MERS-CoV genetic sequences from humans and camels in Egypt, Oman, Qatar and Saudi Arabia point out a close similarity between the virus identified in camels and that detected in human in the same geographic area.

These and other studies also have found MERS-CoV antibodies in camels in Africa and the Middle East and also, preliminary results from an ongoing investigation in Qatar show that people working closely with camels (e.g. farm workers, slaughterhouse workers and veterinarians)

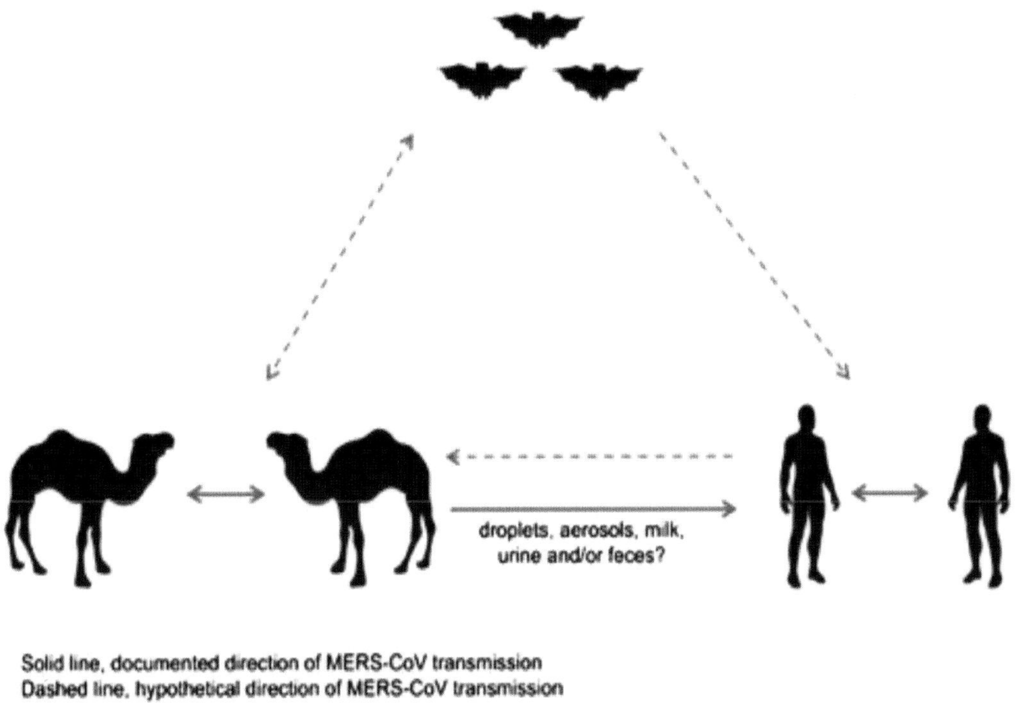

Figure 2. Reported Infection sources and transmission routes of MERS-CoV between bats, camels and human (Source: Taylor and Francis, 2016).

may be at higher risk of MERS-CoV infection than people who do not have regular close contacts with camels and, also health care workers (WHO, 2014d).

MERS coronavirus in dromedary camel

According to Informer East Africa (2016), many outbreak cases of MERS in camels of Kenya is reported and more than 500 camels died due to the disease. An investigation, using real time polymerase chain reaction (RT-PCR) identified MERS-CoV prevalence rate of 3.6% in apparently healthy camels in a slaughterhouse of Egypt. Other research report also indicate that 92% of examined sera collected from camels were reactive to MERS-CoV antibodies and the camels that tested positive were all imported from either Sudan or Ethiopia (Chu et al., 2014).

Studies conducted from 2010 to 2013, in which incidence of MERS was examined in 310 dromedary camels, indicate high titers of neutralizing antibodies to MERS-CoV in the collected serum sample of these animals (Hemida et al., 2013).

A further investigation was conducted on sequenced MERS-CoV on nasal swabs of dromedary camels in Saudi Arabia, result indicate that, MERS-CoV in camels had sequenced exact similarity with previously sequenced human isolates (Briese et al., 2014). The prevalence of MERS-CoV antibodies is significantly higher in older camels when compared with those aged two years or less (Alagaili et al., 2014), which indicates MERS-CoV have been found circulating in dromedary camels for more than 20 years in camel rearing in middle east and African countries (Corman et al., 2014). In addition to the high total prevalence of MERS CoV serum antibody in dromedary camels from Kenya and other African countries, 14.28% of MERS-CoV sero prevalence in dromedary camels from the Canary Islands were also reported by Hemida et al. (2014), this result also included three positive camels that were imported from Morocco to the Canary Islands even though there is no current report from Morocco on the disease.

In contrast to the Middle East and African camel infection prevalence report, currently, there is no published report on MERS-CoV antibodies detection in dromedary camels from Australia, Canada, the United States of America, Germany, the Netherlands or Japan, which will be a research question for researchers indicating that further global epidemiological study on the disease is mandatory.

The investigated high sero prevalence of MERS-CoV in dromedary camel of Africa and the Middle East (Table 1) suggests that animal movement has facilitated the transmission and circulation of MERS-CoV (Briese et al., 2014).

Which is also suggestive of the risk of emerging new outbreak in those countries currently free from MERS-CoV.

Table 1. Sero prevalence of MERS-CoV antibodies in dromedary camel in different countries reporting the disease.

Country	Number of camel tested	Prevalence (%)	Year
Saudi Arabia	9	100	2013
UAE	8	100	2015
Oman	50	100	2015
Jordan	11	100	2013
Qatar	105	97	2014
Egypt	110	98.2	2013
Tunisia	158	54	2009
Ethiopia	31	93	2010-2011
Nigeria	358	94	2010-2014
Somalia	86	83.7	1983-1984
Sudan	60	86.7	1984
Kenya	774	29.5	1992-2013
Canary Island	105	14.3	2013

Source: (Taylor and Francis, 2016).

Prevention and control

Understanding the route of transmission of MERS-CoV and its pattern of transmission is important for proper implementation control and prevention of the disease. Currently, as mentioned above, the pattern of the disease transmission will dictate the methods for prevention (Figure 2). The WHO advises people at risk of MERS-CoV infection to avoid contact with camels, to practice good hand hygiene, and to avoid drinking raw milk or eating contaminated food unless it is properly washed, peeled or cooked (WHO, 2014a). Since most of the cases occur in the health care setting, it is thoughtful that all health care workers practice appropriate infection control measures when taking care of patients with suspected or confirmed MERS-CoV (WHO, 2014b).

Currently, there is no specific drug or vaccine available for treatment of infection caused by MERS-CoV. Therefore, medical care is focused on supportive treatment. Even though, a number of antiviral medicines are currently under study (Zumla et al., 2015), there is no licensed vaccine to prevent MERS-CoV infection. However, one company has developed an experimental candidate MERS-CoV vaccine (Novavax, 2013). Almazán et al. (2013) also developed other candidate vaccines which are being studied as full-length infectious cDNA clone of the MERS-CoV genome in a bacterial artificial chromosome.

CONCLUSION

MERS-CoV is a zoonotic emerging disease with bats and dromedary camels as the important animals mainly involved as source for its emergence, outbreak and epidemiological pattern. Transmission of MERS-CoV from camel to human is well documented and studied by different researchers but is generally not very efficient because transmission route of the virus back from human to camel is still hypothetical. The exact mechanism of transmission is not clear, including whether other intermediate hosts are involved, which will be a risk for new incidence of the disease, especially for those countries in which infection cases were not reported. Currently, the most applicable and commonly used control measures of MERS-CoV spread are strict regulation of camel movement, regular herd examination and isolation of positive camels. Thus, case-control studies of humans with MERS-CoV infection are needed to identify important risk factors and possible chains of transmission from camels and other animals and animal products which are sources of human infections. Similarly, urgent epidemiological studies and molecular detection like sequencing of viral RNA by real-time reverse-transcriptase polymerase chain reaction of MERS-CoV are mandatory to better understand the transmission patterns of MERS-CoV both in human and camel samples, in camel rearing African countries like Ethiopia where camel dependent poor pastoral communities are found, even though current human cases are not reported.

REFERENCES

Aburizaiza AS, Mattes FM, Azhar EI, Hassan AM, Memish ZA, Muth D, Meyer B, Lattwein E, Müller MA, Drosten C (2014). Investigation of anti-Middle East respiratory syndrome antibodies in blood donors and slaughterhouse workers in Jeddah and Makkah, Saudi Arabia, fall 2012. J. Infect. Dis. 209(2):243-246.

Ahsa B (2013). Mucopurulent nasal discharge and lacrymation in dromedary camel naturally infected with Middle East respiratory syndrome coronavirus, Saudi Arabia. Emerg. Infect. Dis. 21:7.

Alagaili AN, Briese T, Mishra N, Kapoor V, Sameroff SC, de Wit E, Munster VJ, Hensley LE, Zalmout IS, Kapoor A, Epstein JH (2014). Middle East respiratory syndrome coronavirus infection in dromedary camels in Saudi Arabia. MBio. 5(2):e00884-14.

Almazán F, DeDiego ML, Sola I, Zuñiga S, Nieto-Torres JL, Marquez-Jurado S, Andrés G, Enjuanes L (2013). Engineering a replication-competent, propagation-defective Middle East respiratory syndrome coronavirus as a vaccine candidate. MBio. 4(5):e00650-13.

Assiri A, Al-Tawfiq JA, Al-Rabeeah AA, Al-Rabiah FA, Al-Hajjar S, Al-Barrak A, Flemban H, Al-Nassir WN, Balkhy HH, Al-Hakeem RF, Makhdoom HQ, Zumla AI, Memish ZA (2013). Epidemiological, demographic, and clinical characteristics of 47 cases of Middle East respiratory syndrome coronavirus disease from Saudi Arabia. Lancet. Infect. Dis.13:752-761.

Assiri A, McGeer A, Perl TM, Price CS, Al Rabeeah AA, Cummings DAT, Alabdullatif ZN, Assad M, Almulhim A, Makhdoom H, Madani H, Alhakeem R, Al-Tawfiq JA, Cotten M, Watson SJ, Kellam P, Zumla AI, Memish ZA (2013). Hospital outbreak of Middle East respiratory syndromell coronavirus. N. Engl. J. Med. 369(5):407-416.

Augustina A, Heather JB,Victor MC , Stefan MK, Michael O, Evans EN, Ebenezer KB, Priscilla A, Olivia A, Benjamin M, Samuel O, Yaw A S, Elisabeth KVK, Peter HCL, Elena VG, Chantal R, Antje S, Florian Gloza-Rausch, Peter V, Marco T, Christian D (2013). Human Betacoronavirus 2c EMC/2012–related Viruses in Bats, Ghana and Europe. Emerg. Infect. Dis. 19:(3).

Azhar E I, El-Kafrawy SA, Farraj SA, Hassan AM, Al-Saeed MS, Hashem AM, Madani TA (2014). Evidence for Camel-to-Human Transmission of MERS Coronavirus. N. Engl. J. Med. 370:2499-2505.

Briese T, Mishra N, Jain K, Zalmout IS, Jabado OJ, Karesh WB, Daszak P, Mohammed OB, Abdulaziz N, Alagaili W, Lipkin I (2014). Middle East Respiratory Syndrome Coronavirus Quasispecies That Include Homologues of Human Isolates Revealed through Whole-Genome Analysis and Virus Cultured from Dromedary Camels in Saudi Arabia. MBio. 5(3):e01146-14.

Chan RW, Hemida MG, Kayali G, Chu DK, Poon LL, Alnaeem A (2014): Tropism and replication of Middle East respiratory syndrome coronavirus from dromedary camels in the human respiratory tract: an in-vitro and ex-vivo study. Lancet. Respir. Med. 2(10):813-22.

Chu DKW, Poon LLM, Gomaa MM, Shehata MM, Perera RAPM, Zeid DA, El Rifay AS, Siu LY, Guan SY, Webby RJ (2014). MERS Coronaviruses in Dromedary Camels, Egypt. Emerg. Infect. Dis. 20(6):1049-53.

Corman VM, Jores J, Meyer B, Younan M, Liljander A, Said MY, Gluecks I, Lattwein E, Bosch BJ, Drexler JF, Bornstein S (2014). Antibodies against MERS coronavirus in dromedary camels, Kenya,1992-2013. Emerg. Infect. Dis. 20(8):1319-1322.

Danielle R, Adney N, van Doremalen A, Vienna R, Brown, Trenton-Bushmaker, Dana S, Wit E, Bowen RA, Munster VJ (2014). Replication and Shedding of MERS CoV in Upper Respiratory Tract of Inoculated Dromedary Camels .Emerg. infect. Dis. 20(12):1999-2005.

Dobson AP (2005). What links bats to emerging infectious diseases. Science 310(5748):628-629.

Drosten C, Seilmaier M, Corman VM, Hartmann W, Scheible G, Sack S, Guggemos W, Kallies R, Muth D, Junglen S, Müller MA, Haas W, Guberina H, Röhnisch T, Schmid-Wendtner M, Aldabbagh S (2013). Clinical features and virological analysis of a case of Middle East respiratory syndrome coronavirus infection. Lancet. Infect. Dis. 13(9):745-751.

Eckerle I, Corman VM, Muller MA, Lenk M, Ulrich RG, Drosten C (2014). Replicative capacity of MERS coronavirus in livestock cell lines. Emerg. Infect. Dis. 20(2):276-279.

Faye B, Bonnet P (2012). Camel sciences and economy in the world: Current situation and perspectives. In: Johnson EH, Mascarina CS, Eds. Proceedings of Emerging Diseases of Camelids, 3rd Conference on the International Society of Camelid Research and Development; Muscat, Oman. pp. 2-15.

George DB, Webb CT, Farnsworth ML, O'Shea TJ, Bowen RA, Smith DL, Stanley TR, Ellison LE , Rupprecht CE (2011). Host and viral ecology determine bat rabies seasonality and maintenance. Proc. Natl. Acad. Sci. 108:10208-10213.

Guery B, Poissy J, el-Mansouf L, Séjourné C, Ettahar N, Lemaire X, Vuotto F, Goffard A, Behillil S, Enouf V, Caro V, Mailles A, Che D, Manuguerra JC, Mathieu D, Fontanet A, van der Werf S (2013). Clinical features and viral diagnosis of two cases of infection with Middle East respiratory syndrome coronavirus: A report of nosocomial transmission. Lancet. 381:2265-2272.

Han HJ, Wen HL, Zhou CM, Chen FF, Luo LM, Liu JW, Yu XJ (2015). Bats as reservoirs of severe emerging infectious diseases. Virus. Res. 205:1-6.

Hemida MG, Chu DK, Poon LL, Perera RA, Alhammadi MA, Hoi-yee Ng, Siu LY, Yi Guan, Alnaeem A, Peiris M (2014). MERS coronavirus in dromedary camel herd. Saudi Arabia. Emerg. Infect. Dis. 20(7):1231-1234.

Hemida MG, Perera RA, Wang P, Alhammadi MA, Siu LY, Li M, Poon LL, Saif L, Alnaeem A, Peiris M (2013).Middle East Respiratory Syndrome (MERS). Coronavirus seroprevalence in domestic livestock in Saudi Arabia. Eur. Surviell. 18:(50).

Hijawi B, Abdallat M, Sayaydeh A, Alqasrawi S, Haddadin A, Jaarour N, Alsheikh S, Alsanouri T (2012). Novel coronavirus infections in Jordan, epidemiological findings from a retrospective investigation. Emhj.19:1.

Holmes D (2014). MERS-CoV enigma deepens as reported cases surge. Lancet 383(9931):1793.

Informer east Africa (2016). Camels in Kenya test positive for MERS virus. J. Med. 365:407-415.

Karesh WB, Dobson A, Lloyd-Smith JO, Lubroth J, Dixon M.A, Bennett M, Aldrich S, Harrington T, Formenty P, Loh EH, Machalaba CC, Thomas MJ, Heymann DL (2012). Ecology of zoonoses: natural and unnatural histories. Lancet 380(9857):1936-1945.

Ki M (2015). MERS outbreak in Korea: hospital-to-hospital transmission. Emrg. Infect. Dis. 37:15-33.

Memish ZA, Al-Tawfiq JA, Makhdoom HQ, Assiri A, Alhakeem RF , Albarrak A, Alsubaie S, Al-Rabeeah AA, Hajomar WH, Hussain R, Kheyami AM, Almutairi A, Azhar EI, Drosten C, Watson SJ, Kellam P, Cotten M, Zumla A (2014). Respiratory tract samples, viral load, and genome fraction yield in patients with Middle East respiratory syndrome. J. Infect. Dis. 292:(10).

Memish ZA, Mishra N, Olival KJ, Fagbo SF, Kapoor V, Epstein JH, AlHakeem R, Al Asmari M, Islam A, Kapoor A, Briese T, Daszak P, Al Rabeeah AA, Ian Lipkin W (2013). Middle East respiratory syndrome coronavirus in bats. Saudi Arabia. Emerg. Infect .Dis.19:1819-823.

Milne-Price S, Miazgowicz KL, Munster VJ (2014). The emergence of the Middle East respiratory syndrome coronavirus (MERS-CoV). Pathol. Dis. 71(12):121-136.

Novavax D (2013). Novavax produces MERS CoV vaccine candidate, A vailable at: http://www.novavax.com/download/releases/2013-0 06%20CoronaV%20 FINAL%20PR.

Oboho IK, Tomczyk SM, Al-Asmari, AM, Banjar AA, Al-Mugti H, Aloraini MS, Alkhaldi KZ, Almohammadi EL, Alraddadi BM, Gerber SI, Swerdlow DL, Watson JT, Madani TA (2014). MERS-CoV outbreak in Jeddah – a link to health care facilities. N. Eng. J. Med. 372:846-854.

Raj VS, Mou H, Smits SL, Dekkers DH, Müller MA, Dijkman R, Muth D, Demmers JAA, Zaki A, Fouchier RAM, Thiel V, Drosten C, Rottier PJM, Osterhaus ADME, Bosch BJ, Haagmans BL (2013). Dipeptidyl peptidase 4 is a functional receptor for the emerging human coronavirus-EMC. respiratory syndrome coronavirus in milk. Emerg. Infect. Dis. 20(7): 1231-1233.

Reusken CB, Haagmans BL, Muller MA, Gutierrez C, Godeke GJ, Meyer B, Muth D, Raj VS, Smits-De Vries L, Corman VM, Drexler JF, Smits SL, El Tahir YE, De Sousa R, van Beek J, Nowotny N, van Maanen K, Hidalgo-Hermoso E, Bosch BJ, Rottier P, Osterhaus A, Gortázar-Schmidt C, Drosten C, Koopmans MP (2013). Middle East respiratory syndrome coronavirus neutralising serum antibodies in dromedary camels: A comparative serological study. Lanc. Infect. Dis.13:859-866.

Reusken CB, Messadi L, Feyisa A, Ularamu H, Godeke G, Danmarwa

A, Dawo F, Jemli M, Melaku S, Shamaki D, Woma Y, Wungak Y, Gebremedhin EZ, Zut It, Bosch B, Bart L. Haagmans BL, Koopmans MPG (2014). Geographic distribution of MERS coronavirus among dromedary camels, Africa. Emerg. Infect. Dis. 20 (8):1370-1374.

Richard LP (2015). Travel alert after eighth camel flu death. The Times. Available at: http://www.thetimes.co.uk/tto/news/world/asia/article4465150.ece

Saad B, Said O (2011). Greco–Arab and Islamic herbal medicine: Traditional system, ethics, safety, efficacy and regulatory issues. Emerg. Infect. Dis. 189(17):117-120.

Saey TH (2013). Scientists race to understand deadly new virus: SARS-like infection causes severe illness, but may not spread quickly. Sci. News183(6):5.

Taylor A, Francis K (2016). Middle East respiratory syndrome coronavirus (MERS-CoV): animal to human interaction Available at: http://www.tandfonline.com/loi/ypgh20?open=109.

Van-Boheemen S, de-Graaf M, Lauber C, Bestebroer TM, Raj VS (2012). Genomic characterization of a newly discovered coronavirus associated with acute respiratory distress syndrome in humans. Molc. Bio. 3(6):2-12.

Van-Doremalen N, Bushmaker T, Karesh WB, Munster VJ (2014). Stability of Middle East respiratory syndrome coronavirus in milk. Emerg. Infect. Dis. 20:1263-1264.

WHO (2015c). Middle East respiratory syndrome coronavirus (MERS-CoV): Fact sheet No. 401.

WHO (World Health Organization) (2013b). The WHO MERS-CoV Research Group. State of Knowledge and Data Gaps of Middle East Respiratory Syndrome Coronavirus (MERS-CoV) in Humans. PLoS. Curr. 5.

WHO (World Health Organization) (2014c). Middle East respiratory syndrome coronavirus (MERS CoV) summary and literature update as of 2014.

WHO (World Health Organization) (2014b). WHO concludes MERS-CoV mission in Saudi Arabia, 2014

WHO (World Health Organization) (2015a). "Middle East respiratory syndrome coronavirus (MERS-CoV)". Retrieved 2015.

WHO (World Health Organization) (2003). Consensus document on the epidemiology of severe acute respiratory syndrome (SARS).

WHO (World Health Organization) (2015b). Middle East respiratory syndrome coronavirus (MERS- World Health Organization CoV) – Saudi Arabia, Disease outbreak news.World Health Organization (2015).

WHO (World Health Organization) (2014d). WHO Risk Assessment. Middle East Respiratory Syndrome Coronavirus (MERS-CoV) 24 April 2014, Geneva.

WHO (World Health Organization) (2014a). Global Alert and Response: Middle East respiratory syndrome coronavirus (MERS-CoV) – update 2014.

World Health Organization(WHO) (2013a). Laboratory testing for novel coronavirus. Interim Recommendations.

Zaki AM, Van- Boheemen S, Bestebroer TM , Osterhaus AD, Fouchier RA (2012). Isolation of a novel coronavirus from a man with pneumonia in Saudi Arabia. England J. Med. 367:1814-20.

Zumla A, Hui DS, Perlman S (2015). Middle East respiratory syndrome. (London, England). Lancet. 386: 995-1007.

Zumla AI, Memish ZA (2014). Middle East respiratory syndrome coronavirus: Epidemic potential or a storm in a teacup? Eur. Respir. Dis. J. 43:1243-1248.

Cross-sectional study on the prevalence and risk factors for major skin diseases of cattle in Hawassa city, Southern Ethiopia

Zekarias Fantaye[1] and Berhanu Mekibib Melake[2*]

[1]Field staff, Ministry of Livestock Development and Fisheries, Ethiopia.
[2]School of Veterinary Medicine, Hawassa University, P. O. Box 05, Hawassa, Ethiopia.

A cross-sectional study was conducted on the major skin diseases of cattle in Hawassa city with the objectives of estimating the prevalence and assessing the effect of different risk factors in the occurrence of these skin diseases in the study area. The study was conducted with thorough physical examination of cattle and laboratory examination of samples collected from all encountered cases. Out of 662 cattle examined for the presence of skin diseases, 146(22.05%) cattle had different skin diseases, namely ring worm (6.2%), lice infestation (6%), tick infestation (5.3%), wart (4.4%), lumpy skin disease (0.6%), mange mites (0.3%) and dermatophilosis (0.2%).There was a significantly higher (p<0.001) prevalence of skin diseases in young (38.5%) than the old (10.3%) animals. However, the other considered risk factors namely; sex, origin and management were not statistically associated with the occurrence of skin diseases. In general, unless feasible control measures are timely implemented the encountered skin diseases can have varied and adverse effect on cattle production, tanning industry and health of the public and concomitantly pose huge economic loss.

Key words: Skin diseases, ring worm, ectoparasites, wart, risk factors, cattle, Hawassa.

INTRODUCTION

The livestock subsector of Ethiopia is the second major sources of foreign currency, through export of live animals and hides and skins (Ayele et al., 2003; Teshome and Derso, 2015). Although the country produces about 2.7 million of hide, 8.1 million of sheepskin and 7.5 million of goatskin per annum for tannery industry, yet as many as one quarter to one – third of all the skins processed at tanneries are unsuitable for export due to various defects (Kassa et al., 1998; Abebayehu et al., 2011). Up to 65% of these defects are believed to occur in the pre-slaughter stage of production while the animal is still alive (Kassa et al., 1998; Wondwossen, 2000). The most common cattle skin diseases reported in Ethiopia are dermatophilosis, lumpy

*Corresponding author. E-mail: berhanumm2002@gmail.com.

skin disease, dermatophytosis, pediculosis, acariasis, photosensitization and warts (Chalachew, 2001; Teshome and Derso, 2015).

Skin diseases are accountable for significant and varied socio-economic impacts. Apart from quality degradation of hides and skin, skin diseases induce associated economic losses due to reduction of wool quality, meat and milk yield, losses due to culling and occasional mortalities related with cost of treatment and prevention of the diseases (Yacob et al., 2008; Salih et al., 2015). In addition, some skin diseases such as ringworm and sarcoptic mites are potential zoonosis (Quinn et al., 2002; McDaniel et al., 2014).

The huge impact of socioeconomic perspective still demands the nationwide detailed investigation of the distribution of important skin diseases and their determinants. Though some research works on bovine skin diseases have been done in some part of the country (Chalachew, 2001; Yacob et al., 2008; Teshome and Derso, 2015), most of them were based on tannery information, some others were focused only on dermatophilosis (Berhanu and Woldemeskel, 1999; Woldemeskel,2000; Woldemeskel and Taye, 2002; Kassaye et al., 2003) and most of them were done in areas other than the current study site and hence there is still information gap in some geographic location and on the remaining skin diseases.

Therefore, this study was conducted to assess the prevalence of major skin diseases of cattle in Hawassa city and to assess the effect of different risk factors associated with these skin diseases.

MATERIALS AND METHODS

Study area

The study was carried out from October 2014 to May 2015 in Hawassa city, which is the capital of south nation nationalities and people regional state (SNNPRS). Hawassa is located at 38°29'E and 7°05'N, 275 Km south of Addis Ababa. The elevation is about 1790 m above sea level and the respective minimum and maximum average temperature is 12 and 28°C. The mean annual rain fall is 960 mm. The short rainy season/'belg' start from February to May and the long rainy season /'meher' start from mid-June to October.

The total livestock population of the zone was 2,172,015 cattle, 858,206 sheep and goat, 155,356 equines and 2,123,579 poultry (CSA, 2017). The two rural villages, Chefe and Dato, are characterized by water lodged and marshy land and are located north east main part of the city following the water course tributary to Lake Hawassa called 'Tikur weha'. The area is known for huge indigenous cattle population and cash crops like Catha edulis (Chat) and 'Enset'.

Study animal and sampling method

The sampling was made first by randomly selecting small-scale rural and urban dairy farms from Hawassa, Chefe and Dato and then the study animals, comprising both sexes, both local and crossbred and different age group were selected using simple random sampling.

Accordingly, a total of 662 cattle, composed of 213 male and 449 female, were selected for physical and laboratory based examinations. Majority (528) of the study animals were cross bred and the rest (134) were local (Zebu) breeds. The age of the animals was estimated based on teeth eruption as suggested by Muylle (2016). The average age of the examined cattle was 2.6 years. For simplicity sake, the study animals were categorized into young (less than 2 years) and adult (above 2 years). The management was classified as poor and better based on the availability of additional feed, shelter and medicament when needed.

Study methodology

History taking and physical examination

History regarding, age, presence of itching, course and progression of the disease, measures taken, if any; the number of animal having the same problem, type of lesion and\or clinical signs observed and their chronology were recorded. The entire skin of the animals was thoroughly inspected and palpated for the presence of papules, vesicles, pustules, erythema, scabs, pigmentation abnormalities, alopecia, tumorous growth and ectoparasites. Distribution of the lesion on the body of the animal and symmetry were also considered.

Samples collection and processing

Depending on the case, appropriate samples were collected for microbiological and parasitological examinations. Lumpy skin disease was diagnosed tentatively based on the characteristic clinical findings and previous serological confirmation made in the area.

Skin scraping: *Skin scraping was collected from representative sites of cases presented with alopecia, Itching and erythematous lesions. Skin scrapings collected from suspected cases were placed in dry clean sterile test tubes. In addition to superficial skin scraping taken from the periphery of the circular lesion, hair specimens were also collected from lesions suspected of dermatophytosis using a pair of forceps. Similarly, for dermatophilosis suspected cases, exudative crusts were also collected by pairs of forceps along with a deep scraping with clean surgical blade. Moreover, the nodular lesions of demodicosis suspected cases were pressed in between two digits until the pus is expressed, the pus was then placed on a slide and crushed in between two glass slides or after placing cover slip (Greiner, 2012; Abu-Samra et al., 2014). The collected samples were properly labeled, packed and transported to the Veterinary Parasitology and Pathology* Laboratory, *Hawassa University for examination.*

Tick and lice collection and examination: Ticks and lice were manually collected by searching on different regions of the animals' body. Various predilections/feeding sites namely; base of the tail, ear, perianal area, sternum, scrotal area and the belly were the targeted sites. The collected ticks and lice were placed in universal bottles, preserved in 70% ethyl alcohol, labeled with the necessary information and transported to the laboratory for further identification.

Laboratory investigation: The squash smears prepared from demodicosis suspected cases were examined for the presence of demodectic mites at 10x magnification of light microscope (Greiner, 2012). Each scraping was transferred to clean and dry petri-dish and examined directly under stereomicroscope for the presence of moving sarcoptic mites. Positive sample was then treated with few drops of 10% KOH and examined based on the standard procedures, mites were picked with dissecting needle along with some content, placed on clean slide, covered with cover slip and examined under 10x magnification to characterize and identify the mites according to their morphology (Urquhart et al., 1996; Greiner, 2012). Exudative crusts and/or deep skin scrapings taken from dermatophilosis suspected cases were moistened with warm saline solution on clean slide, smeared, dried with heat and subjected to Giemsa staining for demonstration of Dermatophilus congolensis (Quinn et al., 2011).The collected ticks and lice were examined under stereomicroscope and identified following the procedures given by Hoogstral (1956) and Walker et al. (2003). Scrapings and hairs collected from ringworm suspected cases were mounted for direct examination of dermatophytes in 25% KOH or NaOH mixed with 5% glycerol, heated for 1 h at 51 to 54°C to emulsify lipids, and examined under 40X magnification for fungal structures (Weitzman and Summerbell, 1995).

Data analysis

Data collected from the field and laboratory examination were recorded, entered in Microsoft Excel spread sheet and analyzed using STATA version 11 (STATA corp., College Station, TX). In the analyses the confidence level was held at 95% and $p<0.05$ was set for establishing significance.

Association with the considered risk factors (age, sex, management system, and origin) was assessed with chi square analysis.

RESULTS

Out of 662 cattle examined for the presence of skin diseases, 146 (22.05%) cattle were positive for different skin problems, namely ring worm (6.2%), lice infestation (6%), tick infestation (5.3%), wart (4.4%), lumpy skin disease (0.6%), mange mites (0.3%) and dermatophilosis (0.2%) (Table 1, Plates 1-3).

The common lice species/genera identified were *Bovicola bovis*, *Linognatus* and *Haematopinus* spps. Moreover, *Rhipicephalus* (*Boophilus*) *decolaratus*, *Rhipicephalus evertsi-evertsi*, *Amblyomma variegatum*, *A. coherence* and *A. lepidium* were the identified tick species.

The variation in the prevalence of skin diseases were statistically significant ($p<0.001$) between age categories, young cattle being more frequently affected (38.5%) than their adult counterparts (10.3%). Hence, young cattle were 5.44 times more likely to have skin diseases than adults (Odds Ratio (OR) =5.44, 95% CI=3.62, 8.18).

However, the other considered risk factors namely; sex, origin and management were not showing statistically significant effect in the occurrence of the problem (Table 2). Age was having statistically significant ($p<0.001$) effect on the occurrence of ringworm, lice infestation and wart. Moreover, the occurrences of wart and lice infestation were significantly influenced by both management and origin of the examined cattle.

DISCUSSION

This study revealed that, skin diseases caused by parasites, bacteria, viruses and fungus were common in Hawassa city in cattle with an overall prevalence of 22.05%. This finding is relatively higher than the report made by Yakob et al. (2008) and lower from that of Teshome and Derso (2015), who reported 15.41 and 27.68% from veterinary clinics of Adama and University of Gondar, respectively. The observed difference among the studies could be partly explained by the difference in the geographic location (that is, ecology and climate), cattle management practice and the study sites preferred for sampling. Although sampling at the veterinary clinics potentially incurs bias, the prevalence current reported and the previous work are still high because of several reasons. The prevailing poor veterinary services, poor animal husbandry, lack of awareness on the problem, the use of communal watering and grazing sites, improper application of acaricides by non-professionals are the major reasons to induce and augment this endemic situation.

Among the different skin diseases, ringworm (aka Dermatophytosis) ranked to be the first with a prevalence of 6.2%. Dermatophytosis in domestic animals is an infection of keratinized tissues by one of the two genera fungi, Microsporum and Trichophyton (Quinn et al., 2002; Kahn et al., 2005). Although information is lacking in Ethiopia, it is believed to pose the greatest economic and human health consequence in most developed countries (Bradford, 1996). In the present study, the prevalence of the disease was significantly higher ($p<0.01$) in animals less than two years of age (12.4%, OR=7.66, 95% CI=3.34, 17.55) than the older age group (1.8%). This variation in the prevalence can be partly explained by the fact that, dermatophytosis in adult and healthy animals is self-limiting but in young and debilitated animals the infection is wide spread and persistent. Moreover, animal susceptibility is determined largely by immunological status, and hence young animals are most susceptible (Radostits et al., 2000; Quinn et al., 2002).

The overall prevalence of cattle skin parasites (11.6%) was markedly lower than the prevalence reported from southern rangelands (73.3%) by Abebayehu et al. (2011). This could be attributed to the differences in the management practice, level of owners' awareness about the problem, ecology and climate of sampling sites. Ticks require moisture and warm environment for survival and the activity of most ticks commences during spring (Mekonnen et al., 2001). It is admitted that tick infestation, perhaps lice and mange mite infestation too, potentially predispose to other skin diseases (Scott, 2007) and hence even low prevalence could not be underestimated.

The prevalence of pediculosis observed in the present study (6%) was in agreement with previous reports made

Table 1. Frequency and prevalence of the observed skin problems of cattle (n=662).

Skin problems	№ of positive cases	Prevalence of positive cases (%)	95% CI
Ringworm	41	6.2	(4.4,8)
Lice Infestation	40	6	(4.2,7.9)
Tick infestation	35	5.3	(3.6,7)
Wart/papilloma	29	4.4	(2.8,5.9)
LSD	4	0.6	(0.01,1.2)
Mange mites	2	0.3	(0.1,0.7)
Dermatophilosis	1	0.2	(0.1,0.4)
Overall skin diseases	146	22.05	(18.89,25.22)

CI=Confidence Interval, LSD=Lumpy Skin Disease.

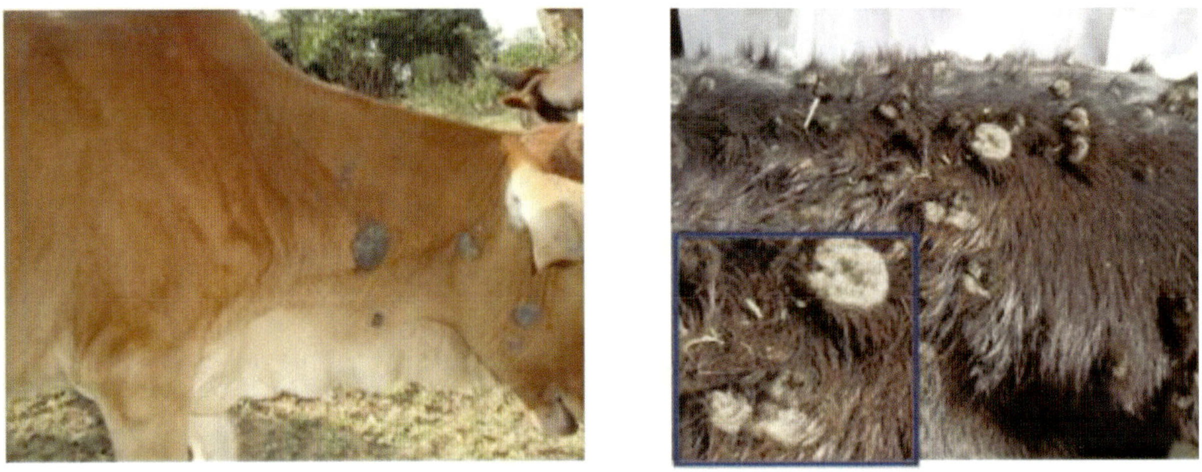

(a) (b)

Plate 1. (a) A case of Wart (bovine cutaneous papilloma): extensive proliferative and keratinized growth on the lateral aspect of the neck, 1year-old, zebu heifer; (b) A case of Dermatophilosis: Crusted and mated hairs on the back of the animal, non-pruritic. Inset: hard, horny and confluent scab.

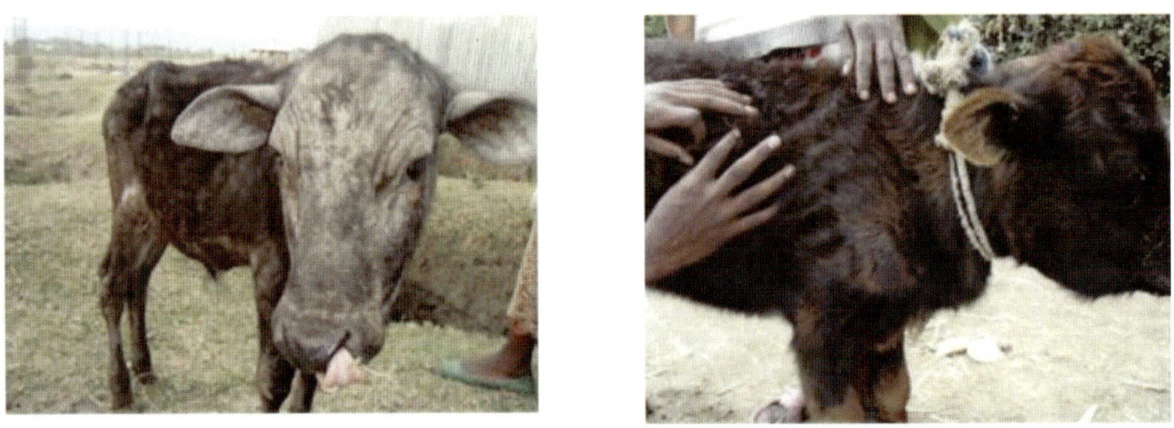

(a) **(b)**

Plate 2. (a) A severe form of Dermatophytosis complicated with mange mite infection: started as ring worm but lately complicated and become prururitic and lichenified. Alopecia, scales, and crusts on the entire body of the animal particularly on the anterior part; (b) Severe pediculosis: a calf with severe lice infestation, faded hairs in normally black hair coat, emaciation and bottle jaw.

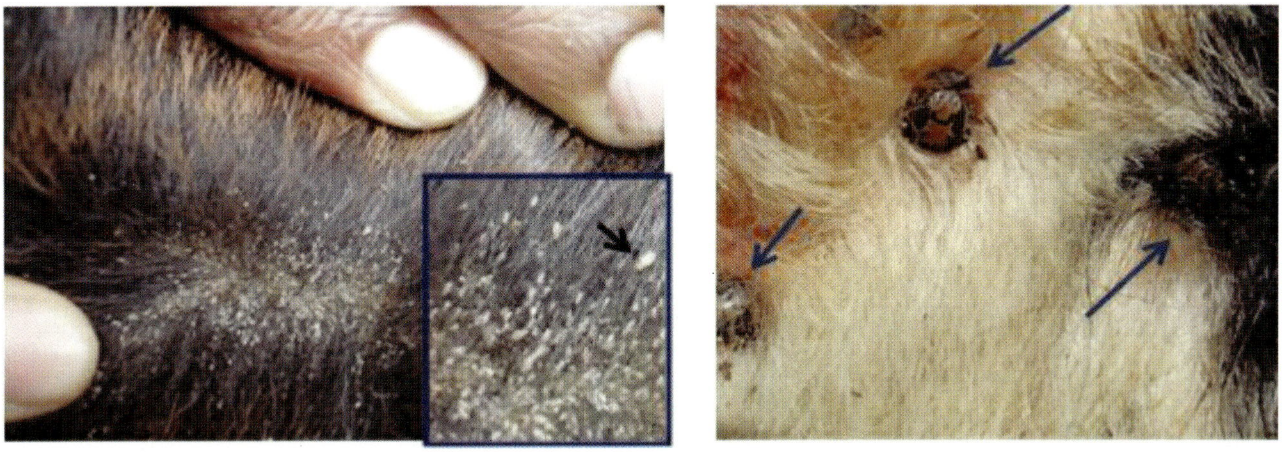

(a) (b)

Plate 3. (a) Closer view of the previous case (Plate 2b). Inset showing several lice (black arrow) and nits; (b) Amblyomma species found attached on the axillary region of a cross bred cattle, look the hyperemia around the attachment sites (arrow).

by Yacob et al. (2008) and Regasa and Abebe (2008), who reported 3.94 and 5.13%, respectively. As previously reported (Regasa and Abebe, 2008; Yacob et al., 2008), no significant sexual predisposition was noted (p>0.05) in the prevalence of lice infestation. Usually mild cases are not considered as, being having any pathogenic effect, but heavy infestations are associated with extensive hide damage and blood loss (Urqhart et al., 1996). All age groups of cattle can be infested with lice, but the heaviest infestations are usually seen on calves, yearlings or in older unthrifty animal. In line with these, young animals were frequently affected (OR=4.77, 95% CI=2.27,10.04) than older animals, this is perhaps because they possess a higher ratio of accessible surface to body volume, inefficient grooming behavior and other defense capabilities (Urqhart et al., 1996; Zewdu et al., 2015). Besides, 2 cases of mange (Demodectic and Sarcoptic, one case each) were also observed in this study. The prevalence of mange (0.3%) obtained in this study was in agreement with previous report made by Regasa and Abebe (2008).

Among all skin diseases encountered in this study, wart was the fourth main skin disease with prevalence of 4.4%. In the present study, the prevalence of the disease was significantly higher (p<0.01, OR=24.72, 95% CI=5.69, 107.34) in animals less than two years of age (9.8%) than the older age group (0.5%). This is because, most virus-induced papilomas are self-limiting and are usually found in young animals (Goldschmidt and Hendrick, 2002), which develop good immunity afterwards.

The prevalence of lumpy skin disease in the current study (0.6%, 4 cases) was lower than the report of Ayelet et al. (2014) and Gari et al. (2010), who reported a prevalence of 13.61% in central Ethiopia (Mojo, Adama, Welenchiti and Wenji) and 8.1% in different agro-climatic zones of Ethiopia, respectively. This difference could be associated with the variation in agro-climatic condition, season and vector population during the study periods. A 6 years retrospective data collected and analyzed by Ayelet et al. (2014) suggest that, outbreaks of lumpy skin disease frequently occur between September and December than in November to June, the period at which the current study was conducted.

In the current study, the prevalence of dermatophilosis was 0.2%. Comparable prevalence ranging from 0.0 to 4.8%, were reported in zebu cattle in different part of the country (Berhanu and Woldemeskel, 1999; Woldemeskel, 2000; Yacob et al., 2008; Meseret and Sefinew, 2011; Teshome and Derso, 2015). This low prevalence could be due to the fact that, the pathogen may not yet established its spore in the premises or the animals were less exposed to the possible predisposing factors such as ticks, insects, thorny bushes, ox-pecker birds, rain, etc. Owing to the difficulty of control and eradication of established dermatophilosis, the current prevalence should not be underestimated. Because of budget and time limitations, this study were conducted mainly during the dry period, hence we couldn't see the effect of season on the prevalence of the different skin diseases including dermatophilosis.

Conclusion

In the study area, different skin diseases were prevalent and among the major diseases affecting cattle production. Compared to the clinical physical examination, assessment at wet blue stage in the tanneries would have indicated more problem/defects that can't be detected while the animal is still alive. The higher prevalence of dermatological problems in

Table 2. Prevalence of different skin diseases in cattle and their variation among/between the categories of the considered risk factors (n=662).

Risk factors		№ of cattle Examined	Ringworm %(№)	Lice %(№)	Ticks %(№)	Dermatophilosis %(№)	Wart %(№)	Mange %(№)	LSD %(№)	Overall %(№)
Sex	Male	213	7(17)	6.6(14)	5.2(11)	0(0)	4.2(9)	0(0)	0.9(2)	23.5(50)
	Female	449	5.3(24)	5.8(26)	5.3(24)	0.2(1)	4.5(20)	0.4(2)	0.4(2)	21.4(96)
Age	Young	275	12.4(34)**	10.9(30)**	6.2(17)	0(0)	9.8(27)**	0.7(2)	0.4(1)	38.5(106)**
	Adult	387	1.8(7)	2.6(10)	4.7(18)	0.3(1)	0.5(2)	0(0)	0.5(3)	10.3(40)
Management	Poor	513	7(36)	7.8(40)**	5.8(30)	0.2(1)	3.1(16)**	0.4(2)	0.4(2)	23.6 (121)
	Medium	149	3.4(5)	0(0)	3.3(5)	0(0)	8.7(13)	0(0)	1.3(2)	16.8(25)
Origin	Chefe	405	6.9(28)	9.1(37)**	6.9(28)	0.2(1)	0.9(4)**	0.5(2)	0.5(2)	24.4(99)
	Dato	50	6(3)	6(3)	4(2)	0(0)	0(0)	0(0)	0(0)	16.0(8)
	Hawassa	207	4.8(10)	0(0)	2.4(5)	0(0)	12.1(25)	0(0)	0.9(2)	18.8(39)

*Statistically significant ($p<0.05$), ** statistically highly significant ($p<0.01$), LSD= Lumpy Skin Disease.

young animals warrant special attentions in the implementation of feasible control and prevention measures at young age categories even before animals reach the age of slaughter.

In general, unless feasible control measures are timely implemented the encountered skin diseases can have varied and adverse effect on the cattle production, tanning industry and health of the public and concomitantly pose huge economic loss. To design appropriate control strategy, further studies should be carried out on the seasonal occurrence and socio-economic impacts of these diseases, on large sample size and wider study sites. Moreover, regular application of acaricides and timely treatment of clinical infectious cases were suggested to reduce further impact.

CONFLICT OF INTERESTS

The authors have not declared any conflict of interests.

REFERENCES

Abebayehu T, Endris F, Berhanu M, Endrias, Z (2011). Study on the prevalence of ectoparasite infestation of ruminants in and around Kombolcha and damage to fresh goat pelts and wet blue (pickled) skin at Kombolch Tannery, Northeastern Ethiopia. Ethiop. Vet. J. 15(2):87-101.

Abu-Samra MT, Shuaib YA (2014). A study on the nature of association between demodex mites and bacteria involved in skin and meibomian gland lesions of demodectic mange in cattle. Vet. Med. Int. 2014:413719.

Ayele S, Assegid W, Jabbar MA, Ahmed MM, Belachew H (2003). Livestock marketing in Ethiopia: A review of structure, performance and development initiatives. Socio-economic and Policy Research Working Paper 52, ILRI (International Livestock Research Institute), Nairobi, Kenya. P 35.

Ayelet G, Haftu R, Jemberie S, Belay A, Gelaye E, Sibhat B, Skjerve E, Asmare K (2014). Lumpy skin disease in cattle in central Ethiopia: outbreak investigation and isolation and molecular detection of the virus. Rev. Sci. Tech. Off. Int. Epiz. 33(3):877-887.

Berhanu D, Woldemeskel M (1999). Bovine dermatophilosis and its influencing factors in central Ethiopia. Transbound. Emerg. Dis. 46(10):593-597.

Bradford P (1996). Large animal internal Medicine, 2nd edition, St. Louis, Mosby year book Inc, USA.

Chalachew N (2001). Study on skin diseases in cattle, sheep and goat in and around Wolayita Soddo, Southern Ethiopia, DVM thesis, AAU-FVM, Debre Zeit, Ethiopia.

Central Statistical Agency (CSA) (2017). Agricultural Sample Survey 2016/17. Federal Democratic Republic of Ethiopia Central Statistical Agency. Volume II, Report on Livestock and Livestock Characteristics, Statistical bulletin 585, Addis Ababa, Ethiopia.

Gari G, Waret-Szkuta A, Grosbois V, Jacquie P, Roger F (2010). Risk factors associated with observed clinical lumpy skin disease in Ethiopia. Epidemiol. Infect. 138:1657-1666.

Goldschmidt MH, Hendrick MJ (2002). Tumors of the skin and soft tissues. In: Meuten DJ (ed) Tumors in Domestic Animals, 4th edition, Iowa State Press, A Blackwell Publishing Company. pp. 45-70.

Greiner E (2012). Diagnosis of arthropod parasites. In: Zajac AM, Conboy GA (Eds) Veterinary clinical parasitology, 8th edition, John Wiley & Sons, Inc. pp. 217-219.

Hoogstral H (1956). Africa Ixoid ticks of Sudan with special reference to equatorial province and preliminary reviews of the genera Boophilus, Margaropus and Hyalomma species, Washington D.C. Department of Navy, Bureau of medicine and surgery. pp. 263-266.

Kahn CM, Line S, Aiello SE (2005). Merck Veterinary Manual. National Publishing Inc., Philadelphia, pp. 1233-1235.
Kassa B, Bisrat M, Asegedech S, Africa J (1998). Control of "Ekeke" skin defects in sheep by insecticides and shearing, EVA proceeding 12th annual conference, Addis Ababa, Ethiopia. pp.104-109.
Kassaye E, Moser I, Woldemeskel M (2003). Epidemiological study on clinical bovine dermatophilosis in northern Ethiopia. DTW. Deutsche tierarztliche Wochenschrift 110(10):422-425.
McDaniel CJ, Cardwell DM, Moeller RBJr, Gray GC (2014). Humans and Cattle: A Review of Bovine Zoonoses. Vector-Borne Zoonotic Dis. 14(1):1-19.
Mekonnen S, Hussein I, Bedane B (2001). The distribution of Ixodid ticks (Acari: Iodidae) in central Ethiopia. Odnderstepoort J. Vet. Res. 68:243- 51.
Meseret A, Sefinew A (2011). Study on clinical bovine dermatophilosis and its potential risk factors in North Western Ethiopia. Int. J. Anim. Vet. Adv. 3(1):33-36.
Muylle S (2016). Estimation of age by examination of the teeth. In: Allen DG, Constable PD, Dart A, Davies PR, Quesenberry KE, Reeves PT, Sharma JM (Eds). The Merck Veterinary Manual, 11th edition, Merck Sharp & Dohme Corp., a subsidiary of Merck & Co., Inc., Kenilworth, NJ, USA. Available at: https://www.merckbooks.com/mvm/pdf/title.pdf
Quinn PJ, Markey BK, Carter ME, Donnelly WJC, Leonard FC (2002). Veterinary Microbiology and Bacterial Disease. Black Well Science, London. P 381.
Quinn PJ, Markey BK, Leonard FC, Hartigan P, Fanning S, Fitzpatrick ES (2011). Veterinary Microbiology and Microbial Disease, 2nd edition,Wiley-Blackwell, UK.
Radostits OM, Gay CC, Blood DC, Hinchcliff KW (2000). Veterinary Medicine. A textbook of diseases of cattle, sheep, pigs, goats and horses, 9th edition, Harcourt publishers limited, London Philadelphia. pp. 701-967, 1476-1478.
Regasa C, Abebe W (2008). Major skin diseases of cattle coming to Nekemte Veterinary Clinic, Western Ethiopia. DVM Thesis, Faculty of Veterinary Medicine, Addis Ababa University, Debre Zeit, Ethiopia, 2003.
Salih DA, El Hussein AM, Singla LD (2015) Diagnostic approaches for tick-borne haemoparasitic diseases in livestock. J. Vet. Med. Anim.Health 7(2):45-56.
Scott DW (2007). Color atlas of farm animal dermatology, 1st edition, Blackwell Publishing Professional, 2121 State Avenue, Ames, Iowa 50014, USA.
Teshome D, Derso S (2015). Prevalence of major skin diseases in ruminants and its associated risk factors at university of Gondar Veterinary Clinic, North West Ethiopia. J.Vet. Sci. Technol. S:S13-002.
Urquhart GM, Armour J, Duncan JL, Dunn AM, Jennings FW (1996). Veterinary parasitology, 2nd edition, Blackwell publisher, UK.
Walker AR, Bouattour A, Camics JL, Estradopena A, Horak IG, Latif AA, Pegram RG, Preston PN (2003). Ticks of Domestics Animals in Africa; a Guide to Identification of species, Bioscience reports, Scotland, U.K. pp.1-27.
Weitzman I, Summerbell RC (1995). The dermatophytes. Clin. Microbiol. Rev. 8(2):240-259.
Woldemeskel M (2000). Dermatophilosis: A threat to livestock production in Ethiopia. DTW. Deutsche tierarztliche Wochenschrift 107(4):144-146.
Woldemeskel M, Taye G (2002). Prevalence of bovine dermatophilosis in a tropical highland region of Ethiopia. Trop. Anim. Health Prod. 34:189-194.
Wondwossen A (2000). Sheep and goat skin diseases control initiatives in Amhara region. Ethiopian veterinary epidemiology newsletter. pp. 1-9.
Yacob HT, Nesanet B, Dinka A (2008). Prevalence of major skin diseases in cattle, sheep and goats at Adama Veterinary Clinic, Oromia regional state, Ethiopia. Revue Méd. Vét.159(8-9):455-461.
Zewdu S, Tsegaye T, Agerie A (2015). Ectoparasites prevalence in small ruminants in and around Sekela, Amhara Regional State, Northwest Ethiopia. Hindawi Publishing Corporation. J. Vet. Med. 2015:216085.

14

Serological prevalence of *Babesia caballi* and *Theileria equi* in camels and donkeys from Karamoja sub-region, North-eastern Uganda

Jesca Nakayima[1]*, Mary L. Nanfuka[2], Daniel Aleper[1] and Duke Okidi[1]

[1]National Livestock Resources Research Institute (NaLIRRI), P. O. Box 96 Tororo, Uganda.
[2]National Animal Disease Diagnostics and Epidemiology Centre (NADDEC). P. O. Box 513, Entebbe, Uganda.

Equine piroplasmosis is a severe disease of horses caused by the intra-erythrocyte protozoan, *Theileria equi* and *Babesia caballi*. *T. equi* and *B. caballi* infections were assessed in serum from camels and donkeys using competitive- enzyme-linked immunosorbent assay (cELISA) assay. A total 110 animals were studied including 25 donkeys and 85 camels from two districts viz. Moroto and Amudat in Karamoja sub-region, North-eastern Uganda. All the (100%) donkeys tested were positive for *Babesia/T. equi* while none of the camels had been exposed to the infection. All animals were negative to *B. caballi* cELISA. Our findings indicated that all donkeys sampled in Karamoja sub-region have been exposed to *T. equi* and this could be prevalent in equine population in Uganda. No exposure status to *B. caballi* was reported. This study represents the first report on the status of *T. equi* and *B. caballi* infection in Uganda.

Key words: Donkey, Camel, *Theileria equi*, *Babesia caballi*, Seroprevalence, cELISA, Uganda.

INTRODUCTION

Equine piroplasmosis (EP) is a tick-borne disease of horses caused by apicomplexan hemoprotozoan parasites *Theileria equi* and *Babesia caballi* of the order Piroplasmida (Wise *et al*., 2013; Scoles and Ueti, 2015; Sumbria *et al*., 2017). The nomenclature was changed from *B. equi* to *T. equi* based on evolutionary, morphologic, biochemical, and genetic evidence (Singla and Sumbria, 2017). The disease is also called biliary fever and affects all equid species including Horses, donkeys, mules and zebras (Friedhoff *et al*., 1990; Schein, 1988). Several genera of tick species including *Hyalomma*, *Rhipicephalus* and *Dermacentor* transmit both these parasites (De Waal, 1992; Sumbria *et al*., 2016a). Clinical signs include fever, anemia, icterus, hepatomegaly, edema, intra-vascular hemolysis, hemoglobinuria and even death (Schein, 1988; Uilenberg, 2006). The disease is distributed in tropical and sub-tropical areas including some temperate zones (Shkap *et al*., 1998; Steinman *et al*., 2012). The equine disease has a worldwide economic importance especially

*Corresponding author. E-mail: jescanl2001@yahoo.co.uk .

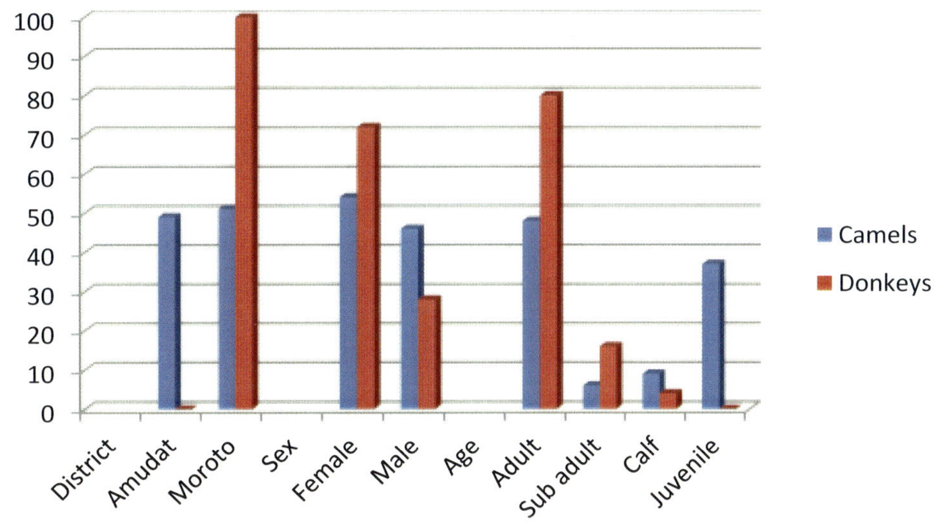

Figure 1. Demographic characteristics of sampled animals.

concerning international movement of horses because carrier horses and infected ticks can be introduced into disease-free countries (Friedhoff *et al.*, 1990; Sumbria *et al.*, 2016b). The vectors of *T. equi* and *B. caballi* are the same (Abedi *et al.*, 2014) although *T. equi* is more virulent than *B. caballi* (Friedhoff *et al.*, 1990; Mehlhorn and Schein, 1998; Posnett *et al.*, 1991). In endemic countries, mixed infections occur (Scoles and Ueti, 2015). Diagnosis depends on clinical observation especially in the acute phase of the disease and is confirmed by microscopic detection of intra-erythrocyte parasites in Giemsa-stained blood smears (Shkap *et al.*, 1998). However, the latent phase of the infection is characterized by low parasiteamia (Kumar *et al.*, 2008; Sumbria *et al.*, 2015) hence the need for more sensitive diagnostics like enzyme-linked immunosorbent assay (ELISA) and polymerase chain reaction (PCR) (Friedhoff and Soule, 1996; Moretti *et al.*, 2010; Alsaad *et al.*, 2012). Ponies, mules and donkeys act as natural reservoirs for disease transmission to the horses (Radostitis *et al.*, 2008).

In Uganda, camels and donkeys are kept in Karamoja and Sebei sub-regions, North-eastern Uganda. They are kept by peasant farmers, pastoralists in this semi-arid region. They are kept for meat, milk, dowry, prestige, and carriage. These animals receive little or no veterinary care. Nakayima *et al.,* (2017) detected helminth parasitosis in these animals in the absence of veterinary intervention. No studies have been undertaken on equine piroplasmosis in Uganda. Therefore, the aims of this work were to determine the infection rate of EP in donkeys and possibly in camels given the fact that they occupy the same ecological setting and could therefore act as accidental hosts. Information from this study will help update current knowledge on the health of camels and donkeys in Uganda for their improved production and productivity.

MATERIALS AND METHODS

Serum samples were collected from Karamoja sub-region in two districts namely: Moroto: N 2° 31' 41.604", E 34° 39' 28.794" and Amudat: N 1° 47' 29.841", E 34° 54' 23.583" districts, Uganda. The study was conducted in March 2016. The camels and donkeys were classified as: Infant, juvenile, sub-adult and adult. Both sexes were sampled (Tables 1 and 2 and Figure 1). Blood was collected from the jugular vein of both camels and donkeys following restraint. 5 ml of blood was collected, 2.5 ml blood was put in anticoagulant ethylene diamine tetra acetic acid (EDTA) vaccutainers for parasitological and DNA analysis while 2.5 ml blood was put in serum tubes. The serum was collected into plain vaccutainer tubes without anticoagulant, serum was separated from blood cells by centrifugation at 2500 rpm for 15 min and stored at -20°C until use in a competitive-ELISA (cELISA) (Kouam et al., 2010) for both *T. equi* and *B. caballi*. The total number of donkeys was 25, while camels were 85 giving a total of 110 animal samples collected. The sample size determination was based on purposive sampling based on the availability of the animals. The age and sex were recorded for each animal. The samples were transferred to the laboratory and stored at -20°C until use. The serum from clinically healthy animals was examined for *T. equi* and *B. caballi* antibodies by two separate cELISA.

ELISA

Commercial cELISA kits were used to analyze sera from donkeys and camels for the presence of antibodies to *T. equi* and *B. caballi* as described by the manufacturer (VMRD Inc., Pullman, WA, USA). The cut-off values for positive infections was 40% of inhibition for both tests, as indicated by the manufacturer (VMRD Inc., Pullman, WA, USA) (Shkap *et al.*, 1998; Kappmeyer *et al.*,1999). Thus samples with %I above 40 are considered as positive, and below 40, considered as negative. The results were expressed as a value of the percent inhibition (%I) according to the following formula:

(%I): %I = 100- {(sample O.D. × 100) / (mean negative control O.D.)}

Microscopic detection of hemoprotozoal parasites depends on morphological and biometrical parameters including the shape, site

Table 1. Infection of camels (Total = 85; all negative for both infections).

Category	Frequency	%
District		
Amudat	42	49
Moroto	43	51
Sex		
Female	46	54
Male	39	46
Age		
Adult	41	48
Sub adult	5	6
Calf	8	9
Juvenile	31	37

Table 2. Infection of donkeys (n=25) (All affected with *Theileria equi,* all negative for *Babesia caballi).*

Category	Frequency	%
District		
Amudat	0	0
Moroto	25	100
Sex		
Female	18	72
Male	7	28
Age		
Adult	20	80
Sub adult	4	16
Calf	1	4
Juvenile	0	0

location and size of parasite in an infected erythrocyte in Giemsa-stained blood smears (Sadeghi Dehkordi *et al.*, 2010). Morphological detection of the parasites could be described as single round, double round, single pyriform and double pyriform with obtuse or acute angle. Microscopically, *B. caballi* is a larger paired pyriform parasite, while *T. equi is a* smaller paired pyriform, rounded and tetrad or Maltese cross arrangement of merozoites (Kuttler, 1988; Levine, 1971).

Statistical analysis

Data were analyzed using SPSS (Version 16). A value of $p < 0.05$ was considered as statistically significant.

RESULTS

110 samples were analyzed with 25 donkeys and 85 camels. All donkeys were positive for *T. equi*. Donkey no. 22 was not done, the sample had dried out. All camels were negative for *Babesia/ T. equi* ELISA. Corrected ODs were calculated from sample ODs and blank ODs (Table 3). Sample Id represents animal species, age, sex and sample number.

All the serum samples from donkeys and camels were negative to *Babesia caballi* Competitive-ELISA. This suggests no history of exposure to this parasite. 110 samples were analyzed with 25 donkeys and 85 camels. Donkey no. 22 was not done, the sample had dried out. Corrected ODs were calculated from sample ODs and blank ODs (Table 4). Sample Id represents animal species, age, sex and sample number.

DISCUSSION

Diagnosis of piroplasmosis can be achieved by clinical observation and confirmed by microscopy (Irwin, 2010). However, given the low sensitivity of parasitological diagnosis, there is need to combine parasitological diagnosis with molecular diagnostics (Abedi *et al.*, 2014; Salib *et al.*, 2013; Baptista *et al.*, 2013; Rosales *et al.*, 2013).

Camels were sampled alongside donkeys. Much as camels are not equines, they could serve as accidental hosts or reservoirs of the parasites since they are in the same ecological setting. However, all camels tested negative to *B. equi* cELISA (Table 3). The serological prevalence of *B. equi* cELISA was 100% in donkeys and 0% in camels (Table 3). Apparently, equine piroplasmids are enzootic in Uganda and their distribution pattern is likely affected by the presence and densities of suitable hosts rather than by ecological conditions. There is a significant correlation between host species and age with the distribution of EP. Horses are more susceptible to the infection than donkeys. Adult animals have a higher risk of infection. All the serum samples from camels and donkeys tested negative to *B. caballi* cELISA (Table 4). This suggests no history of exposure of these animals to this parasite or the fact that the infection is cleared in 1 to 4 years. All the 25 donkey serum samples (100%) were found positive for *T. equi* antibodies (Table 3), *B. caballi* was not detected in the study area (Table 4) while all the 85 camels tested negative to equine piroplasmosis (Tables 3 and 4). A study of equine piroplasmosis in horses in Sudan by Salim *et al.* (2008) recorded 100% prevalence of *T. equi* in Khartoum North (100%) and Atbara (100%); a low prevalence for *B. caballi* was reported and 0% prevalence was detected in Khartoum, Khartoum North, and Kosti areas. The infection rate of EP varies in different countries. Several factors account for this namely: disease management practices, tick vector abundance and climate. Climatic factors influence the habitat of tick vectors like rainfall, humidity and temperature (Oncel *et al.*, 2007). In endemic countries, equines adopt to infection possibly because of the phenomenon of endemic stability. However, stress and immune-suppression could revert otherwise sub-clinical infection to overt disease. *T. equi* infection results into life-long carrier status (Brüning, 1996) while *B. caballi* could persist in subclinical form for at least 1 to 4 years

Table 3. *Babesia / Theileria equi* competitive-ELISA of camel and donkey serum.

S/N	Animal species	Sample ID	Corrected Ods	% Inihibition (%I)	Sample status
1	Donkey	D/A/M/01	0.262	75.40	Positive
2	Donkey	D/A/F/02	0.209	80.38	Positive
3	Donkey	D/SA/F/03	0.159	85.07	Positive
4	Donkey	D/A/F/04	0.218	79.53	Positive
5	Donkey	D/A/F/05	0.196	81.60	Positive
6	Donkey	D/A/F/06	0.395	62.91	Positive
7	Donkey	D/A/F/07	0.252	76.34	Positive
8	Donkey	D/A/F/08	0.572	46.29	Positive
9	Donkey	D/A/F/09	0.275	74.18	Positive
10	Donkey	D/A/M/10	0.173	83.76	Positive
11	Donkey	D/A/M/11	0.167	84.32	Positive
12	Donkey	D/A/F/12	0.291	72.68	Positive
13	Donkey	D/A/F/13	0.244	77.09	Positive
14	Donkey	D/A/F/14	0.232	78.22	Positive
15	Donkey	D/A/M/15	0.159	85.07	Positive
16	Donkey	D/A/M/16	0.147	86.20	Positive
17	Donkey	D/A/F/17	0.247	76.81	Positive
18	Donkey	D/A/F/18	0.241	77.37	Positive
19	Donkey	D/A/M/19	0.17	84.04	Positive
20	Donkey	D/SA/F/20	0.483	54.65	Positive
21	Donkey	D/SA/F/21	0.606	43.10	Positive
23	Donkey	D/A/F/54	0.48	54.93	Positive
24	Donkey	D/A/F/55	0.298	72.02	Positive
25	Donkey	D/SA/F/56	0.507	52.39	Positive
26	Donkey	D/C/M/57	0.328	69.20	Positive

110 samples were analyzed with 25 donkeys and 85 camels. All donkeys were positive for *T. equi*. Donkey no. 22 was not done, the sample had dried out. All camels were negative for *Babesia/ T. equi* ELISA. Corrected ODs were calculated from sample ODs and blank ODs. Sample Id represents animal species, age, sex and sample number.

before being eliminated. This could be attributed to the fact that *T. equi* parasites are not completely eliminated from the blood of equines after treatment or natural recovery (de Waal and van Heerden 1994) as compared to *B. caballi*. Therefore, failure to detect *B. caballi* by ELISA is most probably due to the parasites clearance from the circulating blood by the host or reduction to a level beyond the detection of the host immune response or the diagnostic test. There was a significant difference between donkeys and camels with respect to the seroprevalence of *T. equi* and *B. caballi* ($P<0.05$).

Treatment strategy for piroplasmosis in equines depends on the endemic status of the country. So it is either parasite elimination in disease free countries or resolution of clinical disease in endemic countries. It is not recommended to eliminate the parasite from equids in endemic countries because the animals need endemic stability due to constant exposure to the parasite at low levels (Donnellan and Marais, 2009). Several drugs can be used to treat EP. Generally, *B. equi* has been reported to be more refractory to babesiacidal drugs than *B. caballi*. More common drugs include imidocarb and diminazene. However, donkeys are more susceptible to imidocarb toxicity than horses (Donnellan and Marais, 2009). Imidocarb causes a dose-dependent hepatotoxicity and nephrotoxicity (Donnellan and Marais, 2009). Other drugs could include artesunate, arteether, buparvaquone. Equine piroplasmosis is endemic in Karamoja sub-region and possibly Uganda at large due to the distribution of equine species and the tick vectors.

Conclusion

All donkeys tested positive to *Babesia / T. equi* cELISA while all camels were negative. This exposure status indicates that this piroplasm could be endemic in Karamoja sub-region and in the equine population in Uganda in the absence of veterinary intervention. No exposure status to *B. caballi* was reported. Camels are not accidental hosts or reservoirs of equine piroplasmosis. The results of this study will help inform policy on the improvement of the health and welfare of these animals through veterinary intervention. To our knowledge, this is the first report on epidemiology of

Table 4. *B. caballi* competitive-ELISA of camel and donkey serum.

No.	Animal species	Sample ID	Corrected Ods	% Inihibition (%I)	Sample status
1	Donkey	D/A/M/01	1.115	-2.6	Negative
2	Donkey	D/A/F/02	1.257	-15.7	Negative
3	Donkey	D/SA/F/03	1.292	-18.9	Negative
4	Donkey	D/A/F/04	1.055	2.9	Negative
5	Donkey	D/A/F/05	1.168	-7.5	Negative
6	Donkey	D/A/F/06	1.175	-8.1	Negative
7	Donkey	D/A/F/07	1.138	-4.7	Negative
8	Donkey	D/A/F/08	1.08	0.6	Negative
9	Donkey	D/A/F/09	1.114	-2.5	Negative
10	Donkey	D/A/M/10	1.263	-16.2	Negative
11	Donkey	D/A/M/11	1.248	-14.8	Negative
12	Donkey	D/A/F/12	1.15	-5.8	Negative
13	Donkey	D/A/F/13	1.055	2.9	Negative
14	Donkey	D/A/F/14	1.127	-3.7	Negative
15	Donkey	D/A/M/15	1.181	-8.7	Negative
16	Donkey	D/A/M/16	1.151	-5.9	Negative
17	Donkey	D/A/F/17	1.044	3.9	Negative
18	Donkey	D/A/F/18	1.185	-9.0	Negative
19	Donkey	D/A/M/19	1.27	-16.9	Negative
20	Donkey	D/SA/F/20	1.174	-8.0	Negative
21	Donkey	D/SA/F/21	1.076	1.0	Negative
23	Donkey	D/A/F/54	1.098	-1.0	Negative
24	Donkey	D/A/F/55	1.141	-5.0	Negative
25	Donkey	D/SA/F/56	1.151	-5.9	Negative
26	Donkey	D/C/M/57	1.136	-4.5	Negative

All the serum samples from donkeys and camels were negative to *Babesia caballi* Competitive-ELISA. This suggests no history of exposure to this parasite. 110 samples were analyzed with 25 donkeys and 85 camels. Donkey no. 22 was not done, the sample had dried out. Corrected ODs were calculated from sample ODs and blank ODs. Sample Id represents animal species, age, sex and sample number.

equine piroplasms in Uganda. Molecular studies for accurate diagnosis of equine piroplasmosis are essential for providing baseline information about its epidemiology, distribution, and prevalence in the affected equine population and for effective control measures.

ACKNOWLEDGEMENT

This study was financially supported by the Government of Uganda under National Agricultural Research Organization (NARO).

REFERENCES

Abedi V, Razmi G, Seifi H, Naghibi A (2014). Molecular and serological detection of *Theileria equi* and *Babesia caballi* infection in horses and ixodid ticks in Iran. Ticks Tick Borne Dis. 5:239-244.

Alsaad KM, Hassan SD, Al-Obaidi QT (2012). Detection of *Babesia equi* and *Babesia caballi* antibodies in horses and donkeys in Mosul, Iraq. Res. Opinions Anim. Vet. Sci. 2(4):291-294.

Baptista C, Lopes MS, Tavares AC, Rojer H, Kappmeyer L, Mendonça D, Machado AC (2013). Diagnosis of *Theileria equi* infections in horses in the Azores using cELISA and nested PCR. Ticks Tick Borne Dis. 4:242-245.

Brüning A (1996) Equine piroplasmosis an update on diagnosis, treatment and prevention. Br. Vet. J. 152:139-151.

De Waal DT (1992). Equine piroplasmosis: a review. Br. Vet. J. 148:6-14.

De Waal DT, van Heerden J (1994) Equine babesiosis. In: Coetzer JAW, Thomson GR, Tustin RC (eds) Infectious diseases of livestock with special reference to South Africa. vol. 1. Oxford University Press, Cape Town, South Africa. pp. 293-304.

Donnellan CMB, Marais HJ (2009). Equine piroplasmosis.In Infectious Diseases of the Horse, ed. Mair TS, Hutchinson RE, Equine Vet. J. 333-340.

Friedhoff KT, Soule C (1996). An account on equine babesiosis. Rev. Sci. Off. Int. Epiz.15:1191-1201.

Friedhoff KT, Tenter AM, Muller I (1990). Haemoparasites of equines: Impact on international trade of horses. Rev. Sci. Tech. 9:1187-1194.

Irwin PJ (2010). Canine babesiosis. Vet. Clin. North Am. Small Anim. Pract. 40(6):1141-1156.

Kappmeyer LS, Perryman LE, Hines SA, Baszler TV, Katz JB, Hennager SG, Knowles DP (1999). Detection of equine antibodies to Babesia caballi by recombinant B. caballi rhoptry-associated protein 1 in a competitive-inhibition enzyme-linked immunosorbent assay. J.

Clin. Microbiol. 37(7): 2285-2290.

Kouam MK, Kantzoura V, Gajadhar AA, Theis JH, Papadopoulos E, Theodoropoulos G (2010). Seroprevalence of equine piroplasms and host-related factors associated with infection in Greece. Vet. Parasitol. 169: 273-278.

Kumar S, Kumar R, Gupta AK, Dwivedi SK (2008). Passive transfer of Theileria equi antibodies to neonate foals of immune tolerant mares. Vet. Parasitol. 151:80-85.

Kuttler KL (1988). Chemotherapy of babesiosis. In: Ristic M, (Eds.). Babesiosis of domestic animals and man. Boca Raton, USA; CRS Press. 227-243.

Levine ND (1971). Taxonomy of the piroplasms. Trans. Am. Microsc. Soc. 90(1):2-33.

Mehlhorn H, Schein E (1998). Redescription of *Babesia equi* Laveran, 1901 as *Theileria equi*. Parasitol. Res. 84:467-475.

Moretti A, Mangili A, Salvatori R, Maresca C, Scoccia E, Torina A, Moretta I, Gabrielli S, Tampieri MP, Pietrobelli M (2010). Prevalence and diagnosis of Babesia and Theileria infections horses in Italy: A preliminary study. Vet. J.184:346-350.

Nakayima J, Kabasa W, AleperD, Okidi D (2017).Prevalence of endo-parasites in donkeys and camels in Karamoja sub-region, North-eastern Uganda. J. Vet. Med. Anim. Health 9(1):11-15.

Oncel T, Vural G, Gicik Y, Arslan MO (2007).Detection of *Babesia (Theileria) equi* (Laveran, 1901) in horses in the Kars Province of Turkey. Türkiye Parazitoloji Dergisi 31(3):170-172.

Posnett ES, Fehrsen J, de Waal DT, Ambrosio RE (1991). Detection of *Babesia equi* infected horses and carrier animals using a DNA probe. J. Vet. Parasitol. 39:19-32.

Rosales R, Rangel-Rivas A, Escalona A, Jordan LS, Gonzatti MI, Aso PM, Perrone T, Silva-Iturriza A, Mijares A (2013). Detection of *Theileria equi* and *Babesia caballi* infections in Venezuelan horses using Competitive-Inhibition ELISA and PCR. Vet.Parasitol.196:37-43.

SadeghiDehkordi Z, Zakeri S, Nabian S, Bahonar A, Ghasemi F, Noorollahi F, Rahbari S (2010). Molecular and biomorphometrical identification of ovine babesiosis in Iran. Iranian J.Parasitol. 5(4):21-30.

Salib FA, Youssef RR, Rizk LG, Said SF (2013). Epidemiology, diagnosis and therapy of *Theileriaequi* infection in Giza, Egypt. Vet. World 6(2):76-82.

Salim B, Hassan SM, Bakheit MA, Alhassan A, Igarashi I, Karanis P, Abdelrahman MB (2008). Diagnosis of *Babesia caballi* and *Theileria equi* infections in horses in Sudan using ELISA and PCR. Parasitol. Res.103: 1145-1150

Schein E (1988). Equine babesiosis. In: Ristic M. (Eds.). Babesiosis of Domestic Animals and Man. Boca Raton, USA; CRS Press. pp.197-208.

Scoles GA, Ueti MW (2015). Vector ecology of equine piroplasmosis. Annu. Rev. Entomol; 60:561-580.

Shkap V, Cohen I, Leibovitz B, Savitsky, Pipano E, Avni G, Shofer S, Giger U, Kappmeyer L Knowles D (1998). Seroprevalence of *Babesiaequi* among horses in Israel using competitive inhibition ELISA and IFA assays. Vet. Parasitol. 76:251-259.

Singla LD, Sumbria D (2017). Equine piroplasmosis: Belles-lettres update with special reference to Indian scenario. In: *An Update on Diagnosis and Control of Parasitic Diseases,* Ananda KJ, Pradeep BS, Rakesh RL and Malatesh DS (Eds), Department of Veterinary Parasitology, Veterinary College, Shimoga, KVAFSU,Bidar, Karnataka, India. pp. 372-400.

Steinman A, Zimmerman T, Klement E, Lensky IM, Berlin D, Gottlieb Y, Baneth G (2012). Demographic and environmental risk factors for infection by *Theileria equi* in 590 horses in Israel. Vet Parasitol.187:558-562.

Sumbria D, Singla LD, Kumar S, Sharma A, Dhayia R, Setia RK (2016). Spatial distribution, risk factors and haematobiochemical alterations associated with *Theileria equi* infected equines of Punjab diagnosed by indirect ELISA and nested PCR. Acta Trop.155:104-112.

Sumbria D, Singla LD, Mandhotra A, Randhawa CS (2015).Molecular Detection and Treatment of Equine Piroplasmosis. Philippine J. Vet. Med. 52(2):131-136.

Sumbria D, Singla LD, Sharma A (2016). *Theileria equi* and *Babesia caballi* infection of equids in Punjab, India: a serological and molecular survey. Trop. Anim. Health. Prod. 48(1):45-52.

Sumbria D, Singla LD, Sharma A, Bal MS, Randhawa CS (2017). Molecular survey in relation to risk factors and haemato-biochemical alteration in *Theileria equi* infection of equines in Punjab Province, India. Vet. Parasitol. Reg. Stud. Rep. 8:43-50.

Uilenberg G (2006). Babesia-a historical overview. Vet.Parasitol.138(1-2):3-10.

Wise LN, Kappmeyer LS, Mealey RH, Knowles DP (2013). Review of equine piroplasmosis. J. Vet. Intern. Med. 27(6):1334-1346.

15

Bursa body index as a visual indicator for the assessment of bursa of Fabricius

A. A. Raji[1]*, B. Mohammed[2], S. B. Oladele[2], L. Saidu[3], A. H. Jibril[4] and C. Cazaban[5]

[1]Department of Veterinary Pathology, Faculty of Veterinary Medicine, Usmanu Danfodiyo University, Sokoto, Nigeria.
[2]Department of Veterinary Pathology, Faculty of Veterinary Medicine, Ahmadu Bello University, Zaria, Nigeria.
[3]Veterinary Teaching Hospital, Ahmadu Bello University, Zaria, Nigeria.
[4]Department of Veterinary Physiology, Faculty of Veterinary Medicine, Usmanu Danfodiyo University, Sokoto, Nigeria.
[5]Innovation Strategy Department, Ceva Santé Animale, France.

The objective of the present study was to identify the significance of the Bursal-Body index (BB index) as a tool in assessing the health status of a chicken flock especially those under experimental condition. With the unending debate on the bursa of Fabricius as a diagnostic tool, a total of 135 day-of-hatch Dominant black Cockerel hybrid were housed in six separate houses with positive pressure and filtered airflow. Houses were assigned to the three vaccines (two intermediate (A, and C), and one intermediate plus (B) vaccine strain), a challenge group (D) and control group (E). The birds were vaccinated according to manufacturer's directives on day 17th post hatch; challenge group was inoculated with 0.05 ml of very-virulent isolate of the infectious bursal disease virus (vvIBDV) on the same day. On day(s) 1, 2, 3, 4, 5, 7, 10, 14 and 21 post vaccination/challenge (Dpv/c) three birds were humanely sacrificed from each group with Bursal-Body ratio (BB ratio) and Bursal-Body index (BB index) recorded. The values (>0.7, that is, no atrophy (mild vaccine); 0.3-0.7 (relative or transient atrophy (for intermediate or intermediate plus vaccine) and <0.3 for a strong atrophy (hot vaccine or infection with vvIBDV) were recorded conforming to the first described standard, and there was not a statistical difference (p>0.05) observed between the groups. This indicating that BB index could be used as a tool in assessing the health status of a flock.

Key words: Avian, Bursa of Fabricius, bursal-body index (BB index), infectious bursal disease (IBD).

INTRODUCTION

The bursa of Fabricius (BF) is an organ unique to birds. It BF undergoes striking changes in size during development, growing rapidly during late embryogenesis and for several weeks (8 to 10 weeks) after hatching before regressing in sexually matured adult chicken at age of 6 to 7 months (Fang and Peng, 2014; Olah and Vervelde, 2012; Olah et al., 2014; Schat and Skinner, 2014). As a primary lymphoid organ, it plays a key role in the differentiation of B-lymphocytes (Cazaban et al., 2015:11). Stress related situations, that is, too low or too high temperature, too much or too little ventilation, other diseases (Marek's, Chicken infectious anaemia (CIA),

*Corresponding author. E-mail: abdullahi.raji@udusok.edu.ng.

infectious bursal disease (IBD), Newcastle disease and Avian influenza) (Jungbaeck and Nutolo, 2001), mycotoxins, management system (deep litter or battery cage) can directly impact BF size (van Herdeen et al., 2011).

With the absence of an ideal standard for the bursal size, it is difficult to evaluate and interpret bursa weight under field condition (Cazaban and Gardin, 2012). Although, Glick (1956) and Wolfe et al. (1962) addressed (BF) size and development in meat type and egg type chickens genetic lines kept in good "normal" conditions and considering bursa free form any infection, sex, age and husbandry influences in the bursa weight and Bursa Body weight ratio (B:B ratio), they fail to issue standards (van Herdeen et al., 2011). With a minimum bursa-to-body weight ratio standard of 0.11 proposed for broilers from 7 to 42 days of age by Cazaban et al. (2015), there is the need to update and device means of standardizing this published standard considering the genetic selection in the poultry today (Cazaban and Gardin, 2012).

The objective of the study was to evaluate the changes in the bursa using BB index, a method developed to overcome the shortfalls of the earlier protocols used in assessing the bursa in some available vaccines in Nigeria and a Nigerian field isolate of the very virulent infectious bursal disease virus (vvIBDV) in cockerels.

MATERIALS AND METHODS

Birds

Two hundred (200) Dominant-Black hybrid commercial day-old cockerels were sourced from reputable hatchery (Terudee Hatchery, Oyo State, Nigeria). The chicks were hatched on the same day and came from the same breeder flock. The breeder flock was vaccinated against infectious bursal disease (IBD) with an intermediate live IBD vaccine at 4 and 10 weeks and inactivated IBD vaccine at 16 weeks. After quality sorting on arrival at the poultry experiment pens of the Avian medicine unit of Ahmadu Bello University, Zaria, and a total of 135 one-day-old chicks were used in the study.

Housing

The birds were housed in the standard avian research facility that mimics field conditions. The birds were placed in a 30 m^2 naturally ventilated. They were raised in the 30 m^2 houses for 17 days (rearing period), and then, from 17th day of age onward they distributed into 5 houses at 3 birds/m^2. They were fed starter from 1 to 21 days of age and grower-finisher feed from 22 days to the end of the study (38 days). Standard lighting period was observed throughout the period of the study.

Vaccination and medication

As a tradition of the hatchery, the chicks were vaccinated against Marek's disease at the hatchery via subcutaneous injection and were vaccinated against infectious bronchitis by aerosol spray. Coccidiostat was incorporated in the grower feed. No other medications were given for the remainder days of the study.

Experimental design and sampling

Guideline protocols of the Avian Medicine Unit standard research facility of the Veterinary Teaching Hospital, Ahmadu Bello University, Zaria was strictly adhered to. Observatory procedure of clinical signs and mortality was carried out daily throughout the period of the study. One hundred and thirty five (135) cockerels were randomly divided into five groups, with each group containing 27 birds each. Each of the group received different treatment; three were vaccinated with 2 intermediate vaccines, and 1 intermediate plus vaccine of the IBDV. The two remaining groups received 0.05 ml of vvIBDV isolate and 0.05 ml of distilled water respectively. The groups were housed in different houses and assigned A, B and C for the vaccinated (A, and C for intermediate and B for intermediate plus); D for the challenge and E for control groups. A total of 27 cockerels, 3 from each group were randomly sampled on day(s) 1, 2, 3, 4, 5, 7, 10, 14 and 21 post vaccination or challenged as follows: Necropsies were conducted at the avian pathology necropsy room of the veterinary pathology department postmortem room of Ahmadu Bello University, Zaria where all the measurements were taken.

Body weight and bursa weight were used to calculate the bursa-body (BB) ratio according to the following formula:

BB ratio = [bursa weight (g)/body weight (g)] × 1000

Bursa-body (BB) index was calculated according to the following formula:

BB index = BB ratio of infected (or vaccinated) birds/ BB ratio of the controls

Each of the BF was cut longitudinally into 2 parts and placed in a 20 ml bottle containing 10% neutral buffered formalin for histopathology and histopathological lesion score using Williams and Davison (2010) criteria with a scoring range of 0 to 5 (0, normal bursal follicle architecture and 5, complete loss of bursal).

Statistical analysis

BB indexes were subjected to statistical analysis between the sampling groups over the period of study using the ANOVA test at a confidence level of 5% (P = 0.05). Tukeys post hoc test was employed to determine differences between groups.

RESULTS

Clinical signs and mortality

Clinical signs were recorded in the challenge (infected) group at day one post challenge (1Dpc). Severe depression, ruffled feathers, anorexia and diarrhoea, characterised by whitish colour were observed in birds in the challenge group, with an increase in birds exhibiting clinical signs. Mortality began on 3Dpc, peaked on 4Dpc, and declined on 5Dpc. At 6Dpc, recovery was observed.

Lesions of the BF

Gross lesions were observed as early as 1Dpc in the challenge group. Slight oedema, hyperaemia and gelatinous yellowish transudate covering the serosal

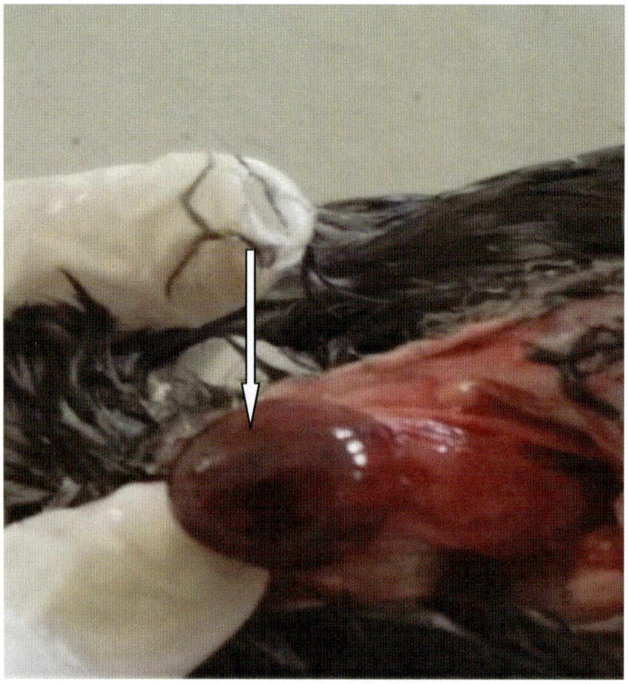

Figure 1. Severe bursal haemorrhage (white arrow) 3 Dpv/c in the challenge group.

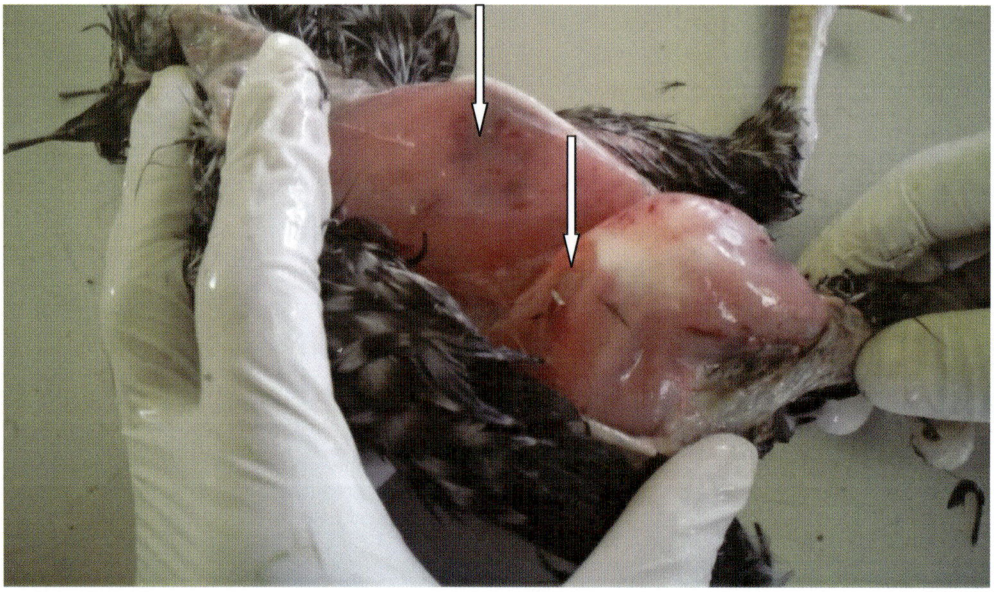

Figure 2. Severe petechial and ecchymotic haemorrhages on the breast and thigh muscle (white arrows) 3 Dpv/c in the challenge group.

surface; on mucosal surfaces, the BF as well as the thigh and breast muscle showed mild petechial haemorrhages. The thymuses were also haemorrhagic on 1Dpc. Bursal haemorrhages; ecchymotic haemorrhages and severe BF congestion (Figure 1) were observed at 3Dpc in the sacrificed and dead birds. At 5 Dpc, mild haemorrhages were observed in the bursae and thigh (Figure 2) of both sacrificed and dead birds, the spleen was also enlarged. The bursae have atrophied to about 1/3 of its size when compared with the control. No relevant gross pathology

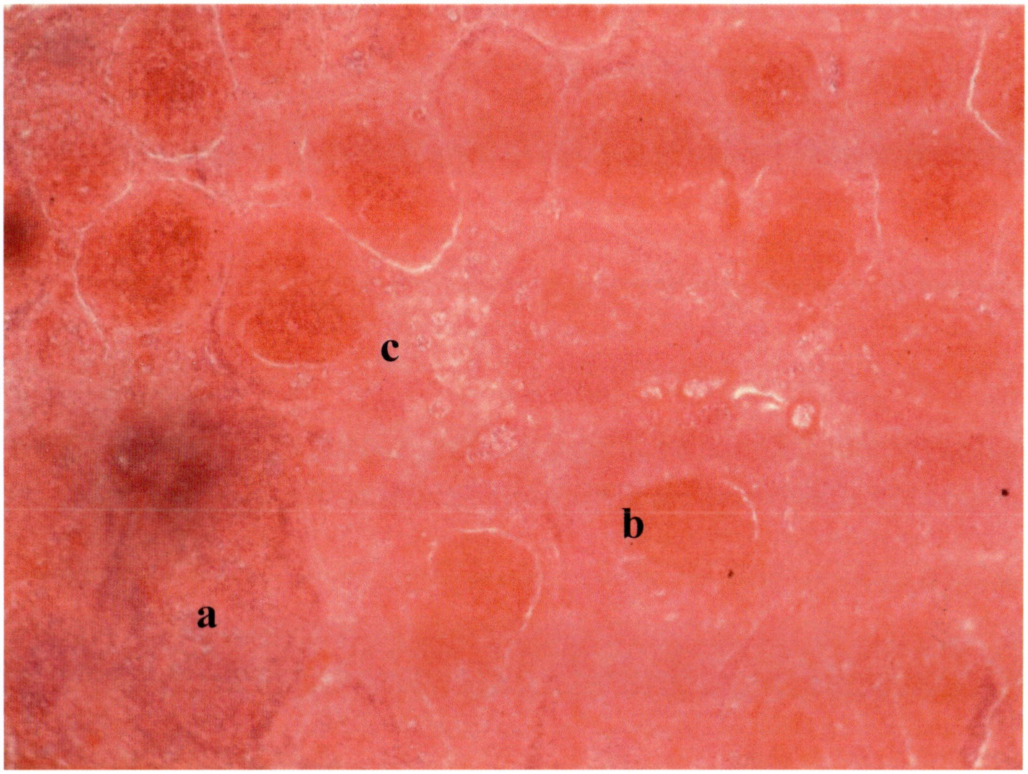

Figure 3. Bursa of Fabricius from Challenge group 5 Dpv/c; lymphoid follicular necrosis (a); Follicular focal haemorrhages (b); marked oedema in the interstitial connective tissue (c). H&E stain × 200.

was observed in birds in the control group.

Microscopically, lymphocytic depletion and haemorrhagic interfollicular interstitium in the medullary areas of the bursal follicles at 1Dpc were observed in the challenge group. Groups B and C presented haemorrhagic follicles at day-one post vaccination (1Dpv) (Figure 3). On days-three, post vaccination and challenge (3Dpv/c), challenge (D) group and group A presented necrosis and depletion of lymphocytes in the follicular medullar and cortex. At 5 Dpv/c, lymphoid necrosis was also observed in the challenge group, progressing to areas of coagulative necrosis within the follicles forming cystic areas (Figure 4) on 21Dpc. Moderate to marked atrophy of BF was observed in groups C and A respectively. Histopathologic lesions scores observed in the challenge group ranged from 4 to 5.

Morphometric of the bursa of Fabricius

Although the mean BF weight increased as birds grew older, however, the vaccinated groups were not able to reduce the bursal weight significantly when compared to the challenge and control groups. However, the challenge group when compared to the control group presented a significant variation in the BF weight on days 10, 14, and 21pv/c.

The BB ration showed a non-significant difference ($p>0.05$) between the groups (Table 1). On 21Dpv/c, all groups revealed a lower BB ratio, with the challenge group exhibiting an early reduction in the BB ratio on day 3 through days 21 post challenge.

The BB index values recorded on 7Dpv/c gave values of <0.3 in the challenge group, indicating strong atrophy; 0.3 to 0.7 in the vaccinated groups, indicating relative transient atrophy (Table 2). The standard is presented in Table 3.

DISCUSSION

For over 50 years bursa of Fabricius has become a major organ (lymphoid organ) of debate since its discovery by Hieronymus Fabricius *ab aquapendente* in the late 16th to early 17th century (Madej et. al., 2012). There exists agreed physiologic pattern of development; colonisation and migration of bursal lymphocytes (B-lymphocytes) in the bursa of bursa of Fabricius, its usage as a tool in diagnosis of infectious bursal disease (IBD) especially bursal size remains unending. Bursal weight, bursal body ratio and bursal diameter were some of the parameters used by Glick in 1956 to study normal bursal regression.

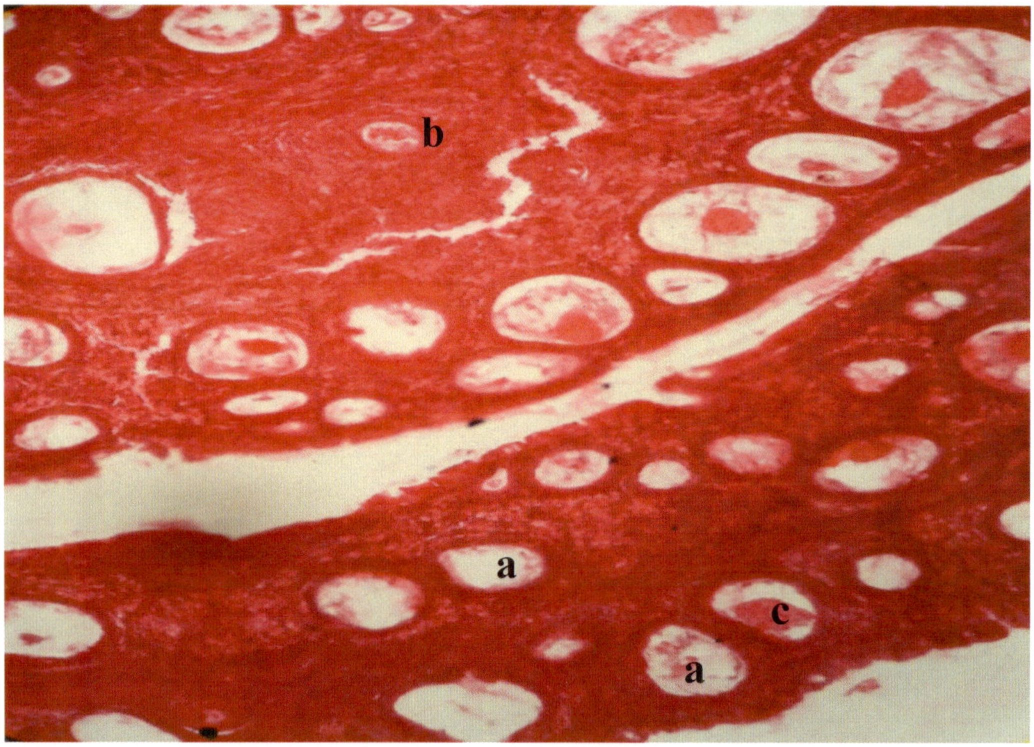

Figure 4. Bursa of Fabricius from MB® group 21Dpv/c: Vacuolar degeneration of the epithelium (a); Follicular atrophy and vacuolar degeneration of the medullary area (b); Follicular necrosis (c). H&E stain × 400.

Table 1. Mean bursa body weight ratio of different treatment and control groups.

Time	A	B	C	D	E
1Dpv/c	4.89±0.53	5.62±1.48	4.35±0.83	5.98±0.31	4.71±1.38
2Dpv/c	6.85±0.48	5.22±1.36	5.80±0.22	6.23±0.91	6.06±1.68
3Dpv/c	6.65±0.93	5.31±1.48	4.31±0.57	2.49±0.28	5.98±1.55
4Dpv/c	4.69±0.80	6.08±1.56	4.37±0.46	1.27±0.13	1.27±0.18
5Dpv/c	6.70±0.22	5.60±1.47	6.45±1.06	1.82±0.37	6.28±1.53
7Dpv/c	2.34±0.08	4.37±1.09	6.19±0.79	1.18±0.09	5.90±1.47
10Dpv/c	1.93±0.38	2.49±0.96	5.68±1.86	0.86±0.24	4.48±1.06
14Dpv/c	1.44±0.22	1.25±0.34	5.73±0.53	1.36±0.15	6.20±1.51
21Dpv/c	1.36±0.16	1.25±0.67	1.13±0.29	1.39±0.24	1.42±0.28

Dpv/c, Day(s) post vaccination or challenge.

But this extensive study of his and that of Jolly in 1914 faced with varying challenging factors ranging from breed type, sex, housing, stress and disease.

Although specific pathogen free (SPF) pullets would have been better for the purpose of this study; however, the cockerels (chicks) used were acquired from an independent, reliable and reputable hatchery where vaccination programme against Marek's disease and infectious bronchitis are routinely administered to day-old-chicks (DOCs). These vaccines have no effect on the integrity of the BF, and the use of the chicks reflected or mimics field conditions.

Vaccine selection was based on commonly available vaccine and as used on poultry farm with little modification. Of the two types of vaccines used in this study, one of the intermediate vaccine produced a moderate to marked reaction on the BF, whereas, the intermediate plus vaccine produced a non-to-mild reactions on the BF. The lesions observed were expected when live IBD vaccine is administered leading to impact

Table 2. Mean (± SEM) value of Bursal Body Index (BB index) of different treatment.

Groups	Bursa Index								
	1Dpv/c	2Dpv/c	3 Dpv/c	4 Dpv/c	5 Dpv/c	7Dpv/c*	10Dpv/c	14Dpv/c	21Dpv/c
A	1.04±0.60	1.13±0.65	1.11±0.64	3.69±2.13	1.07±0.62	0.40±0.23	0.43±0.25	0.23±0.13	0.96±0.55
B	1.19±0.69	0.86±0.50	0.89±0.51	4.79±2.76	0.89±0.52	0.74±0.43	0.55±0.32	0.20±0.12	1.61±0.93
C	0.92±0.53	0.96±0.55	0.72±0.42	3.44±1.99	1.03±0.59	1.05±0.61	1.27±0.73	0.92±0.53	0.79±0.46
D	1.27±0.73	1.03±0.59	0.42±0.24	1.00±0.58	0.29±0.17	0.20±0.12	0.19±0.11	0.22±0.13	0.98±0.56

SEM = Standard error mean; N=3; Dpv/c= Day(s) post vaccination or challenge. A and C = intermediate vaccines; B = intermediate plus vaccine; D = challenge (Infected) group; 7Dpv/c*= BB index calculation day.

Table 3. Standards of the BB index used in classifying IBD viruses, or conventional live IBD vaccines.

BB index	Conclusion
>0.7	Physiological variability = no atrophy Mild vaccines
0.3-0.7	Relative and transient atrophy Intermediate vaccines
<0.3	Intermediate plus vaccines Strong atrophy; Hot vaccines

BB index = BB ratio of infected (or vaccinated) birds / BB ratio of the controls.

on the BF size (Jungbaeck and Nutolo, 2001). Mazeriegos et al. (1990) showed that intermediate vaccine varied in their pathogenicity. They divided intermediate vaccines into 3 pathogenic categories based on bursal damage, bursal B/W and histopathological findings; low or mild pathogenic, moderate pathogenic and highly pathogenic. In line with this result, intermediate vaccine used in group "A" showed to be highly pathogenic.

Furthermore, no clinical signs and mortality were observed in the vaccinated and non-vaccinated (control group (group E)); however the challenge group (D) presented clinical signs exhibited by birds infected with vvIBD virus.

The presence of histopathological lesions on the BF confirmed the pathogenicity of the field IBD virus field isolate used. Although the scoring pattern followed that of Williams and Davison, (2010); it was compared with the European pharmacopoeia lesion scoring because of the live attenuated IBD vaccines used in this study, with lesion of 4 and 5 recorded in the challenge group.

With values of BF weight and size steadily increasing prior to vaccination and challenge as a result of variables due to continues genetic selection through output in egg and carcass. This variability as described by Cazaban and Gardin (2012) was observed during the course of this study.

Following infection or vaccination, the BF goes through several stages; (1) Acute inflammation stage, where bursa is getting larger, and lasts for about 4 days post infection (dpi); (2) Sub-acute stage where BF quickly regresses and gets back to its original size at around 5 dpi and the final stage; (3) Which is the relevant stage to record bursal atrophy, and calculate BB ratio and BB index (which is the main target of this study). As in the previous and only study on BB index by Cazaban and Gardin (2012), the relevant schedule to start recording BB index is from 7 dpi onwards (and say up to 14dpi). The sizes recorded in this study presented the picture of the vaccine virus strain used and likewise the strain of the field virus. The challenge virus isolate gave value of <0.3 BB index indicative of a hot vaccine or vvIBDV infection, whereas the intermediate and intermediate plus vaccines gave a value of between 0.3 to 0.7 which is indicative of the administration of either of the vaccines used.

Conclusively, this study has confirmed that BB index can be used in assessing the BF status (in vaccination or infection) as the BF histopathologic lesion scoring scale is used in designing the safety of live IBD vaccines.

REFERENCES

Cazaban C, Gardin Y, Kaewpoowat N (2012). The BB Index Assists on Assessing Flock Health (Part 2). Chick Program Online 41:5.

Cazaban C, Gardin Y (2012). Bursa of Fabricius is a visual indicator (Part 1). Chick Program Online 40:5.

Cazaban C, Masferrer NM, Pascual RD, Espadamala MN, Costa T, Gardin Y (2015). Proposed bursa of fabricius weight to body weight ratio standard in commercial broilers. Poult. Sci. 94(9):2088-2093.

Fang J, Peng X (2014). Developmental changes in cell proliferation and apoptosis in the normal duck bursa of Fabricius. J. Vet. Sci. 15(4):465-474.

Glick B (1956). Normal growth of the bursa of Fabricius in chickens. Poult. Sci. 35:843-851.

Jungbaeck C, Nutolo S (2001). The degree of bursa damage as a possible parameter to define the virulence of IBDV vaccine strain. Proc. II. International symposium on infectious bursal disease and chicken infectious anaemia. Rauischholzhause. Germany. pp. 460-474,

Madej JP, Chrzazstek K, Piasecki T, Wieliczk A (2012). New Insight into the Structure, Development, Functions and Popular Disorders of Bursa Fabricii. Anat. Histol. Embryol. 42:321-331.

Mazeriegos LA, Lukert PD, Brown J (1990). Pathogenicity and immunosuppressive properties of infectious bursal disease "Intermediate" strains. Avian Pathol. 9:395-405.

Olah I, Vervelde L (2012). Structure of the avian lymphoid system. In: Avian Immunology. Davison F, Kaspers B, Schat KA (Eds.). London: Academic Press. pp. 13-50.

Olah I, Nagy N, Verwelde L (2014). Structure of the Avian Lymphoid System. in Avian Immunology, 2nd Edition. Schat KA, Kaspers B, Kaiser P (Eds.). Elsevier Ltd. Publishing, San Diego, CA. pp. 11-44

Schat KA, Skinner MA (2014). Avian Immunosuppressive Diseases and Immune Evasion. in Avian Immunology, 2nd Edition. Schat KA, Kaspers B, Kaiser P (Eds.). Elsevier Ltd. Publishing, San Diego, CA. pp. 275-297

Van Herdeen K, Cazaban C, Alva B (2011). The Relevance of Bursa Size in Modern Poultry Production. August 2011. Pluimvee Poult. Bull. pp. 24-26.

Williams AE, Davison TF (2010). Enhanced immunopathology induced by very virulent infectious bursal disease virus. Avian Pathol. 34(1):4-14.

Wolfe HR, Sheridan SA, Bilstad NM, Johnson MA (1962). The growth of lymphoid organs and the testes of chickens. Anat. Rec. 142:485-493.

Tick resistance of two breeds of cattle in Wolaita Zone, Southern Ethiopia

Desie Sheferaw

Faculty of Veterinary Medicine, Hawassa University, P.O. Box 5, Hawassa, Ethiopia.

The objective of this study was to evaluate total tick burden and resistance differences of local indigenous breeds and Holstein-crosses (50%). Longitudinal study method was employed to assess the mean monthly half-body regions of total tick burdens. The mean monthly half body regions of total tick count on local indigenous cattle and Holstein-crosses (50%) were 75.2 and 201.7, respectively. The monthly mean half-body region of total tick count on the Holstein-crosses (50%) was significantly ($p<0.05$) higher than that of the indigenous breed throughout the study months. From 4425 collected adult ticks, *Boophilus decoloratus* (47.50%), *Amblyomma gemma* (21.06%), *Amblyomma variegatum* (18.31%), *Amblyomma cohaerens* (4.97%), *Amblyomma lepidum* (3.75%), *Rhipicephalus evertsi evertsi* (2.87%), *Rhipicephalus muhsamae* (0.79%) and *Rhipicephalus guilhoni* (0.75%) were the tick species identified in descending order. Among the tick species identified, seasonal variation was observed in four species, namely: *A. variegatum*, *A. gemma*, *A. lepidum* and *R. evertsi evertsi*. Animal health extension especially on tick control strategy should be in place in order to improve animal productivity.

Key words: Burden, Holstein-cross (50%), indigenous, resistance tick, Ethiopia.

INTRODUCTION

Ticks are globally important in livestock production, because of their economic and health implications (Jongejan and Uilenberg, 2004). It has been estimated that about 80% of world's cattle are infested with ticks (Minjauw and McLeod, 2003). According to CSA (2010), there are about 723,343 heads of cattle in Wolaita of which 3825 are Holstein-crosses. The total cattle population of Wolaita accounts for 7.46% of the Southern Region. Crossbred cattle are being introduced into Wolaita during the working phase of Wolaita Agricultural Development Unit project as a means of milk production to satisfy the protein demand of the human population. Resistance of cattle to tick infestation was reported to consist of innate and acquired components (Wikel and Whelen, 1986).

According to Utech et al. (1978) high levels of host resistance to ticks are primarily associated with zebu cattle, but a proportion of resistant individuals can occur in all breeds. Hence the objective of this study was to assess total tick burden difference, which is one of an indicator for tick resistance differences, of indigenous and Holstein-crosses (50%) in Kokatie, area.

*Corresponding author. E-mail: mereba480@gmail.com.

MATERIALS AND METHODS

Study area

The study was carried out in Kokatie PA of Sodo-Zuria district, (Figure 1) which is 2083 to 2213 m above sea level, and located between 6°52'01.9" to 6°52'42.6" N and 37°47'06.9" to 37°48'55.3" E. The vegetation of the study area is predominantly eucalyptus tree, natural grasses, tuft of grasses and some bushes. The area is characterized by bimodal rainfall, long rainy period (June to October) and short rainy period (March and April). Moreover, it is one of the areas that are densely populated.

Experimental animals

The experimental animals were selected from two breeds of cattle that were kept under backyard and/or traditional management system. From these, thirty two animals, sixteen indigenous and sixteen Holstein-crosses (50%), were selected through purposively sampling method for this field experimental study. Then the selected animals were grouped into two according to their breed types: Group I indigenous cattle and Group II Holstein-crosses (50%). The study animals were not treated with acaricide throughout the study periods and for about two months before the start of the study.

Study design and methodology

A longitudinal study method was employed in which monthly half-body regions total tick burden were taken regularly for eight consecutive months, August to March. During these eight study months, adult ticks were collected from the animals into universal sample bottles containing 70% ethanol following the procedure described by Okello-Onen et al. (1999). Then samples were transported to Hawassa University Veterinary Medicine Parasitology Laboratory and identified following the standard identification procedures described by Hoogstraal (1956), Okello-Onen et al. (1999) and Walker,(2003). Rainfall, humidity and temperature data of the study months were taken from Sodo meteorological station. The study considered 95% level of significance and 5% desired absolute precision.

Data analysis

The data collected were analyzed by descriptive statistics; and log transformed data were analyzed with t-test and repeated measure of variance using SPSS 16.5 software.

RESULTS

Tick burden

The overall mean half body regions of total tick count on the indigenous and Holstein-crosses (50%) were 75.2 and 201.7, respectively. The trend of mean monthly half-body regions total tick count of the indigenous and Holstein-crosses (50%) are shown on Figure 2. Repeated measure of collected data analysis showed that, there was a significant ($p<0.05$) variation in the mean monthly half-body region of tick burdens between the two breeds of cattle, indigenous and Holstein-crosses (50%) (F= 370.61, P> 0.000, Partial η squared= 0.925; 95% CI=1.766 to 1.833 for indigenous breed and 2.209 to 2.275 for Holstein-crosses 50%). Within the breeds there was significant ($p<0.05$) variation in the mean monthly tick burden of half-body regions in both breed (F= 4.585, P< 0.001 and Partial η squared = 0.132), due to the interaction of breeds with months. The seasonal tick burden of half body region on both breeds is shown in Figure 3. The analysis for presence or absence variation in the two breeds of cattle half-body region tick burden is shown in Table 2. Humidity and rainfall had positively influenced (t = 10.28, P = 0.000; t = 9.71, P = 0.000) on the half-body regions total tick burden of both breeds (Figure 4), while the temperature had negatively affected (t = -9.74, P = 0.000) the half-body regions total tick burden of both breeds as shown in figure 5. That is why about 80.76% of the overall total tick burden differences were observed between the study months (F = 125.95, P = 0.000 and partial η squared = 0.8076).

Tick species identification

A total of 4425 adult ticks were collected from half body regions of the study animals, and a total of three genera of ticks were identified. From the identified genera, a total of eight species of ticks were identified, namely: *B. decoloratus* (47.5%), *A. gemma* (21.1%), *A. variegatum* (18.3%), *A. cohaerens* (5.0%), *A. lepidum* (3.8%), *R. evertsi evertsi* (2.9%), *R. muhsamae* (0.8%) and *R. guilhoni* (0.8%). Among these eight tick species six of them were identified as the major tick species in the study area: *A. variegatum*, *A. gemma*, *A. cohaerens*, *A. lepidum*, *B. decoloratus* and *R. evertsi evertsi* (Table 1).

DISCUSSION

The mean monthly half-body region of total tick count on the Holstein-crosses (50%) was significantly ($p<0.05$) higher than that of the indigenous breed throughout the study months (F= 370.61, P= 0.000, Partial η squared= 0.925). This variation is clearly shown in Figure 2 that showed the trends of half body region of total tick counts. This finding agreed with Ali and de Castro (1993) who reported that Horro breed carried fewer total tick burdens than Horro X Holstein. Aragaw (1994), Yohualashet et al. (1995) and Solomon and Kaaya (1996) also reported better control of tick burdens in the local zebu than Holstein crosses.

At Abernossa ranch, Arsi breed was found to be highly tick resistant, followed by Boran breed, but Boran X Holstein was the least resistant (Solomon and Kaaya, 1996). Moran et al. (1996) also observed that pure Ankole cattle of Burundi were more resistant than Ankole X Holstein. In this study, mean monthly Log_{10} (x+1) of total tick burden was statistically significant and observed

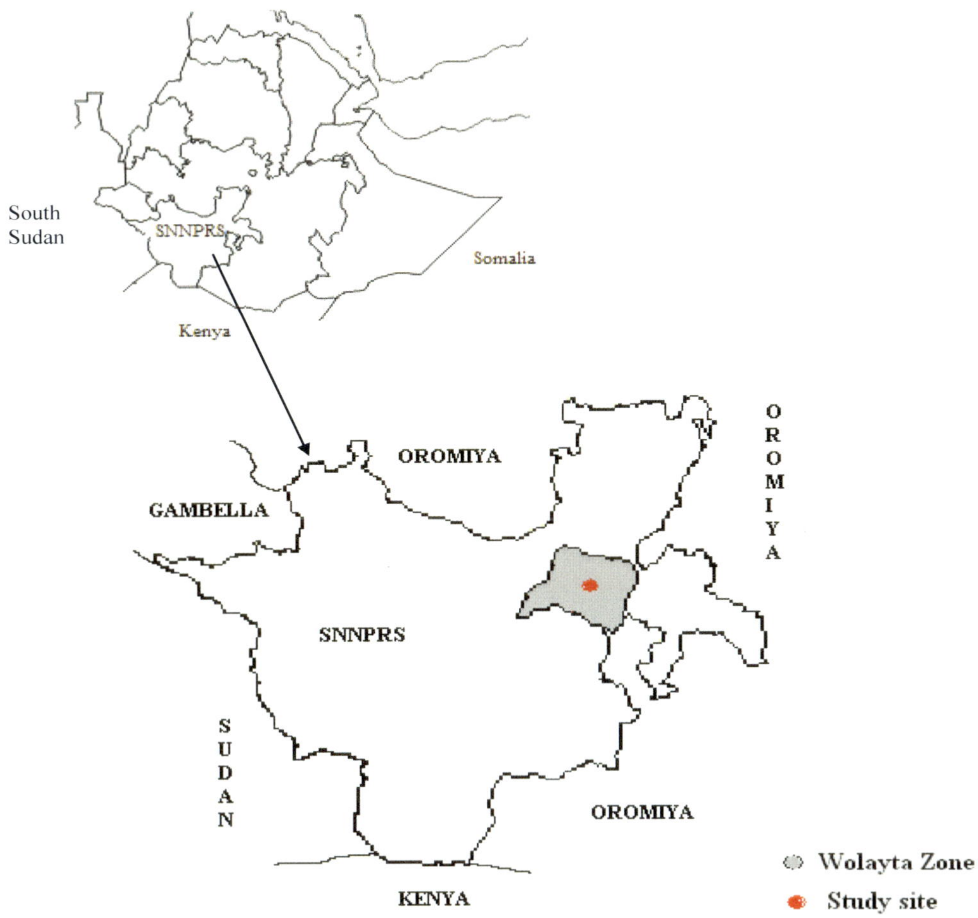

Figure 1. Map of SNNPRS to show the study site

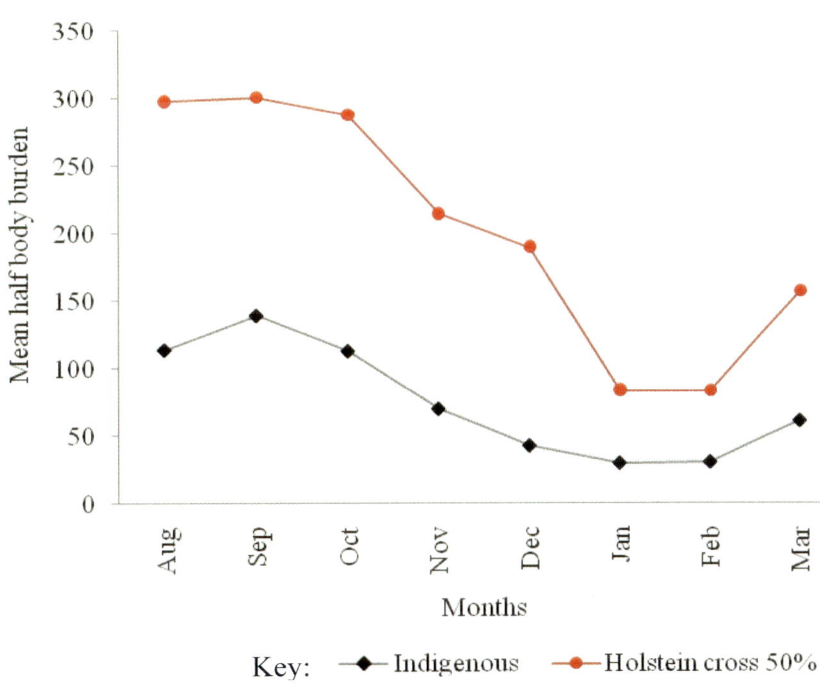

Figure 2. Pattern of mean monthly half-body tick burden of the Indigenous and Holstein crosses 50%.

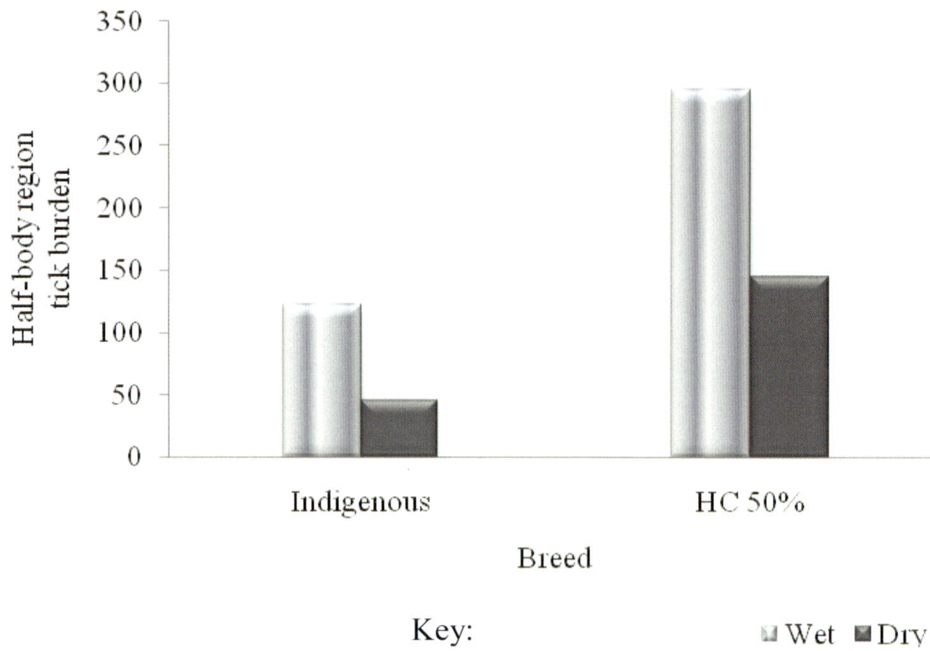

Figure 3. Wet and dry periods mean half-body regions total tick burden of indigenous and Holstein-cross (50%) cattle breed.

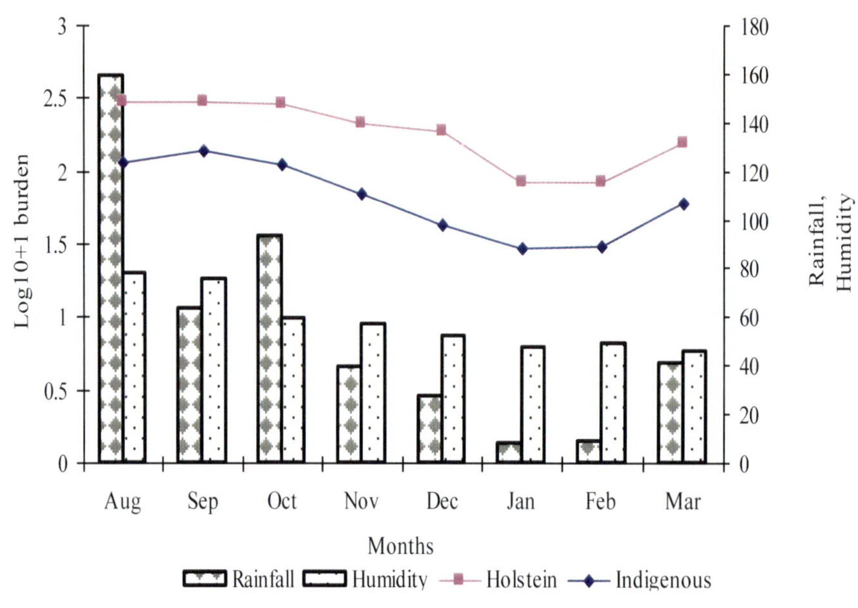

Figure 4. Trends of mean $\log_{10}(X+1)$ half body tick burden of the breeds, rainfall and humidity.

higher in Holstein-crosses (50%) than on the indigenous breed throughout the study months. Even with the various temperatures, rainfall and humidity had no change in the mean half body region tick burden. Gene expression studies strongly indicated that both immune and non-immune mechanisms are associated with tick resistance in cattle (Porto et al., 2011).

Tick counts positively correlated to coat characteristics in cattle (Marufu, et al., 2011; Verissimo et al., 2002); and also it was observed that cattle with shorter and smoother coats carried lower tick counts (Marufu, et al., 2011). Generally it is believed that cattle breeds with short hairs exposed the ticks to harmful climatic conditions and to predators like birds (Tatchell, 1987; Taylor, 2006;

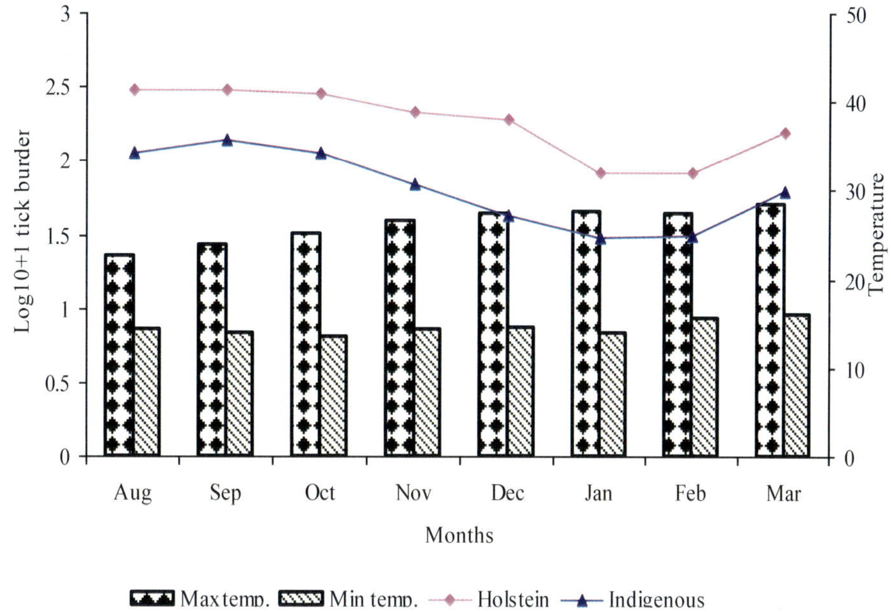

Figure 5. Trends of mean $\log_{10}(X+1)$ tick burden of the breeds and temperature.

Table 1. Comparison of the two breeds of cattle half-body regions tick burden [$Log_{(X+1)}$]

Breed	Log transformed mean of half-body tick burden (Mean count)	Std. Err	95% CI	t-value	P-value
Indigenous	2.78 (601.8)	0.015	2.74-2.81	17.66	0.000
HC 50%	3.20 (1613.4)	0.019	3.16-3.24		
Total	2.99 (1107.6)				

Table 2. Seasonal variation of the major tick species identified during the study period ($Log_{10}(X+1)$

Tick spp.	Season	Mean	Std. Error	t – value	P > |t|	[95% CI]	Significance
AV	Wet	4.304	0.594	4.3993	0.000	3.130 - 5.478	* * *
	Dry	1.565	0.187			1.195 - 1.936	
AG	Wet	2.261	0.173	-5.7173	0.000	1.919 - 2.603	* * *
	Dry	4.493	0.350			3.801 - 5.185	
AC	Wet	0.667	0.141	-1.2189	0.224	0.388 - 0.946	NS
	Dry	0.928	0.161			0.609 - 1.246	
AL	Wet	0.377	0.090	-2.3018	0.022	0.198 - 0.556	* *
	Dry	0.826	0.173			0.484 - 1.168	
BD	Wet	7.884	0.319	1.0566	0.292	7.253 - 8.516	NS
	Dry	7.348	0.394			6.568 - 8.128	
RhE	Wet	0.725	0.115	4.1495	0.000	0.497 - 0.953	* * *
	Dry	0.196	0.054			0.088 - 0.303	

NB. Equal variances assumed. (AV =*A. variegatum*, AG =*A. gemma*, AC = *A. cohaerens*, AL = *A. lepidum*, BD = *B. decoloratus*, RhE = *Rh. evertsi evertsi* NS = Not significant). * * * = Highly significant and * * = Significant)

Marufa et al., 2011). According to de Castro (1991) observation *Bos indicus* naturally self-groom and groom each other frequently and thoroughly. It is already known that grooming is a means by which the host can express resistance; fewer ticks were seen on those animals that were able to groom (Minjauw and de Castro, 2000; Brossard, 1998).

Tropical cattle breeds are known to possess short hair to overcome heat stress. And those animals with shorter hairs tend to have lower tick counts compared to those with longer hairs, since long hairs create favourable conditions for tick survival (Taylor et al., 1995; Marufa et al., 2011). Moreover, longer coat hairs may protect ticks from the animal's self-grooming that enables them to remove ticks attached to the coat (Machado et al., 2010). *B. indicus* were reported to be more innately resistant to *B. microplus* infestation (Wikel and Whelen, 1986).

Among the tick species identified seasonal variation was observed in four species, namely: *A. variegatum*, *A. gemma*, *A. lepidum* and *R. evertsi evertsi* (Table 2). This result is in a general agreement with observation of Kaiser et al. (1991) who reported that all stages of *Rh. evertsi evertsi* were less active during dry season. There was a significant seasonal variation of *A. variegatum* ($t = 10.2719$, $P = 0.05$ at $\alpha = 0.05$) in the study area, which was with highest mean count during wet period.

This finding is in agreement with that of Gebre et al. (2000) and Solomon (1993) observations at Sebeta and Abernossa, respectively. They recorded highest counts of *A. variegatum* in July and April, which coincide with the rainy months for the areas. Moreover, Hoogstraal (1956), Morel (1980), Petney et al. (1987), Yohualashet et al. (1995), Mattioli et al. (1997), Bekele (2002) and Assefa (2004) observed the seasonal fluctuation of this tick species with a relative rise in numbers during the short and long rains. The life-cycle of this tick species is most closely linked to rainfall. The adults were aroused by rain in the rainy months, in which by that time most had apparently found a host (Kaiser et al., 1988). In Ethiopia Pegram et al. (1981) observed that the onset of feeding activity of adult coincides with the start of wet season. From de Castro (1994) survey in western Ethiopia females, *A. variegatum* were mostly present in rainy time during collections of tick species.

The mean distribution of *A. gemma* ($t= 5.7173$, $P< 0.05$) and *A. lepidum* ($t= 2.3018$, $P< 0.05$) were significantly and seasonally varied. These ticks were highly prevalent during dry period, and they are xerophilous African species of *Amblyomma* (Morel, 1980). This finding is in a general agreement with Petney et al. (1987). There was a significant seasonal variation of *Rh. e. evertsi* ($t = 4.1495$, $P= 0.000$) with the highest collection of the adult in wet period (95% CI 0.497 to 0.953 and 0.088 to 0.303 during wet and dry periods, respectively). This finding is in line with Kaiser et al. (1991) who showed that all stages of this tick were less active during dry season. In fact according to Pegram et al. (1981), de Castro (1994) and Bekele (2002) it appears to occupy a wide range of climatic and ecological conditions with rain occurring in most of the year, and throughout the year.

CONCLUSION AND RECOMMENDATION

Ticks burden of Holstein-crosses (50%) was significantly higher than the local indigenous breed in all the seasons. So to increase cattle productivity in the study area and elsewhere in the country, consideration of the breed type would be helpful. But for this purpose, animal health extension work, especially on breed use for strategic tick control could be important.

ACKNOWLEDGEMENT

The author would like to Wolaita Sodo Regional Veterinary Laboratory. The encouragement as well as material support given by Ato Bergudie Bancha is highly appreciable.

REFERENCES

Ali M, de Castro JJ (1993). Host resistance to ticks (Acari: Ixodidae) in different breeds of cattle at Bako, Ethiopia. Trop. Anim. Health prod. 25(4): 215-222.

Aragaw K (1994). Study on host resistance to natural infestation in Friesian and indigenous zebu cattle, DVM thesis, Addis Ababa University, Faculty of Veterinary Medicine, Debre-Zeit. pp.1-34.

Assefa B (2004). A survey of ticks and tick-borne blood protista in cattle at Asela, Arsi Zone. DVM Thesis, Faculty of Veterinary Medicine, Addis Ababa University, Debre Zeit. pp. 25-36.

Bekele T (2002). Studies on seasonal dynamics of ticks of Ogaden cattle and individual variation in resistance to ticks in eastern Ethiopia. Zoonoses Public Health 49(6):285-288.

Brossard M (1998). The use of vaccines and genetically resistant animals in tick control. Revue scientifique et technique-Office international des épizooties 17:188-193.

CSA (2010). Federal Democratic Republic of Ethiopia. Central Statistical Agency, Agricultural Sample Survey Report on Livestock and Livestock Characteristics. Volume II, 2009/10. Statistical bulletin 468, Addis Ababa, Ethiopia. Available at: http://www.sciepub.com/reference/216283

de Castro JJ (1991). Resistance to ixodid ticks in cattle with an assessment of its role in tick control in Africa. Breeding for disease resistance in farm animals. CABI, Wallingford, UK. pp. 244-262.

Gebre S, Nigist M, Kassa B (2000). Seasonal variation of ticks on calves at Sebeta in western Shewa Zone. Ethiop. Vet. J. 7(2):17-30.

Hoogstraal H (1956). African Ixodoidea. Vol. I. Ticks of the Sudan (with special reference to Equatoria Province and with Preliminary Reviews of the Genera Boophilus, Margaropus, and Hyalomma). African Ixodoidea. Vol. I. Ticks of the Sudan (with special reference to Equatoria Province and with Preliminary Reviews of the Genera Boophilus, Margaropus, and Hyalomma).

Jongejan F, Uilenberg G (2004). The global importance of ticks.

Parasitology 129(Suppl):S3˜S14.
Kaiser MN, Sutherst RW, Bourne AS (1991). Tick (Acarina: Ixodidae) infestations on zebu cattle in northern Uganda. Bull. Entomol. Res. 81(3):257-262.
Kaiser MN, Sutherst RW, Bourne AS, Gorissen L, Floyd RB (1988). Population dynamics of ticks on Ankole cattle in five ecological zones in Burundi and strategies for their control. Prevent. Vet. Med. 6(3):199-222.
Latif AA, Walker AR (2004). An introduction to the biology and control of ticks in Africa. ICTTD-2 project. pp.1-29.
Machado MA, Azevedo AL, Teodoro RL, Pires MA, Peixoto MG, de Freitas C, Prata MC, Furlong J, da Silva MV, Guimarães SE, Regitano LC (2010). Genome wide scan for quantitative trait loci affecting tick resistance in cattle (Bos taurus× Bos indicus). BMC Genomics 11(1):280.
Marufu MC, Qokweni L, Chimonyo M, Dzama K (2011). Relationships between tick counts and coat characteristics in Nguni and Bonsmara cattle reared on semiarid rangelands in South Africa. Ticks Tick-borne Dis. 2(3):172-177.
Mattioli RC, Janneh L, Corr N, Faye JA, Pandey VS, Verhulst A (1997). Seasonal prevalence of ticks and tick-transmitted haemoparasites in traditionally managed N'Dama cattle with reference to strategic tick control in the Gambia. Med. Vet. Entomol. 11(4):342-348.
Minjauw B, De Castro JJ (2000). Host resistance to ticks and tick-borne diseases: its role in integrated control. Breed. Dis. Resist. Farm Anim. 153-169
Minjauw B, McLeod A (2003). Tick-borne diseases and poverty: the impact of ticks and tick-borne diseases on the livelihoods of small-scale and marginal livestock owners in India and eastern and southern Africa. Tick-borne diseases and poverty: the impact of ticks and tick-borne diseases on the livelihoods of small-scale and marginal livestock owners in India and eastern and southern Africa. Available at: https://www.cabdirect.org/cabdirect/abstract/20063155090
Moran MC, Nigarura G, Pegram RG (1996). An assessment of host resistance to ticks on cross-bred cattle in Burundi. Med. Vet. Entomol. 10: 12-18.
Morel P (1980). Study on Ethiopia ticks (Argasidae, Ixodidae) Republic of France, Ministry Of foreign affairs, French Vet Mission, Addis. CJEVT 12:332.
Okello-Onen J, Hassan SM, Essuman S (1999). Taxonomy of African ticks: an identification manual. International Centre of Insect Physiology and Ecology (ICIPE). Available at: https://www.cabdirect.org/cabdirect/abstract/20023066680
Pegram RG, Hoogstraal H, Wassef HP (1981). Ticks (Acari: Ixodoidea) of Ethiopia. I. Distribution, ecology and host relationships of species infesting livestock. Bull. Entomol. Res. 71(3):339-359.
Petney TN, Horak IG, Rechave Y (1987). The Ecology of the African vectors of heartwater, with particular reference to *Amblyomma hebraeum* and *Amblyomma variegatum*. Onderstepoort J. Vet. Res. 54: 381-395.
Porto Neto LR, Jonsson NN, Michael J, D'Occhio MJ, Barendse W (2011). Molecular genetic approaches for identifying the basis of variation in resistance to tick infestation in cattle. Vet. Parasitol. 180:165-172
Solomon G (1993). Resistance of three breeds of cattle to ticks and tick-borne diseases at Abernossa ranch, Ethiopia, Proceeding of the seventh Ethiopian Veterinary Association Conference. pp. 78-99.
Solomon G, Kaaya GP (1996). Comparison of resistance in three breeds of cattle against African Ixodid ticks. Exp. Appl. Acarol. 2(4): 223-230.
Tatchell RJ (1987). Interactions between ticks and their hosts. Int. J. Parasitol. 17(2):597-606.
Utech KBW, Wharton RH, Kerr JD (1978). Resistance to Boophilus microplus (Canestrini) in different breeds of cattle. Aust. J. Agric. Res. 29(4):885-895.
Verissimo CJ, Nicolau CV, Cardoso VL, Pinheiro MG (2002). Haircoat characteristics and tick infestation on gyr (zebu) and crossbred (holdstein x gyr) cattle. Archivos de zootecnia 51(195).
Walker AR (2003). Ticks of domestic animals in Africa: a guide to identification of species. Edinburgh: Bioscience. pp. 3-210
Wikel SK, Whelen C (1986). Ixodid-host immune interaction. Identification and characterization of relevant antigens and tick-induced host immunosuppression. Vet. Parasitol. 20(1-3):149-174.
Yohualashet T, Gebreab F, Wakijira A, Tsega T (1995). Preliminary observation on ticks: Seasonal Dynamics and Resistance of Three Indigenous and Three Cross-Bred Cattle in Ethiopia. Bull. Anim. Health Prod. Afr. 43(2):105-114.

17

Tsetse density and bovine trypanosomosis in selected sites of Konta, Ethiopia

Anteneh Wondimu*, Endeshaw Reta and Asnake Fekadu

Haramaya University College of Veterinary Medicine, P. O. Box 138 Dire Dawa, Ethiopia.

A cross-sectional study was conducted in selected sites of Southern Nation, Nationalities and People Regional State (SNNPRS) of Konta, Ethiopia. The purposes of study were to determine the apparent density of tsetse flies and prevalence of bovine trypanosomosis. Ngu traps for entomological survey were deployed at grazing and watering points of animals in the village of Dolba (Kerara Peasants Association, PAS) and near Gojeb River. Assessment of tsetse indicated the presence of *Glossina pallidipes* with the apparent density 8.45% flies/trap/day. Other biting flies (tabanids) were also caught along with tsetse that transmits trypanosomes mechanically. For parasitological study, a total of 400 blood samples were collected from randomly selected animals and examined for the presence of trypanosomes and indicate overall prevalence of trypanosomosis in study cattle as 12%. The dominant trypanosome species were found *Trypanosoma conglonse* 29 (60.4%) followed by *Trypanosoma vivax* 14 (29.2%), *Trypanosoma bruci* 3 (6.25%) and mixed infection (*T. congolonse* and *T. vivax*) of 2 (4.2%). Based on these results it is concluded that trypanosomosis is a major constraint of livestock production in the study area.

Key words: Konta, Southern Nation, Nationalities and People Regional State (SNNPRS), Tsetse, Trypanosomosis, trypanosome, prevalence.

INTRODUCTION

Trypanosomosis is serious constraints to livestock production and agricultural development in Ethiopia. A total of 14.8 million cattle, 6.12 million sheep and goats, 1 million camels and 1.23 million equine are at risk of contracting trypanosomes (MoA, 1995). Trypanosomosis is a wide spread and economically important disease in human and animals (Sumbria and Singla, 2016). It is caused by protozoan parasites belonging to the family trypanosomatidae genus *Trypanosoma*, which inhibits the blood plasma, various bodies' fluids and tissue of the host (Singh and Singla, 2012). The species of *Trypanosoma* known to exist in Ethiopia, which are pathogenic to cattle and small ruminants, are: *Trypanosoma vivax*, *Trypanosoma congolense* and *Trypanosoma bruci*. They are distributed mainly in tsetse belt of the country (south west and southern parts) between 33°and 38°E and 5° to 12°N. *T. vivax*, also found in area outside of the belt, where it can possibly

*Corresponding author. E-mail: anteneha7@gmail.com.

transmitted by mechanical vectors of biting flies like tabanus and stomoxy (Eneyew, 1997).

The most important trypanosome species affecting cattle are: *T. congolense, T. vivax* and *T. brucei*, which are generally termed as Nagana (Jordan, 1986; Langridge, 1976) and *T. eqiperdum* for equines (Dagnachew and Shafo, 1981). In 1962, the cattle survey in southern Ethiopia, by the livestock division, established that bovine trypanosomosis was a major cattle disease in the Omo valley. It was stated that the problem of trypanosomosis is the main cause of decline in the number of cattle and particularly draught oxen (Abebe and Jobere, 1996).

Trypanosomosis depends on the distribution of the vectors, the virulence of parasite and the response of the host (Langridge, 1976). Tsetse flies are the major and true cyclical vectors. They are blood feeding insects that belongs to phylum arthropoda, class insecta family muscidae sub family glossinidae and genus *Glossina*. Today five species of glossina have been identified in Ethiopia: *Glossina submorsitans* and *Glossina palldipus* (savanna groups), *Glossina fuscipes* and *Glossina tacnoidus* (Riverine groups) and *Glossina longipennis* (Langridge, 1976). In the area of tsetse transmitted trypanosomosis which affects cattle production, trypanocidal drugs, both prophylactic and curative drugs and other tsetse control methods such as insecticide application on the back of animals are the most widely used methods of trypanosomosis control.

Trypanosomosis is the most serious disease of cattle, which cause great socio-economic losses in SNNPR. The socio-economic impact of trypanosomosis is reflected on direct losses such as mortality, morbidity, reduction in milk and meat production, and still birth (Leak et al., 1993). Thus, trypanosomosis is one of the causes for food in security in the Omo-Ghibe belt as well as the tributaries of Gojeb Rivers, where wide grazing land which favors animal production is located. Therefore, the objectives of the current study were: To assess the apparent density and distribution of tsetse and other biting flies and prevalence of bovine trypanosomosis Konta special districts.

MATERIALS AND METHODS

Study area

The present study was conducted in 5 selected peasant association (PAs) namely Biteti, Chida, Kecharoba, Kerara, and Mareka in Konta special woreda of SNNPRS which is located 498 km south of Addis Ababa. The area has humid, sub-humid climate with a moderately hot temperature and reliable annual average rain fall of 1200 mm. The annual temperature and altitude ranges from 12 to 24°C, 1062 (Gojeb river) to 1542 (Kerara PAs) m.a.s.l. respectively. Livestock species are cattle, sheep, goats, mule and donkey. The predominant species in the area is cattle which are estimated at 20,985 in the study area 5 PAs. Livestock management system is mixed farming system. The animals in the area mainly depend on communal grazing fields and watering points are at Gojeb River and its tributaries (Konta Woreda Agricultural Office).

Study population and design

Cross-sectional survey was conducted from January 2009 to March 2010 on indigenous cattle. They were kept under traditional extensive husbandry system with communal herding and watering in small and big rivers.

Sampling method and sample size determination

The sampling method applied in the present study was a simple random sampling and the sample size was approximated by using formula given in Thrusfield (1995) using 95% confidence interval and expected prevalence of 50%.

$$n = \frac{1.96^2 \text{ (Pex (1-Pex))}}{d^2}$$

Where, n = sample size; Pexp = expected prevalence; d^2 = desired absolute precision.

Accordingly, the estimated sample size was 384 animals; however, to increase the precision 16 cattle were added and a total of 400 cattle were sampled.

Entomological survey

Tsetse population and other flies were sampled using NGU traps deployed for 24 h at two sites and baited with acetone and 3 weeks old cow urine (Brightwell et al., 1992). All odors were placed on the ground about 15 cm up wind of the traps. The traps polls were greased to avoid the entry of insect predators like ants. Fly challenge has been taken as the product of the relative density of tsetse flies, their trypanosome infection rate and the proportion of feed that they have taken from domestic livestock. Site selection was done to include suitable tsetse habitats like savannah area, river valley, livestock grazing area and watering points and vicinity to assumed wild game reserve areas.

Parasitological survey

Blood samples were collected randomly from ear vein by using sterile blood lancet and capillary tubes. A capillary tube were filled with blood from animals to ¾ of their height and sealed at one end with crystal seal. The capillary tubes were loaded on the microhaematocrit centrifuge symmetrically and centrifuge at 1200 rpm for 5 min (Murray et al., 1977). Packed cell volume (PCV) was determined using haematocrit reader (Woo, 1969). After the PCV was read, capillary tubes were broken 1 mm below the buffy coat to include the RBC layer and the content were expressed on microscopic slide and mixed and cover with a 22 × 22 mm cover slip and examined under 40x objectives (Murray et al., 1977). From positive samples thin blood smears were made, fixed with methanol for 5 min and stained with geimsa solution for 30 min and examined using oil emersion under 100 x objectives to identify the species of trypanosomes.

Data management and analysis

Data collected from vector fly and trypanosomosis infection survey were entered into Microsoft excel spread sheet and analyzed using

Table 1. Tsetse flies and tabanides catches during the study period.

Altitude (m.a.s.l)	Traps deployed site description	No. of traps	Tsetse spp. flies/trap/day	Biting flies spp. flies/trap/day		
			G. pallideps	Tabanus	Stomoxys	Haematopota
1062	Drainage lines of the Gojeb river*	8	9.5	0.5	1.875	0.375
1546	bush**, acacia and short grass	8	7.4	0.125	0.875	0.25

*, Trap positioned at watering; **, trap positioned at grazing area.

Table 2. Species of trypanosomosis involved in disease process in each PAs.

Pas	Animals		Trypanosomosis species				Prevalence (%)
	Examined	Infected	T.c	T.v	T.b	Mixed	
Biteti	84	10	5	5	0	0	11.9
Kecharoba	76	11	5 (45.5%)	3 (27.3%)	2 (18.2%)	1 (9.0%)	14.5
Kerara	80	7	3 (42.8%)	2 (28.6%)	1 (14.3%)	1 (14.3%)	8.75
Chida	81	12	9 (75.0%)	3 (25.0%)	0	0	14.8
Mareka	79	8	6(75.0%)	2 (25.0%)	0	0	10.1

T.c, Trypanosoma congolense; T.v, Trypanosoma vivax; T.b, Trypanosoma brucei.

statically software program SPSS. Descriptive statics like percentage can be used to determine prevalence of trypanosomosis and chi- square (χ^2) used to evaluate the associations with different risk factors. In the analysis, confidence level was held at 95% and p<0.05 was set for significance.

RESULTS

Hematological findings

Considering anemia as one of the major signs of a herd infected with trypanosomosis, the anemic status of sampled animals was assessed by measuring the mean packed cell volume. The range of PCV value in parasitaemic was 12 to 30% and aparasitaemic 18 to 40%. Out of total 48 trypanosome positive cattle, 87.5% had PCV value was less than 26 and 12.5% of positive were found having normal PCV (Table 4).

Entomological survey

Tsetse flies found during the survey were only *G. pallidipes*. This species were registered at suspected fly habitat of kerara PAs and around Gojeb River which is watering points for farmers near and away from the river. Biting flies like tabanides also caught along with tsetse flies. The mean catch of *G. pallidipes* at kerara PAs was 7.4 flies/trap/day whereas around Gojeb River was 9.5 flies/trap/day and an overall apparent density was 8.45 flies /trap/day. A total of 167 flies were caught out of which *G. pallidipes* accounted 80.8% and tabanide accounted 13.2%. *G. pallidipes* were abundant at high gallery forest and valley flanks along the drainage lines of the river which is 59.3% whereas 43.7% flies were caught at Kerara PAs which tsetse are more suspected habitat were the vegetation dominated by thorny bush, short grass and dispersed acacia species (Table 1).

Parasitological survey

Overall trypanosome prevalence cattle in the 5 PAs were 12%. The dominant trypanosome species was *T. congolense* (60.8%) followed by *T. bruci* 3 (6.25%), *T. vivax* (29.17%) and mixed infection (*T. bruci* and *T. vivax*) 4.2% (Table 2). Almost similar prevalence of trypanosomosis was registered at the different study sites Table 3.

DISCUSSION

The disease trypanosomosis is the main important livestock constraint impeding the agricultural activity and livestock productivity. It was stated that trypanosomosis is the main cause of decline in the number of cattle and particularly draught oxen (Abebe and Jobre, 1996). The overall trypanosome prevalence in study area was 12% (Table 3). This result was comparable with works different scholars: Twelde (2001) who reports (15%) at Keto settlement area south western Ethiopia; Habtewold (1993 and 1995) at Humbo larena of Wolaita zone (9.3%) and at Konso wereda (11.5%). But, slightly lower than the finding of Afework (1998) at Pawe, North-west Ethiopia (17.2%), Abebe and Jobere (1996) for tsetse infested

Table 3. Prevalence of trypanosomosis in selected PAs of Konta special Woreda.

Name of surveyed PAS	No. of samples	Total positive	Prevalence (%)
Biteti	84	10	11.9
Kecharoba	76	11	14.4
Kerara	80	7	8.75
Chida	81	12	14.8
Mareka	79	8	10.12
Total	400	48	12

Table 4. Hematological findings.

PAs	Sample size	Mean PCV value (%)	% Cattle with PCV<26	% Cattle with PCV ≥ 26	Range
Biteti	84	24.96	48.81	51.19	14-36
Kecharoba	76	24.75	56.58	43.42	12-38
Kerara	80	24.33	62.50	37.50	17-40
Chida	81	25.90	29.63	70.37	13-37
Mareka	79	27.97	26.57	73.42	18-38

area of Ethiopia (17.67%). The study result also revealed that majority of infection (60.4%) were due to *T. congolense* a comparable results was reported by different researches who reported *T. congolense* in different parts of Ethiopia: Muturi (1999) at Merab Abaya, south west Ethiopia (66.1%), Afework et al., (2001) at Pawe, North west Ethiopia (60.9%) and Abebe and Jobre (1996) for tsetse infested area of Ethiopia (58.5%).

The results of present study showed an overall apparent density of *G. pllidipes* 8.45 flies/trap/day (Table 1) which was greater density than 1.9 and 1.0 in the late and dry season, respectively, reported by Masangi (1999) in the south rift valley of Ethiopia. This could suggest an absolute increase in the number of tsetse flies due to favorable environment has enough moisture, vegetation growth and suitable habitat or spread of flies from the rivers where they usually inhibit during day season to more open areas there by increasing relative density.

The present findings indicated that the tsetse fly distribution along the two altitudinal level (1062 m.a.s.l) was different from another (1546 m.a.s.l) irrespective of the areas indicating that the catch was decreasing with the increasing altitude (Table 1). This was in agreement with the previous work done in Ethiopia by Verysen et al., (1999) who found a significant high catch (over 93%) in altitude between 1100 and 1400 m.a.s.l level in the southern rift valley of Ethiopia.

Present finding reported 1.5% of the parasitaemic and 53.75% of the aparasitaemic animals PCV values was greater than or equal to 26% this result was in agree well with the result obtained by Rowland's et al. (2001) at Ghibe valley in the south western Ethiopia, in which he indicated that as the proportion of samples detected parasitaemic increased, PCV value decreased.

CONCLUSION AND RECOMMENDATIONS

The results of the present study revealed that trypanosomosis is the most important problem for agricultural activity and animal production at study area of Konta special wereda in SNNPRS. One species tsetse flies *G. pallidipes* and biting flies such as tabanids were caught in the study area. Based on the conclusions made above the following recommendations are forwarded:

1. Designing and implementing of control strategies of trypanosomosis focusing on applying integrated approach (vector control and chemotherapy).

2. Further studies on the epidemiological aspects and development of drug resistance in pathogenic trypanosome are required.
3. Awareness creation about the disease and its transmission.

REFERENCES

Abebe G, Jobere Y (1996). Trypanomosis: A threat to cattle production in Ethiopia Revue de Médecine Vétérinaire 147(12):897-902.
Afework Y (1998). Field investigation on the appearance Drug resistant population of Trypanosomes in Metekel District, North-west Ethiopia. MSc thesis, Addis Ababa University and Freie University Berlin.

Afework Y, Clausen PH, Abebe G, Tilahun G, Dieter M (2001). Appearance of multiple drug resistant trypanosome population in village cattle of Metkel District. North West Ethiopia. Livestock community and environment. Proceedings of the 10th Copenhagen Denmark. pp. 1-2.

Brightwell R, Dransfield RD, Korku CA, Golder TK, Tarimo SA, Mugani D (1992). A new trap for *Glossina Pallidipes*. Trop. Pest Manag. 33:151-159.

Dagnchew Z, shafo K (1981). An investigation of dourine in Arsi administrative region. Ethiope. Vet. Bull. 4:3-9.

Eneyew M (1997). Bovine Trypanosomiasis in south Gonder administrative Zone bordering Lake Tana, Ethiopia in the apparent absence of glossina J. Ethiop. Vet. Assoc. 1(1):19-34.

Habtewold T (1993). Bovine Trypanosomiasis in wolita: prevalence and assessment of drug efficacy. AAU, Faculty of Veterinary Medicine, Debre Zeit, DVM Thesis.

Habtewold T (1995). Community based tsetse and trypanosomosis control pilot programme using deltamethrin in Konso, Southern, Ethiopia. Proceeding of 11th Conference of the Ethiopia Veterinary Association, Addis Abeba, and Ethiopia. pp. 57-65.

Jordan AM (1986). The role of tsetse in Africa animal trypanosomomsis. In Livestock production in tsetse affected area of Africa. Proceedings of a meeting held in Nairobi, (ILCA/ILRAD). pp. 37-41.

Langridge W (1976). A tsetse and trypanosomosis survey of Ethiopia. Ministry of agricultural of Ethiopia. Addis Abeba, Ethiopia. pp. 96-98.

Leak SGA, Mulatu W, Authie E, d'Iletern GDM, Peregrine AS, Rowlands GJ, Trail JCM (1993). Epidemiology of bovine trypanosomosis in the Ghibe valley, South west Ethiopia. Acta Trop. 53:124-133.

Ministry of Agriculture (MoA) (1995). Ethiopia Ruminant Livestock Development Strategy Addis Abeba, Ethiopia. pp. 112-113.

Msangi S (1999). Distribution, Density and Infection rates of tsetse flies in selected sites of Southern Rift valley of Ethiopia. MSc thesis, Addis Ababa University Faculty of Veterinary Medicine, Ethiopia.

Murray M, Murray PK, McIntyre WI (1977). An improved parasitological technique for the diagnosis of Africa trypanosomosis. Trans. R. Soc. Trop. Med. Hyg. 71:325-326.

Muturi KS (1999). Epidemiology of bovine trypanosomosis in selected sites of the southern rift valley of Ethiopia. MSc Thesis, Addis Ababa University.

Rowlands GH, Leak SGA, Peregrine AS, Nagda SM, Mulatu W, d'Iteren GDM (2001). The incidence of new and the prevalence and persistence of recurrent trypanosome infection. Acta Trop. 79(2):149-163.

Singh V, Singla LD (2012). Trypanosomosis in cattle and buffaloes from latent carrier status to clinical form of disease: Indian scenario. In: *Integrated* Research Approaches in Veterinary Parasitology, Shanker D, Tiwari J, Jaiswal AK and Sudan V (Eds), Bytes & Bytes Printers, Bareily. pp. 10-18.

Sumbria D, Singla LD (2016). Human atypical trypanosomosis in Indian subcontinent. *Veterinaria* 4(1):7-10.

Tewlde N (2001). Study on the occurrence of the drug resistant Trypanosomes in cattle in the farming tsetse control area (FITCA) project in western Ethiopia MSc thesis, Addis Ababa University and Freie Universitat, Berlin.

Thrusfield MV (1995). Veterinary Epidemology. 2nd edition. Blackwell Science, Oxford. P 83.

Vreysen MJ, Mebrate A, Menjeta M, Bancha B, Woldeyes G, Musie K, Bekele K, Aboset G (1999). The Distribution Relative abundance of tsetse flies in the southern rift valley of Ethiopia: *International Scientific council for Trypanosomosis Research and control* (ISCTRC). 120:202-213.

Woo PJK (1969). The hematological centrifugation technique for the detection of trypanosomes. Can. Vet. J. 200(47):921-923.

Health and welfare status of donkeys in and around Hawassa Town, Southern Ethiopia

Agegnehu Ashinde*, Abebaw Gashaw and Nejash Abdela

School of Veterinary Medicine, College of Agriculture and Veterinary Medicine, Jimma University, Jimma, P. O. Box. 307, Jimma, Ethiopia.

A cross-sectional study was conducted from November 2016 to April 2017 with the objective of assessing the welfare situation and identifying major health problem of donkeys in association with risk factors identification using physical examination and questionnaire survey in and around Hawassa town, Southern Ethiopia. Three hundred and eighty four donkeys were physically examined for health related and management problems and three hundred and eighty four donkey owners and cart drivers were interviewed for awareness and welfare assessment in the study area. Out of the total 384 donkeys, the prevalence of wound, lameness, skin problem, other illness signs, eye problem, dental problem and change on visible mucous membrane were found in 47.7, 38.8 36.2, 14.3, 9.4, 7.6 and 6.3%, respectively. Statistically significant ($p<0.05$) association was observed between the occurrence of wound and age, type of work, duration of work and body condition of the study animals. The prevalence of wound in old age groups, poor body conditioned animals, donkeys that transport construction material and those working for more than 10 h were 76.6, 74.6, 71.2 and 93.8%, respectively. Furthermore, the welfare problems association with donkey users' ownership status, age, and educational status were assessed and 51.3% of cart drivers' owners, 47.1% young drivers and 62.2% had educational status under grade four and have little experience on handling working donkeys. Out of 384 respondents, 63.2% were not aware of common animal welfare freedoms. The health and welfare problems of cart pulling donkeys in the study area were created and complicated with multiple influential factors. The whole community should participate on awareness creation, introduction of improved design of harnesses and carts, also training on animal welfare to owners should be given to reduce health and welfare problems on donkeys.

Key words: Donkeys, health problems, risk factors, welfare, wound.

INTRODUCTION

The donkey (*Equus asinus*) is believed to be the first member of the Equidae family that was domesticated (Rossel et al., 2008). The world donkey population is estimated to about 44 million; half is found in Asia, just

*Corresponding author. E-mail: agegnehuashinde@gmail.com.

over one quarter in Africa and the rest mainly in Latin America (Fielding and Starkey, 2004). Ethiopia has the largest population of donkeys in Africa and the second largest donkey population in the world next to China (Kumar et al., 2014).

Equines are important animals to the resource poor communities in rural and urban areas of Ethiopia, providing traction power and transport services at low cost. The use of equines in door-to-door transport service also provides urban dwellers with the opportunity of income generation. The majority of the income generation product of equines mainly comes from donkeys (Biffa and Woldemeskel, 2006; Tesfaye et al., 2016; Abdela et al., 2017; Genetu et al., 2017). Donkeys are one of the most important domestic animals most intimately associated with humans. They contribute a lot through their involvement in different social and economic sectors (Ayele et al., 2006). The donkey is harder than the horse, survives with much less attention, drives sustenance from poor quality food and can tolerate considerable heat and dehydration. This makes it a suitable animal for harsh environments and difficult working conditions. Its main role is that of a beast of burden, typically transporting materials such as grains, fuel wood, water, crop and building materials (Kiros et al., 2016).

Since these animals are working animal, they are always expected to undergo suffering in their day to day life due to stress, strain due to overwork, fatigue due to working with poor health, feed, nutrition and drinking water. Pains are due to unscientific ill-fitting equipments, harness devices, poorly designed agricultural equipments and carts. Non availability of proper veterinary care, working under hot and dusty environment, lack of proper shelter, care and management, crude castration, restraining and tethering devices, walking long distances and overloading, poor handling during loading and unloading and inhumane slaughter is common. Most of the animal owners are not even aware of animal welfare practices and as a result, animals have to undergo significant suffering due to improper handling, transport and husbandry practices (Biswas et al., 2013).

The animal welfare is being compromised due to several constraints such as poverty and lack of knowledge. Research conducted in Ethiopia demonstrated that improvements in the welfare of donkeys had significantly improved their work output which in turn improved livelihood situations of the poorest communities in the rural and peri-urban areas (Smith, 2003). The welfare of working donkeys in developing countries is therefore crucially important, not only for the health and survival of those animals, but also for the livelihoods of those people dependent on them (Wilson, 2002; Pearson and Krecek, 2006).

The causes of poor welfare outcomes frequently identified for working animals include poor nutrition, poor harness design and use, overwork and inappropriate management practices, such as beating and working animals at too young an age. Additional related problems include wounds, lameness, colic in equids and preventable infectious disease. Initiating factors are usually multi-layered. They include traditional or cultural beliefs and economic constraints. Cultural factors can include traditional beliefs in harmful practices such as nostril-slitting and firing. Economic factors commonly constrain marginalized communities from accessing resources such as feed and water, good harnessing and carts, quality shoes, shelter, and health care for their working animals, which all have a direct impact on animal welfare (Rahman and Reed, 2014).

As any other animals, donkeys are vulnerable to a variety of disease of biological origin, nutritional diseases and other miscellaneous cause that leads them to ill health, suffering, considerable loss of work output and reduced longitivity (Gebreab and Fanta, 2007). In countries like Ethiopia they are subjected to a variety of health disorder including multi-parasitism, back sore and other wounds due to different causes, hoof problems, colic, various infectious diseases such as strangles, tetanus and others. Feed shortage and disease are the major constraints to productivity and work performance of equines. The major and common clinical manifestations of disease which affect organs of support are lameness, failure of support, insufficiency of movement and deformity (Amene et al., 2015).

They are brutally treated, made to work overtime without adequate feed or healthcare. They suffer from lack of shelter from sun, rain or biting insects at markets or working sites. These have a potential to negatively affect their welfare and quality of life. This was justified by low number of donkeys presented annually to the clinic compared to other domestic animals; 270 donkeys vs. 20,000 head of other domestic animals such as cattle, between 1987 and 1988 (Yilma et al., 1991).

According to recent central statistical agency (CSA, 2013), there are about 2.03 million horses, 7.43 million donkeys, 0.4 million mules, and about 1.16 million camels in the sedentary areas of the country. In Ethiopia the use of donkeys as pack animal or for pulling cart has enabled small scale farmers to participate in the market economy. Donkeys are used for fetching water, for household shifting, for carrying the sick to hospital, for carrying sick calves, for transportation, and for pulling materials needed for construction. Probably one of the most important limitations is the general lack of information on the proper management and welfare problems of donkeys, which leads them to receive minimum care. Donkey has spent hundreds of years being used by man but, despite that only little attempt has been made to study any aspect of this animal until recently and particularly in countries where they are most important (Amene et al., 2015).

Even though donkeys are used as the source of income generation and provides invaluable and cheap energy for the whole communities in the study area, their health and welfare situation are compromised through poor husbandry practices, lack of animal welfare knowledge, problem of the daily income of drivers, absence of legislation policy for working animal and poor design harness material. In Hawassa and its surrounding, large population of cart pulling donkeys are found, but their health and welfare situation show that they suffer from multi-factor life threatening problems. Therefore this study was planned with the following objectives: to assess welfare situation of cart pulling donkeys in Hawassa town and also to identify major health problems and associated risk factors of the Donkeys in the study area.

MATERIALS AND METHODS

Study area

The study was carried out in and around Hawassa Town, Southern Nations, Nationalities and Peoples of Southern Ethiopia. Hawassa is situated at 275 km South of Addis Ababa (the capital of Ethiopia) at latitude between 6°83' to 7°17' N and longitude 38°24' to 38°72' E on the escarpment of the Great Rift Valley along the Addis Ababa Moyale highway. The altitude ranges from 1650 to 1700 m above sea level. The annual average rainfall and temperature are 955 mm and 20.3°C, respectively. Hawassa is the capital of South nation, nationalities and people region (SNNPR) and has eight sub cities, namely Addis Ketema, Mehal, Menariya, Misrak, Hayk Dar, Behal Adarash, Tabor and Hawela Tula sub cities. The population of donkey (Equus asinus), mule (Equus hemonious) and horse (Equus cabalis) of Hawassa city are 13961, 369, and 5161, respectively (CSA, 2008). A total of five areas of Hawassa were included in the study (Aroge Gebeya, Adis Gebeya, Atena Tera, Alamura Sefer and Hawela Tula Gebeya).

Study animals and sampling procedure

Working donkeys (384) which were used for cart pulling to transport different material were sampled. Working donkeys of all age groups from different localities in and around Hawassa city were randomly selected for the study. The breed of the donkeys were local breed called Abyssinia type with the characteristic feature of short, compact, lower feed requirement and easily manageable. The assessment of welfare and health was done with the corresponding risk factors such as age, behavior, body condition, lameness, harnessing condition, wound distribution and types of wound. Animals were physically examined for their health and problems associated to welfare and owners or cart drivers were interviewed with structured/semi-structured questionnaires.

Sample size and sampling method

A total of 384 donkeys were randomly selected for physical examination and questionnaire survey. The sample size has been determined according to the formula given by Thrusfield (2007) based on expected prevalence of 50%. Based on simple random sampling methods and 95% confidence interval with required 5% precision, the sample size was determined as:

$$N = Z^2 \times Pexp\,[1-Pexp] / d^2$$

Where, N= required sample size, Z= the Z-value at 95% confidence level, Pexp=expected prevalence=50%, and d= required precision.

Study design and methodology

A cross sectional study was carried out on cart pulling donkeys found in five selected areas of in and around Hawassa city. The sites were selected purposively based on their accessibility, easy of logistic and number of donkey populations in the area. The sites were Aroge gebeya, Adis gebeya, Atena tera, Alamura sefer and Hawela Tula gebeya. Donkeys were randomly selected, all are indigenous breeds irrespective of age, sex and body condition score to investigate the health and welfare situation and associated risk factors.

Data collection

Direct assessment

A structured direct assessment format was developed and data was collected by direct physical examination of the animals. Prior to the assessment, consent was obtained from animal's owners or users after explaining the objective of the study. If the animal owner is not willing, then opportunity was given to the next willing animal owner. The same procedure was continued steadily until the sample size was attained throughout the study period. All sampled animals were physically restrained by animal owner and causal worker. Mouth was thoroughly examined for the presence of any feed pack on teeth. If there is feed pack, the tooth is removed so as not to interfere with age estimation and also cause abnormal teeth identification.

Information regarding general health parameters such as: type of wound, anatomical distribution of wound/physical injuries, lameness, skin problems, problems of visible mucus membrane, and eye conditions and other signs of illness were properly recorded on data collection format. Assessment was carried out at field level, market and around homestead on the day time. Animals were allowed to stand for maximum 10 min after being held by head collar and lead rope assessment began, without causing major disturbance to donkey routine work.

Age determination

Age of the animal was estimated based on the observation of the animal's front teeth (Incisors) (Crane, 1997). Accordingly, the study animals were categorized into three age groups as less than 5 years, 5 to 10 years, and above 10 years. Dental abnormalities were also observed and recorded. But for the ease of study simplification and absence of donkeys that are too old, this study took three age categories as <5, 5-10 and >10 that are considered as young, adult and old, respectively.

Wound assessment

Body lesions were then recorded with regard to type of wound and anatomical location as wither sore, back sore, tail and tail base

Table 1. Age, body condition score and behavior of study animal (n=384).

Variable		Frequency	Percentage
Age	Less than 5 years	51	13.3
	Between 5 to 10 years	218	56.8
	Above 10 years	115	29.9
BCS	Poor	63	16.4
	Medium	186	48.4
	Good	135	35.2
Behavior	Anxious	7	1.8
	Friendly approach	120	31.3
	Friendly not approach	13	3.4
	Depressed	87	22.7
	No response	142	37
	Tail tuck	9	2.3
	Biting	6	1.6

BCS: body condition score.

sore, girth sore, neck sore, chest sore, mouth-commissure sore, head sore, and other sore in study animal.

Body condition of animal

Body condition score was done according to the criteria described by Pritchard et al. (2005) and animals were examined from all sides. The donkey body condition was scored as 0 to 5 (0 = very thin, 1 = thin, 2 = fair, 3 = good, 4 = fat and 5 = very fat). However, for the purpose of data analysis, body conditions 0 to 5 were categorized into three distinct groups: categories 0, 1 and 2 were grouped as "poor", category 3 was defined as "medium" and body condition scores 4 and 5 were categorized as "Good".

Demeanor of the animal

The behaviors of all animal sampled were assessed as anxious, friendly approach, not friendly approach, depressed, no response, tail tuck and biting which involve an observation of general alertness versus unresponsiveness to the environment to correlate these behaviors with physical problem and diseases (Morka et al., 2014).

Indirect welfare assessment

Semi-structured questionnaire was developed to collect data on the major constraints health and welfare considering use of donkeys, veterinary service, disease management system, management practice (feeding, watering, health care, shelter and resting time), working nature (duration on work, weight carried, length of journey covered, nature of working environment), educational status, and age of donkey cart drivers and other people working on animal. Accordingly, 384 people were interviewed to generate information which was missed during direct assessments of the animal.

Data management and analysis

The data collected from the 384 donkeys and interviews made with 384 drivers were entered into Microsoft excel spread sheet and analyzed using SPSS version 20 statistical software. Descriptive statistics were used to quantify the problems and Chi-square (χ^2) was used to determine the association of the problem with the risk factors. In all calculations, the confidence interval was set at 95% and statistical significant differences were considered as $p<0.05$.

RESULTS

Direct assessment results

The direct assessment data was collected by assessing age, work type, body condition, different wound types, distribution of wound, behavior, causes of lameness, origin of lameness, degree of lameness, dental problem, skin problem, mucous membrane problem, and other illness signs observed from the examined donkeys. For the 384 studied animals, results for the distribution of age, body condition and behavior are illustrated in Table 1.

During the study period, the donkeys were thoroughly examined for type of wound and distribution of wound. Out of 384 donkeys sampled, 183 of them were found to be wounded; the overall prevalence of wound was 47.7% (Table 2).

Out of 183 wound exposed donkeys, 56.3% were found with abrasion, 24% were positive with laceration, 13.7% had puncture, and 6% were affected with incision wound (Figure 1).

From the examined donkeys, many health problems were identified with thorough examination of the sampled animal. Out of 384 examined for other illness signs,

Table 2. Wounds identified during the study period and their anatomical distribution.

Wound distribution	Frequency	Percentage	Overall prevalence (%)
Wither sore	48	8.7	
Back sore	62	11.2	
Tail/Tail base sore	17	3.1	
Girth/Belly sore	23	4.2	
Chest sore	16	3	
Ribs/Flank sore	32	5.8	
Loin sore/croup sore	7	2.26	47.7
Knee sore	4	0.72	
Hock sore	4	0.72	
Mouth-commissure sore	28	5.07	
Foreleg other than knee	5	1	
Hindquarter other than hock	3	0.5	
Lip lesion	6	1.1	
Head sore	4	0.72	

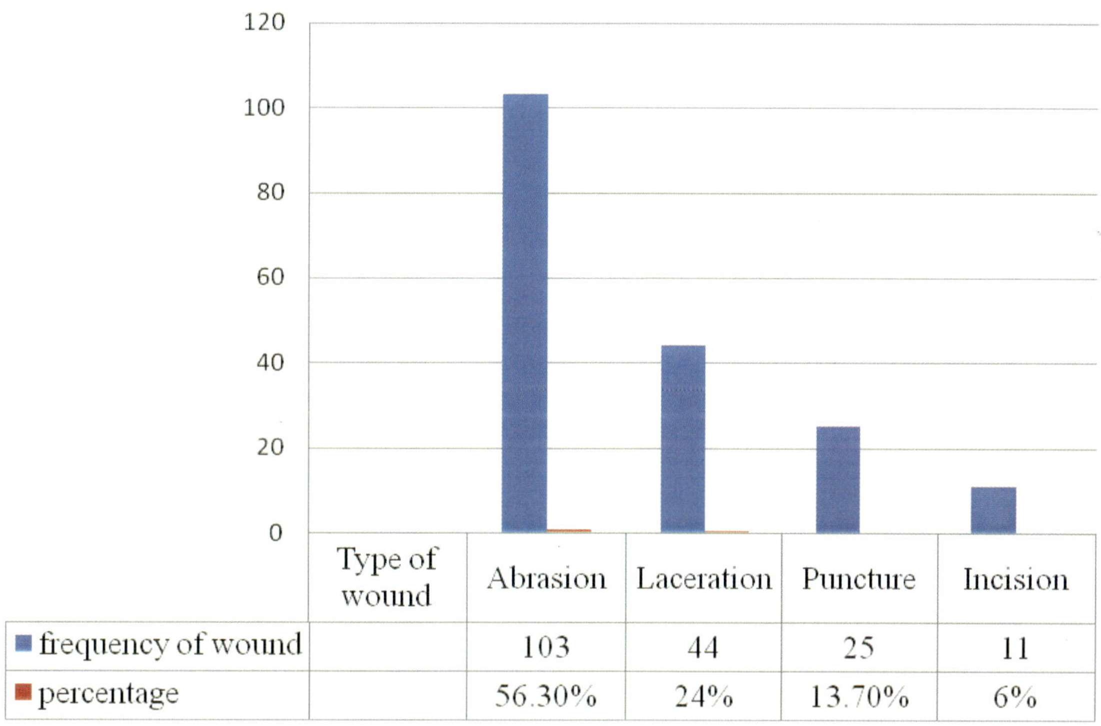

Figure 1. Wound type identified during study period.

14.3% (55) donkeys were positive for other illness signs. For the dental problem examined, 7.6% (29) donkeys had dental problem. The abnormality on visible mucous membrane was found in 6.3% (24) donkeys.

Eye problems were found in 9.4% (36) donkeys. The skin problem was one of the major finding constraints. Out of 384 examined donkeys, 139 (36.2%) were affected. In the study area, donkeys have crucial importance to the transportation of goods. However, lameness is the main problem affecting transport services of the donkeys in the study area. From the total examined donkeys, 38.8% (149) were found with lameness problem. Table 3 illustrates the other illness signs, dental problem, skin problem, eye problem, change on visible

Table 3. General health problem encountered.

Encountered health problem	Number affected	Prevalence (%)	Overall prevalence (%)
Other illness signs			
Coughing	12	3.1	
Discharges from nostril	11	2.9	
Fever	3	0.8	
Listlessness	2	0.5	
Constipation	7	1.8	14.3
Diarrhea	6	1.6	
Refuse to move	8	2.1	
Refuse to eat	4	1	
Swollen belly	2	0.5	
Dental problem			
Overbite problem	9	2.3	
Periodental disease	13	3.4	7.6
Diastema	7	1.8	
Visible mucous membrane			
Pale	11	2.9	6.3
Congested	13	3.4	
Eye problem			
Lacrimination	17	4.4	
Inflammation	9	2.3	9.4
Loss of vision	2	0.5	
Swelling	8	2.1	
Skin problem			
Rough hair coat	73	19	
Alopecia	16	4.2	
Sarcoid	4	1.0	
Habronemiasis	7	1.8	36.2
Ectoparasites	21	5.5	
Loss of elasticity	18	4.7	
Degree of lameness			38.8
Low grade	67	17.4	
Moderate grade	58	15.1	
High grade	24	6.3	
Causes of lameness			
Hoof problem	77	51.7	
Wound	32	21.5	
Fracture	37	24.8	
Arthritis	3	2	
Origin of lameness			
Above knee	55	37	
Below knee	56	37.5	
Above hock	16	10.7	
Below hock	22	14.8	

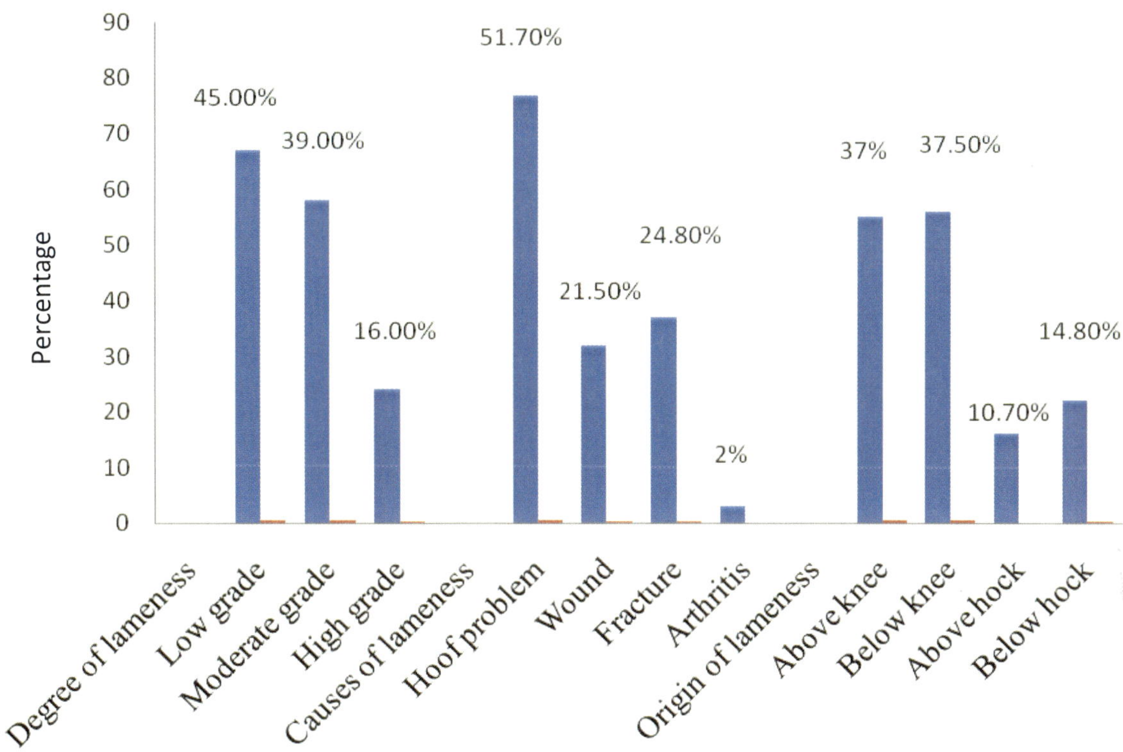

Figure 2. Grade of lameness, factors that cause lameness and origin of lameness.

mucous membrane problem, degree of lameness and origin of lameness, and causes of lameness. In Figure 2, the grade, causes of lameness and origin of lameness are shown.

The prevalence of wound associated with different age groups were examined and the statistical association reflects that the donkeys between five and up to 10 years had high prevalence of wound than the age groups of below five and above 10 year (χ^2 =10.745, P-value=0.005). The prevalence of wound with body condition of the donkeys are highly significant in poor body conditioned donkeys (χ^2=21.971, P=0.00). Also, there was a statistically significant association observed (χ^2=63.883, P-value=0.000) for prevalence of wound with the type of work animal used. The prevalence of wound is strongly associated (χ^2=89.817, P-value=0.000) with duration on work and the donkeys worked above 10 h (Table 4).

Result of questioner survey

Out of a total of 384 interviewed, 51.3% (197) of the respondents are owners of donkeys and 48.7% (187) respondents were not the owners. Age distribution of drivers was 47.1% (181) young, 44.8% (172) adult, and 8.1% (31) old. The drivers educational status were 62.2% (239) below grade four, 32.8% (126) between grade 5 and up to 8, and 5% (19) above grade eight. The survey of experience of working year using this animal were 29.7% below one year, 35.9% one to two years and 34.4% above two years (Figure 3).

Out of the total respondents, 63.2% (243) were not aware of animal welfare, 27.9% were not aware of freedom from thirst and hungry, and 8.9% were not aware of freedom from injury and disease. The animal welfare knowledge source was veterinarian (16.7%), radio programme (9.6%), their friends (3.4%) and world animal day (7%). The drivers' responses about care for sick animal were 43.2% (166) taken to Government Veterinary Clinic or private clinic, 34.4% (132) given traditional medication and 22.4% (86) left to self-healing. Out of the total respondents, 90.4% (347) owners were forced to use their donkeys that had wound and only 9.6% (37) owners use their donkeys after wound healed. In the study area, 81.6% (313) did not get any training or consultation about animal welfare from Veterinarian and only 18.4% (71) cart drivers were trained on animal welfare and management. The opinion of respondents about responsibility for donkey health and welfare assessed and their response were 42.4% veterinarian, 32% owner, and 25.6% government. Also, respondents reflects different standing on severe diseased or old

Table 4. Prevalence of wound based on the age group, BCS groups, type of work, and duration on work and harnessing condition.

Category	Number of examined	Number of affected	Prevalence (%)	χ^2	p-value
Age of animal					
below 5 years	51	29	7.6		
Between 5 and 10 years	218	88	22.9	10.745	0.005
Above 10 years	115	66	17.2		
BCS					
Poor	63	47	74.6		
Medium	186	78	41.9	21.971	0.000
Good	135	58	43		
Type of work					
Multipurpose	140	78	55.7		
Construction material	104	74	71.2		
Wood and charcoal	48	9	8.8	63.883	0.000
Flour from mill house and farm products	64	14	21.9		
Garbage	28	8	28.6		
Duration on work					
Less than 6 h	45	10	22.2		
6 up to 10 h	259	98	37.8	89.817	0.000
Above 10 h	80	75	93.8		
Harness condition					
Tire rope	166	80	48.2	0.034	0.854
Mill rope	218	103	47.2		

donkey not used for work purpose: out of 384 respondents, 62.5% (240) owners showed their response to leave out of home and 37.5% (144) owners keep their severed diseased or old aged donkeys not used for work purpose at their home (Table 5).

The questionnaire survey result of 384 donkeys drivers and owners interviewed from five selected areas indicated that all animal owners do provide water and feed to donkeys at home and working places, out of 384; only 70.3% (270) provide shelter to donkeys at their home and 29.7% (114) of the owners of cart donkeys in and around Hawassa city reflected that they could not provide shelter at home specially at night and they keep their donkeys in fenced compound without any shade paying off fee; this is due to the fact that the owners do not have their own house and live in rented homes as a result of this, donkeys were exposed to different welfare problems. 41.4% fed their donkeys three times per day and 58.6% fed their donkeys twice in day. The owners fed their donkeys depending on the income they got daily and availability of feeding material (Table 6).

DISCUSSION

In Hawassa, all donkeys are kept to transport different materials in order to insure their owners' daily income. This study is in agreement with reports by Usman et al. (2015), Solomon et al. (2013) and Pritchard et al. (2005) describing that equids are mainly kept for transport purposes and only rarely as source of meat or milk. The current study revealed that 100% of the owners were using their animals for transportation or carrying load for more than 6 h a day in average which is in agreement with Biswas et al. (2013) and Panwar et al. (2008).

In this study area, 47.7% donkeys population had overall prevalence of wound, 56.3% were found with abrasion, 24% were positive with laceration, 13.7% had puncture and 6% were affected with incision wound. Similarly, the finding of Fikru et al. (2015) reported that 50.6% of abrasion wound was examined from the same study area. During the study period, the wound was classified depending on the anatomical distribution and result indicated that the high frequency of back, wither, ribs/flank, mouth-commissure, tail/tail base and chest wound were examined. The current study agreed with those of Helen (2001) who reported similar situation in the Northern Ethiopia and this higher prevalence of wound at the back region could be due to improper harnessing that cause injuries in working donkeys. Similarly, the present result also agrees with the previous report of Mandefro (2008), in which, those ill-fitting and

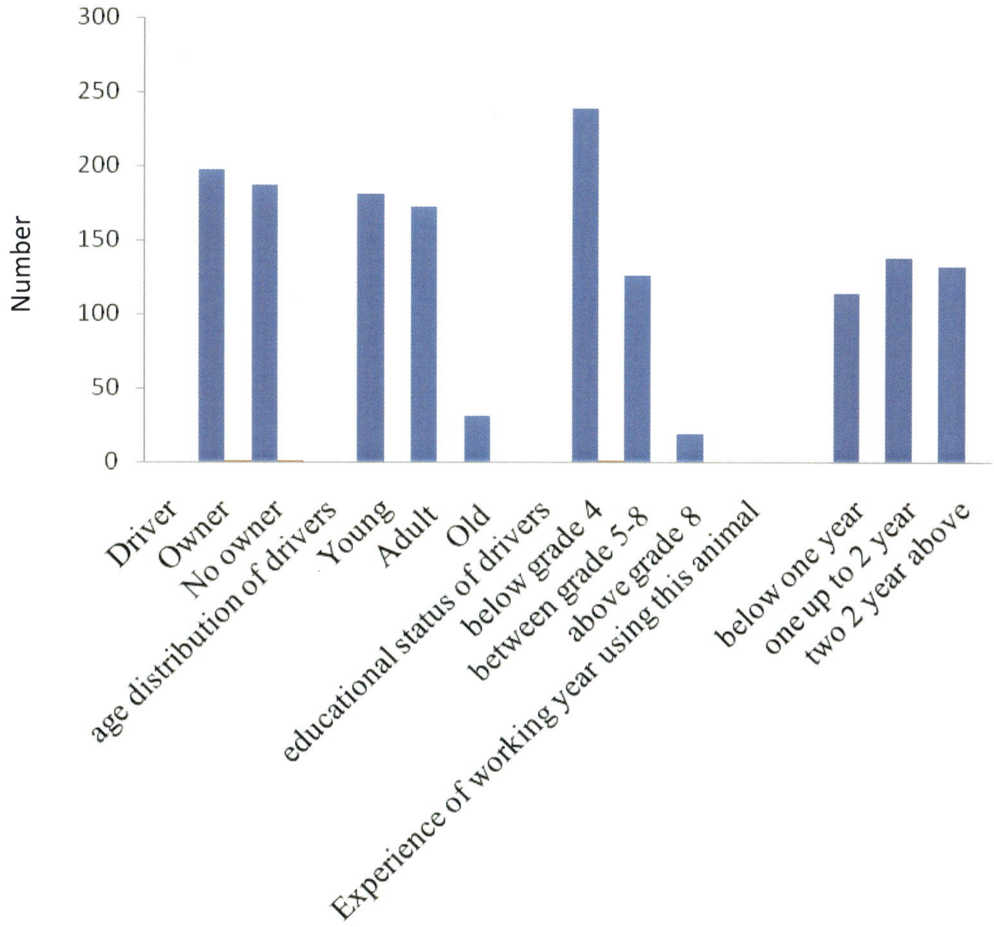

Figure 3. General status of cart drivers.

improperly made tail straps that usually has sharp edge, causes lesions on the underneath of the base of tail of working donkeys.

In current study, wound had higher prevalence than the reports of Morka et al. (2014) in and around Nekemte Town, East Wollega Zone (38.4%) and lower prevalence of donkey wound than the result of Fikru et al. (2015) and Biffa and Woldemeskel (2006) who revealed 63.4 and 79.4%, respectively. These differences might be due to variation in care for animal health, management practices, the weight of load and the work type of the donkeys in the region. All the donkeys examined for the present study were used for cart pulling purpose in the study area.

The current study revealed that higher prevalence of wound was examined in above 10 year old donkeys (48.1%) than other age groups. This finding is in line with those of Tesfaye et al. (2016) who reported 69.2% wound in older age groups than other age groups. This study agreed with reports of Biffa and Weldemeskel (2006) in Hawassa who reported that older equines had greater wound risk than other age group. This might be due to more exposure to work and carrying heavy load over a long distance, less owners' attention to wound management and also the immune defense mechanism also reduce with age advancement.

There was significant association between prevalence of wound and body condition (P=0.000) with 74.6% of poor body conditioned donkeys affected with wound. This result was found to be in agreement with the reports of Abdela et al. (2017), Tesfaye et al. (2016), Tsega et al. (2016) and Henneke et al. (1983) who reported strong association between prevalence of wound body condition. These might be due to dehydration which decreases the elasticity of the skin in poor body condition animals and the prominence of bones leading to easy skin injury.

In this study, the prevalence of wound and type of work donkeys regularly involved has significant association (p=0.000). The donkeys commonly used for transporting construction materials were found to be wounded (71.2%) than donkeys transporting other materials. This

Table 5. Responses of welfare knowledge of cart drivers (n=384).

Welfare issues	Frequency	Percentage
Owner's welfare knowledge		
Not aware	243	63.2
Freedom from thirst and hungry	107	27.9
Freedom from injury and disease	34	8.9
Freedom from pain and discomfort	0	0
Freedom to express normal behavior and enough space to move	0	0
Freedom from fear and distress	0	0
Awareness source		
Veterinarian	64	16.7
Radio programme	37	9.6
Their friends	13	3.4
World animal day	27	7
Care for sick animal		
Taking to vet clinic or private clinic	166	43.2
Traditional medication	132	34.4
Leave to self-healing	86	22.4
The owners use their animal while wounded		
No	37	9.6
Yes	347	90.4
Trained or consulted by veterinarian		
Not trained	313	81.6
Trained	71	18.4
Responsible for donkey		
Veterinarian	163	42.4
Owner	123	32
Government	98	25.6
Decision on severe diseased or old donkey not used for work purpose		
Leave out of home	240	62.5
Keep at home	144	37.5

is due to the transportation of highly loaded metals, sand, cement, stones and woods from far distance for long time without rest. This study is not in agreement with those of Tesfaye et al. (2016) in Mirab Abaya, Gamo Gofa and Kumar et al. (2014) in Mekele who reported that the highest prevalence was recorded in charcoal transporting donkeys (52.1%). This may be due to burning characters of charcoal and wider surface area of sack that lay on the back of the donkeys in which the whole surface not covered by proper harness leads to at least injury in one area of the anatomical location.

In the present study, the prevalence of skin and skin associated problems were found with overall prevalence (36.2%). These findings are higher than Mulisa et al. (2015) in Wolaita zuria (12.6%), Kumar et al. (2014) in Mekelle city (23.7%) and Tesfaye et al. (2016).

In the current study, eye problem and dental problem were identified as the health problem of the studied animals in the study area with overall prevalence, eye problem (9.4%) and dental problem (7.7%). This result disagrees with those of Tesfaye et al. (2016) in Mirab Abaya, Gamo Gofa zone with prevalence with unilateral eye problem (5.4%), bilateral eye problem (11.4%) and dental problems (11.5%). But these outcomes are lower

Table 6. Response of the respondents to the way of management; (n=384)

Respondent knowledge	Frequency	Proportion (%)
Feeding time		
Before loading	83	21.6
After loading	104	27.1
Both before and after loading	197	51.3
Feeding material		
Concentrates	283	73.7
Concentrates and sugar cane	55	14.3
Concentrates, grass and sugar cane	46	12
Feeding condition		
Separately feeding	271	70.6
Feeding with other animal	113	29.4
Feeding frequency		
Twice per day	225	58.6
Three times per day	159	41.4
Watering frequency		
Once per day	40	10.4
Twice per day	325	84.6
Three times per day	19	5
Presence of rest in week		
One day in week	273	71.1
Two day in week	77	20
No rest in week	34	8.9
Shelter		
Absent	114	29.7
Present	270	70.3

than that in the report of Kumar et al. (2014) in Mekelle city; 19.3% eye problem and 16.2% dental problem and higher than the report of Abutarbush et al. (2014) with 4% problem in Jordan. These differences might arise due to difference in topographical nature and misuse, low level of donkey health care keeping characteristics, feeding characteristics and age of working donkey.

The present study revealed that 77.6% of respondent provide care for their donkeys (43.2% taken to government veterinary clinic or private clinic and 34.4% traditional medication) and 22.4% left to self-healing. Also, most of the owners are forced to use their donkeys having wound (90.4%). The result is closely related with those of Tesfaye et al. (2016) in Mirab Abaya that showed 84.2% of the respondents provide care for their sick animal out of which 48.3% took donkey to nearby veterinary clinic.

In this study, the owners fed their donkeys depending on the income they got daily and availability of feed. The responses for supply water to animal were 10.4% once in day, 84.6% twice in day and 5% three times in day. The result of the study shows that 51.3% fed their donkeys both before and after loading at home and working places. However, in the report of Tesfaye et al. (2016), 48.3% provided feed before loading only.

The current study indicated that 70.3% provide shelter to donkeys at their home and 29.7% of the owners keep their donkeys in fenced compound without any shade paying off fee. This result agree with those of Morka et al. (2014) with 76.6% providing shelter to equine at home and 23.6% of the owners of cart horses in Nekemte town reflected that they could not provide shelter at home especially at night and they release them to the street or forest after work. This is due to the fact that to cover a wide range of role of equine, the owners do not have their own house and live in rented homes as a result of this, animals were exposed to predators', environmental factors, car accident and easily stolen by thieves.

Conclusion

The present study revealed that the cart pulling donkeys in and around Hawassa were faced the multi-factorial health and welfare problems. Poor design wood worked carts, no standard in harnessing equipment, absence of approved policy in working animals, poor animal welfare knowledge, dependence of daily income source on cart work, overloading, overworking and work types were major factors causing health and welfare problems. In the current study, abrasion, laceration, puncture and incision were the identified wound types. Furthermore, the distribution of wound on different body parts were assessed and back sore, wither sore, mouth-commissure sore, tail/tail base sore, ribs/flank sore, chest sore and girth/belly sore were the major wounds examined on working donkeys. Lameness problem, skin problem, other illness signs, and dental problems frequently occurred in donkey's health situation in this study area. Lack of awareness of animal welfare knowledge and less attention to husbandry practices to feeding management, housing condition, watering the donkeys, and heath care of animals were indicators of the minimum understanding of the health and welfare of this study population. These situations strongly call for awareness creation on animal welfare by government and charity organizations interested in animal welfare. The country should also have policy on working animal handling and management. The standardized harnessing equipment should be available in market. Moreover, the donkey sanctuary model carts should be used for all cart pulling donkeys.

REFERENCES

Abdela N, Teshome E, Hassan A, Deressa FB (2017). Prevalence and associated risk factors of equine wound in and around Asella town, South Eastern Ethiopia. J. Vet. Med. Anim. Health 9(4):63-71.

Abutarbush SM, Alqawasmeh DM, Shaheen ZH, Anani SF, Ledger MP (2014). Equine Diseases and Welfare in Jordan: A Retrospective Study (1261 cases). Jordan J. Agric. Sci. 10(3).

Amene F, Hiwot T, Teshome W (2015). Epidemiology of Lameness among Cart Pulling Donkeys in Hawassa City Administration, Southern Ethiopia. Acad. J. Anim. Dis. 4(2):52-59.

Ayele G, Feseha G, Bojia E, Joe A (2006). Prevalence of gastro-intestinal parasites of donkeys in Dugda Bora District, Ethiopia. Livest. Res. Rural Dev. 18(10):14-21.

Biffa D, Woldemeskel M (2006). Causes and factors associated with occurrence of external injuries in working equines in Ethiopia. Int. J. Appl. Res. Vet. Med. 4:1-7.

Biswas P, Dutt T, Patel M, Kamal R, Bharti PK, Sahu S (2013). Assessment of pack animal welfare in and around Bareilly city of India. Vet. World 6(6):332-336.

Crane M (1997). Medical. In: Svendsen, E. (ed) The professional hand book of the donkey. 3 ed. w140 by London: Whittet Books LTD. P 29.

Central Statistical Agency (CSA) (2013). Federal Democratic Republic of Ethiopia Central Statistical Agency. Agricultural Sample Survey (2012/13 [2005 E.C). Volume II, Report on Livestock and Livestock Characteristics. Statistical Bulletin 570. Addis Ababa, Ethiopia. Available at: http://www.iiste.org/Journals/index.php/JBAH/article/view/23252/23708

Central Statistical Agency (CSA) (2008). Federal Democratic Republic of Ethiopia. Central Statistical Agency, Agricultural sample survey report on livestock and livestock characteristics. Volume II, 2007/08. Addis Ababa, Ethiopia. Available at: http://www.instepp.umn.edu/sites/default/files/product/downloadable/Ethiopia_2007-08_Vol2.pdf

Fielding D, Starkey P (2004). Donkeys, people and development: Resource books in the animal traction network for Eastern and Southern Africa (ATNESA), ACP-EU Technical Centre for Agricultural and Rural Cooperation (CTA), Wageningen, Netherland.

Fikru A, Tadese A, Gebreegziabher Z (2015). Prevalence of Equine Wound and Associated Risk Factors in and around Kombolcha Town, North Ethiopia. J. Vet. Sci. Technol. 6:234.

Gebreab F, Fanta A (2007). Saddle harness development and trial. In Fifth International Colloquium on Working Equines. The future for working equines. Addis Ababa, Ethiopia, 30 October-2 November, 2006. The Donkey Sanctuary. pp. 41-47.

Genetu H, Yohannes G, Abdela N, Ibrahim N (2017). Prevalence of Wounds and Associated Risk Factors in Working Equines in Jimma Town of Oromia Region, South-Western Ethiopia. Acad. J. Anim. Dis. 6(2):23-29.

Helen B (2001). The Gharry horses of Gonder. Draught Animal News. Centre for Tropical Veterinary Medicine: University of Edinburgh, Scotland. 35:23-24.

Henneke D, Potter G, Kreider J, Yeates B (1983). Relationship between body condition score, physical measurement and body fat percentage in mares. Equine vet. J. 15(4):371-372.

Kiros A, Gezahegn M, Aylate A (2016). A cross sectional study on risk factors associated with lameness of working donkeys in and around Hawassa, Ethiopia. J. Anim. Health Prod. 4(3):87-94.

Kumar N, Fisseha KK, Shishay N, Hagos Y (2014). Welfare Assessment of Working Donkeys in Mekelle City, Ethiopia. Glob. Vet.12(3):314-319.

Mandefro A (2008). A study on harnessing problems of working donkeys in Sidama zone. DVM Thesis, Addis Ababa University, Faculty of Veterinary Medicine, Debre-Zeit.

Morka A, Adisalem H, Bojia E, Eyob H, Bedasso M (2014).Health and Welfare Assessment of Working Equine in and Around Nekemte Town, East Wollega Zone, Ethiopia. *Amer-Euras.* J. Sci. Res. 9(6):163-174.

Mulisa M, Tamirat H, Ayalew N, Teka F (2015). Assessment on Working Donkey Welfare Issue in Wolaita Soddo Zuria District, Southern Ethiopia. Glob.Vet 14(6):867-875.

Panwar S, Tripathi H, Bhanja SK, Kumar S (2008) Animal welfare practices followed by pack animal owners- an investigative study. Centaur 25(1):7-19. Available at: http://www.veterinaryworld.org/Vol.6/June%20-%202013/Assessment%20of%20pack%20animal%20welfare%20in%20and%20around%20Bareilly%20city%20of%20India.pdf

Pearson RA, Krecek RC (2006). Delivery of health and husbandry improvements to working animals in Africa. Trop. Anim. Health Prod. 38(2):93-101.

Pritchard JC, Lindberg AC, Main DC, Whay HR (2005). Assessment of the welfare of working horses, mules and donkeys, using health and behavior parameters. Prev. Vet. Med. 69:265-283.

Rahman AS, Reed k (2014). The management and welfare of working animals: identifying problems, seeking solutions and anticipating the future. Revue Scientifique et Technique International Office of Epizootics 33(1):197-202.

Rossel S, Marshall F, Peters J, Pilgram T, Adams MD, O'Connor D (2008). Domestication of the donkey: Timing, processes, and indicators. Proceed. Natl. Acad. Sci. 105(10):3715-3720.

Tesfaye S, Deressa B, Teshome E (2016). Study on the Health and Welfare of Working Donkeys in Mirab Abaya District, Southern Ethiopia. Acad. J. Anim. Dis. 5(2):40-52.

Smith D (2003). Final technical report R7350: Use and management of donkey by poor society's peri-urban areas of Ethiopia. Available at: http://www.napier.ac.uk/research-and-innovation/research-search/outputs/r7350-final-technical-report-use-and-management-of-donkeys-by-poor-societies-i-peri-urban

Solomon M, Matusala M, Rahmeto A (2013). Management practices and welfare problems encountered on working equids in Hawassa town Southern Ethiopia. J. Vet. Med. Anim. Health 5(9):243-250.

Thrusfield M (2007). Veterinary Epidemiology. Third Edition, Blackwell Science Ltd, Oxford. pp. 244-259.

Tsega AM, Worku Y, Tesfaye T, Nazir S (2016). Prevalence of wound and associated risk factors of donkeys in Merawi District, North Western Ethiopia. J. Anim. Res. 6(5):765-771.

Usman S, HaimanotDisassa TK, Kebede TZ (2015). Health and welfare related assessment of working equine in and around Batu Town, East Shoa, Central Ethiopia. Nat. Sci. 13(10):1-8.

Wilson RT (2002). Specific welfare problems associated with working horses. In: Waran, N (ed.): The welfare of horses. Dordrecht: Kluwer Academic Publishers. pp. 203-218.

Yilma J, Feseha G, Svendsen E, Mohammed A (1991). Health problems of working donkeys in Debrezeit and Menagesha Regions of Ethiopia. In: D. Fielding and R.A. Pearson (Editors). Donkeys, Mules and Horses in Tropical Agricultural Development, CTVM, Edinburgh. pp. 151-155.

19

Prevalence and species of major gastrointestinal parasites of donkeys in Tenta Woreda, Amhara Regional State, Ethiopia

Temesgen Kassa Getahun* and Tihune Zeleke Kassa

Ethiopian Institute of Agricultural Research, Holeta Agricultural Research Center, P.O. Box 31, Holeta, Ethiopia.

A cross sectional study was carried out from January 2014 to May 2015 in Tenta Woreda, Amhara regional state, Ethiopia to identify the species and determine the overall prevalence of gastrointestinal (GI) parasites of donkeys. A total of 300 fecal samples were collected from randomly selected donkeys and examined with flotation, sedimentation, McMaster and Baerman fecal examination techniques. The overall prevalence was found to be 72.33. The major GI parasites identified based on qualitative faecal examination techniques were Strongyles spp. (57.2%), *Parascaris equorum* (11.2%), *Strongyloides* spp. (10.4%), *Gastrodiscus aegypticus* (5.1%), *Oxyrus equi* (2.7%), *Fasciola* spp. (2.0%) and *Anoplocephal* spp. (2.6%). The prevalence in female and male animals was 58.5 and 41.5%, respectively. There was a statistically significant difference (p<0.05) for the prevalence and mean epg count of strongyles and *P. equorum* among different age groups. Accordingly, the prevalence as well as mean epg count was higher in young than adults and old age groups. Further analysis of positive samples using coproculture revealed the occurrence of *Strongylus vulgaris* (27.7%), *Strongylus edentates* (16.6%), *Strongylus equinus* (4.8%), *P. equorum* (11.2%), *Trichostrongylus axei* (8.3%) *Strongyloides westeri* (9.5%), *Dictyocaulus arnfieldi* (7.5%), *Oxyuris equi* (6.5%) and *Triodonthophorus tencollis* (1.3%). There was concurrent infection of donkeys with a maximum of two different GI parasites with prevalence of 33.48%. The findings of the present study clearly suggest that GI parasites of donkeys in the study area are still widespread and economically important constraints for the productivity and use of donkeys in rural towns. Hence, further and strengthened intervention is highly recommended taking into account the importance of these animals to the economy.

Key words: Coproculture, donkeys, egg per gram of faeces (epg), faeces, GI parasites, prevalence, Tenata, Ethiopia.

INTRODUCTION

Donkeys (*Equus asinus*) are among the early-domesticated equines that have been existing, dating back to the time of early men (Saul et al., 1997). Today, there are more than 40 million donkeys distributed

*Corresponding author. E-mail: Temesgen.kassa@yahoo.com.

throughout the world (FAO, 2013). In Africa, the donkey population is estimated to be 13 million (Starkey and Starkey, 2013) and Ethiopia has about four million donkeys or 32% of all the donkeys in Africa and 10% of the world population (Alemu et al., 2004). Donkey in Ethiopia is most commonly found in the dry and mountainous areas. There is one equine for every four people in the agricultural sector and for every five persons of the total population (Yilma et al., 1991).

Despite the increase in mechanization throughout the world, donkeys are still well deserving of the name beasts of burden. Their prominent position in the agricultural systems of many developing countries is shown by the wide spread use of donkeys in rural and urban areas. It is suggested that donkeys can play a great role in the frame works of food security and social equity of high food insecure countries (Pearson and Krecek, 2006).

The low level of development of road transport and rough terrain of Ethiopia make donkeys the most valuable, appropriate and affordable pack animals under the small holder farming system (Gebrewold et al., 2004). Donkeys appear to be an effective entry point for assisting women in domestic responsibilities (Marshall and Ali, 2004) and also in areas where draft power is a constraint to crop cultivation; a pair of well-conditioned donkeys could be used as an alternative draft power sources for secondary and tertiary land preparation (Abayneh et al., 2002).

Certain impediments hinder the maximum utilization of these animals to their potential. The most important ones are parasitic disease (Chhabra et al., 2011; Sumbria et al., 2014; Sumbria et al., 2016), especially gastrointestinal parasites, harness sores; infectious disease likes strangles and poor management system of these animals (Ministry of Agriculture and Rural development, 2012). Donkeys harbor a large quantity of parasite that prevail in the GIT including round worms (families: Stronglidae, oxyuridae, Trichostronglidae and Ascaridae), flat worms (Fasciolidae) and tapeworm (family: Anoplocephalidae) which damage the intestine depend on the species and number present, nutrition, age and natural defense of the individual equine (Pereia and Vianna, 2006). In donkeys, infection with endoparasites is responsible for problems including poor body condition, reduced power output, diarrhea, colic, emaciation, impaired growth, poor reproductive performance, short lifespan and predisposition to other infectious diseases (Elisabeth and Sevendesen, 1997; Fikru et al., 2005).

Studies on endoparasites including haemoprotozoa in working donkeys across several countries of the world have disclosed the involvement of several species (Sotiraki et al., 1997; Wells et al., 1998; Matthee et al., 2002; Mushi et al., 2003; Uslu and Guclu, 2007; Sumbria et al., 2015). These investigations have revealed that in developing countries where nutrition and hygiene are generally poor, GI parasites are highly prevalent and are the major problems of donkeys. In Ethiopia where the health care is minimal, especially for equines, the prevalence, species composition and epidemiology of GI parasites affecting donkeys have not been investigated in detail (Getachew et al., 2009, 2010).

However, the available information suggests that gastrointestinal GI parasites are the main reasons for early demises of donkeys in the country (Yoseph et al., 2001; Fikru et al., 2005; Ayeleet al., 2006). Despite their invaluable contributions, donkeys in Ethiopia are the most neglected animals, accorded low social status. Apart from few studies in other parts of Ethiopia, there is no previous information on GI parasites of donkeys in Tenta woreda, Amhara Regional State, Ethiopia

Hence, the objectives of this study were to determine the overall prevalence of GI parasites of donkeys in Tenta woreda Amhara Regional State, Ethiopia. Besides, the level of infection based on the mean epg count and the relationship between measurable parameters and GI parasites were assessed.

MATERIALS AND METHODS

Study area

The present study was conducted in Tenta Woreda, Amhara Regional State, Ethiopia from January 2014 to May 2015. The livestock resources of the region consist of cattle, goats, sheep, camel, poultry and equines. Tenta is a town located in South Wollo Zone of the Amhara Region. It has a latitude and longitude of 11° 19′N 39°15′E / 11.317° N 39.250°E, with an elevation of 2972 m above sea level.

Study animals

Animals used in this study were systematically selected 300 donkeys from Tenta woreda Amhara Regional State, Ethiopia maintained under traditional small holder extensive management production system. The animals were owned by the individual farmers for the purpose of packing to generate income and for household use. Though selected animals represented different age and sex groups, but donkeys were randomly selected irrespective of age, sex and body condition scores and color.

Sample size determination

Sample size was calculated with an expected prevalence of 77.3% from the previous research work on prevalence of GIT parasite in similar highland area, South Wollo (Alemayehu and Etaferahu, 2013). The desired sample size for the study was calculated using the formula given by Thrusfield (2007) with 95% confidence interval and 5% absolute precision.

$$n = \frac{1.96^2 Pexp\ (1\text{-}Pexp)}{d^2}$$

Where, Pexp = expected prevalence; d= absolute precision; n=sample size. Accordingly, a total of 300 donkeys were used in this study.

Table 1. Overall prevalence.

Parasite	Number positive	Prevalence (%)	Standard error	[95% Confidence interval]
Strongyles	138	57.2	0.0291536	[0.49-0.60]
Oxyrus equi	8	6.5	0.0169264	[0.06-0.13]
Parascaris equorum	27	11.2	0.0095369	[0.01-0.05]
Strongyloides spp.	25	10.4	0.0163485	[0.05-0.12]
Faciola spp.	6	4.0	0.0082881	[0.01-0.04]
Gastrodiscus aegypticus	15	8.1	0.0128976	[0.03-0.08]
Anoplocephala spp.	2	2.6	0.0048184	[-0.01-0.01]

Study design and sampling strategy

A cross sectional study was conducted from January 2014 to May 2015 in Tenta Woreda, Amhara Regional State, Ethiopia to identify, assess and determine the prevalence of the GI parasites. Sampling method followed was a household based systematic random sampling in which the study animals were randomly selected from respective village of the district and from the selected village, the house were also randomized systematically in every second household.

Age and body condition estimation

During sample collection, various potential risk factors including sex, age, and body condition score of donkey was recorded. The age of the selected donkeys was determined from birth records of owners and by dentition (Crane and Svendsen, 1997). Body condition score (BCS) was subjectively estimated based on the guides published (Svendsen, 1997). Accordingly, donkeys were grouped into three age categories: donkeys from 1-3 years of age were classified as young; 3-10 years were considered as adult; and those beyond 10 years were classified as old. These age classes were based on age of first work, productive age and the life span of Ethiopian donkeys (Svendsen, 1997; Yosef et al., 2001). Regarding BCS, the studied animals were grouped poor, moderate, ideal, fat and obese (NEWC, 2005).

Sample collection and examination

Faecal sample collection

Fecal samples were collected from donkey per-rectum from fresh deposits using plastic rectal gloves. Each sample was labeled with the animal number, date of collection, age, sex, BCS, number of animal owned and place of collection in edible pen. The collected samples were kept in icebox, having adequate ice and able to close tightly and transported to Woreda laboratory. The samples were kept in plus four refrigerators if immediate processing was not possible, but it had been processed within 48 h.

Faecal sample examination

Microscopic faecal examination was done by different qualitative and quantitative faecal examination technique for the presence of parasitic eggs and identification of larvae.

Qualitative faecal examination was carried out by sedimentation and floatation technique. For identification of parasite to species level, fecal samples were cultured and the larvae were recovered using Baerman apparatus technique and then identified under lower power microscope (10x objectives) based on the shape, relative size and shape of larvae's tail and under oil emersion (100x objectives) based on number of gut cells (Kaufmann, 1997). The floatation fluid used in the study was supersaturated solution of sodium chloride (Nacl) salt prepared in the laboratory. The procedure given by Gutpa and Singla (2012) was followed for the above parasitological methods.

Egg counts were also conducted using McMaster age counting technique. Severity of infection as obtained from the number of eggs per gram of faeces was determined less than or equal to 500 eggs/g of faeces regarded as mild infection; 500-1000 eggs/g of faeces as moderate infection; and above 1000 eggs/g of faeces as severe infection (Urquhart et al., 1996).

Data analysis

The entire collected row data were entered into Microsoft Excel spread sheet and coded. Statistical analyses were performed using STATA, version 11 software packages. Percentage was used to calculate prevalence. Additionally Chi-square was used to calculate degree of association between risk factors and prevalence of gastrointestinal parasites. In the analysis, a difference was taken as significant at a p-value less than 0.05 and the confidence level was held at 95%

RESULTS

Coproscopical examination

The present study revealed an overall prevalence of 72.33%. The parasites encountered in the study period includes: *Strongyles*, *Oxyrus equi, Parascaris equorum, Fasciola* spp., *Gastrodiscus aegypticus*, *Strongyliodes* spp. and *Anoplocephala* spp. (Table 1).

Quantitative faecal examination

The McMaster technique applied to determine the number of GI parasites egg per gram of feces revealed minimum and maximum epg value of 0 to 9000. Likewise, the study showed that the mean epg and prevalence of

Table 2. Mean epg and prevalence in different age groups.

Parasites	Mean faecal egg count(epg)			Prevalence (%)		
	Young	Adult	Old	Young	Adult	Old
Overall egg count	442	530.754	410	10.5	79.8	9.7
Strongyles	359.09	213.24	355.26	91	74	7.9
Fasciola spp.	75	300	0	0.9	1.9	0
Parascaris equorum	750	314.58	225	13.8	11.5	10
Oxyuris eaui	50	175	0	2.6	0	0
Strongyloides spp.	100	290	383.3	11.2	11.5	1.6
Gastrdiscus aegypticus	100	233.33	160	4.3	2.9	0
Anoplocephala spp.	0	0	150	0.9	0	0

Table 3. Eggs per gram of faeces in different age groups.

Level of infection	Percent		
	Mild infection	Moderate infection	Sever infection
Young	45.7	20	2.9
Adult	43.3	16.9	9.5
Old	45.6	22.8	8.8

Table 4. Intensity of infection of GI parasites on the basis of epg.

Degree of severity	Number of donkey	Percentage (%)	Standard error	[95% Confidence interval]
Mildly infected	130	44.4	0.0290741	[0.39-0.50]
moderately infected	54	18.4	0.0226901	[0.14-0.23]
Heavily infected	25	8.5	0.0163485	[0.05-0.12]

strongyle type nematode is significantly greater than the other GI parasites (Table 2).

The study showed that young donkeys were with greater proportion of mild, moderate and heavy level of epg than both young and old age donkeys (Table 3)

Intensity of infection

Based on the result of epg counts in the study area, 130 (44.4%) were mildly infected, 54 (18.4%) were moderately infected and 25 (8.5%) were severely infected (Table 3).

Larvoscopic examinations

Identification of L3 of GI parasites isolated by Baerman technique from coprocultured faeces showed the predominance of *Strongylus vulgaris, Strongylus edentatus* and *Parascaris equorum* than the other GI parasites (Table 4 and 5). Infections with one species of helminthes were more common, 139 (66.52%) than infections with two, 70 (33.49%) species of helminthes (Table 6).

Analysis of risk factors

Analysis of different risk factors showed that age and body condition score was significantly associated with the risk of infection with GI parasites ($p<0.05$), whereas sex of the animal was not significantly associated with GI parasite infection(Table 7).

The prevalence of GI parasites in both body condition groups (good and poor) was determined in larvoscopy. The larvoscopy results revealed that, the prevalence of GI parasites in moderate body condition donkeys were *Dictyocaulus arnfieldi* (50%) which was the top species of parasites and the least were *Triodontophorus tenuicollis* and *Anoplocephala* spp. (0%). In ideal body condition, *T. tenuicollis* (100%) was the highest. Similarly, in poor body condition animals, the highest prevalent parasites was *Anoplocephala* spp. (100%) and least was *T. tenuicollis*

Table 5. Species of GI parasites identified from coprocultured faeces of donkey in Sendafa district, Oromia Regional State, Ethiopia.

Species of parasite	Number positive	Prevalence (%)	Standard error	[95%Confidence Interval]
Strongylus vulgaris	84	27.7	0264639	[0.23-0.34]
Strongylus edentatus	43	16.6	0.0207083	[0.11-0.19]
Strongylus equinus	11	4.8	0.011124	[0.02-0.06]
Dictyocaulus arnfieldi	16	7.5	0.0132966	[0.03-0.08]
Tricostrongylus axie	21	8.3	0.0150951	[0.04-0.10]
Strongyloides westeri	25	9.5	0.0136811	[0.03-0.08]
Triodonthophorus tencollis	1	1.4	0.003413	[0.003-0.01]
Cythostomum spp	17	7.9	0.0095369	[0.01-0.04]
Parascaris equorum	27	11.2	0.0095369	[0.01-0.05]
Oxyrus equi	8	6.5	0.0169264	[0.06-0.13]

Table 6. Concurrent infections.

Concurrent infection	Number of positive donkeys	Percentage (%)
One species	139	66.52
Two species	70	33.48

Table 7. The relative prevalence among the sex category.

Parasites	Total	Sex	
		Female	Male
Strongyles	159	95(59.9%)	64(40.3%)
Parascaris equorum	27	14(51.9%)	13(48.1%)
Oxyuris equi	8	4(50%)	4(50%)
Fasciola spp.	6	4(66.7%)	2(33.3%)
Anopleocephalus spp.	2	2(100%)	0
Gastrodiscus aegyrticus	15	9(60%)	6(40%)

Table 8. Prevalence between body conditions.

Species of parasite	Poor	Moderate	Ideal	X^2value	p-value
Strongylus vulgaris	59.5	36.9	3.6	33.511	0.000
Strongylus edentateus	55.8	41.9	2.3	14.264	0.003
Strongylus equinus	45.5	44.5	0	4.115	0.249
Strongyloides westeri	52.0	48.8	0	9.077	0.028
Parascaris equorum	51.9	44.4	0	8.23	0.042
Triodontophorus tenuicollis	0	0	100	28.397	0.000
Dictyocaulus arnfieldi	43.8	50.0	6.2	3.486	0.323
Gastrodiscus aegypticus	66.7	33.3	0	6.887	0.076
Anoplocephala spp.	100	0	0	3.073	0.381
Trichonema spp.	70.6	29.4	0	9.065	0.028
Trichostrongylus axei	57.1	33.3	9.5	4.72	0.254

(0%). There was statistically significant difference ($p<0.05$) in prevalence of *S. vulgaris, S. edentates Strongyloides westeri, P. equorum, T. tenuicollis* and *Trichonema* spp. between the body conditions as examined by larvoscopy (Table 8).

The prevalence of GI parasites in different age groups

Table 9. Age wise prevalence.

Species of parasite	Age group			X^{2-} value	p- value
	Young (%)	Adult (%)	Old (%)		
Strongylus vulgaris	14.3	61.9	23.8	2.458	0.293
Strongylus edentatus	7.0	79.0	14.0	2.630	0.268
Stronglus equinus	9.1	63.6	27.3	0.478	0.787
Stronyloides westeri	8.0	64.0	28.0	1.467	0.480
Oxyuris equi	12.5	75.0	12.5	0.256	0.880
Parascaris equorum	92.6	7.4	0	95.013	0.000
Triodontophorus tencollis	0	0	100	7.644	0.022
Dictyocaulus arnifieldi	18.8	43.8	37.5	5.013	0.082
Fasciola spp,	0	83.3	16.7	0.950	0.622
Anoplocephala spp,	0	50.0	50.0	1.308	0.520
Cythostomum spp,	11.8	58.8	29.4	1.172	0.557
Gastrodiscus aegypicus	0	86.7	13.3	2.945	0.229
Trichostrongylus axei	9.5	61.9	28.6	1.467	0.480

revealed that *P. equorum* (92.6%) was the highest and *G. aegypticus, T. tenuicollis, Anoplocephala* spp. and *Fasciola* spp. (0%) the lowest in the young. In old age, the highest was *T. tenuicollis* (100%) and the lowest was *P. equorum* (0%). In adults, *G. aegypticus* (86.7%) and *T. tenuicollis* (0%) were the highest and lowest, respectively. There was statistically significant difference ($p<0.05$) in prevalence of *P. equorum* between different age groups (Table 9).

DISCUSSION

The coprological examination done in this study using floatation and sedimentation method revealed an overall GI parasite prevalence of 72.33% in the study area, which was relatively lower than some of the earlier reports of 98.2% by Ayele et al. (2006), 84.4% by Gulima (2006), 96.9% by Ibrahim et al. (2011) and 92.71% by Mezgebu et al. (2013) at and around Gonder, Hawassa Town, Dugda Bora district and Awi Zone, respectively. This difference could be attributed to the variation in sampling time as seasonality. Additionally, accessibility of donkeys to grazing land, deworming habit of the donkeys and giving supplementary feed to these animals affect its occurrence.

The prevalence of strongyles was 57.2%. This figure was much lesser than the earlier finding of Zerihun et al. (2009), Yoseph et al. (2001), Muleta (2005), Fikru et al. (2005) who reported prevalence of 100, 100, 100 and 98.2% in Sululta and Gefersa, Wonchi, highlands of Wollo province and western highlands of Oromia, respectively. This is most probably attributed to the difference in the study area or due to nutritional status of the animal in the respective study area which can influence the level of immunity to be infected by the parasite. Additionally, it could be affected by deworming strategy and accessibility to veterinary clinic.

The prevalence of 11.2% *P. equorum* recorded in the current study is lower than the previous reports of Fikru et al. (2005), Ayele et al. (2006) and Zerihun (2008) who reported 43, 17.3 and 42.8% in Western highlands of Oromia, Dugda Bora district, and highlands of Wollo provinces, respectively. These differences in prevalence might be due to the variation in the length of the study period, the season of the study period, ecology of the study area, intervention with anthelminthic (deworming) and the ecological and climatic differences among localities. The prevalence and mean epg of *P. equorum* was significantly ($p<0.05$) higher in young donkeys than the other age groups. This is most probably due to the fact that young donkeys have less immunity against *P. equorum* infection than both adult and old donkeys. This agrees with the earlier report by Zerihun (2008) in central Showa, Ethiopia. However, this finding contrast the research of Ayele et al. (2006) and Getachew et al. (2009) who reported absence of statistically significant differences in the prevalence of *P. equorum* among donkeys of different age groups that may reflect differences in the study design and geographic locations.

The prevalence of 4% for *Fasciola* spp. recorded from intervention area in the current study is higher than the previous report by Ayele et al. (2006) who reported 1.5% in Dugda Bora district. This higher prevalence suggests that *Fasciola* spp. is common in highlands where donkeys share the same grazing area with ruminants that are considered as primary hosts of liver fluke and favorable ecological conditions which allow multiplication and spread of intermediate snail host in both study districts as has been reported by Getachew et al. (2010). As compared to other reports in the central highlands of Ethiopia (Yoseph et al., 2001) in Wonchi (Muleta, 2005),

South and North Wollo zones) lower prevalence of *Fasciola* was recorded. This lower prevalence might be due to the differences in season of sample collection and effect of deworming.

Lower prevalence of *Anoplocephala* spp, 2.6% recorded in this study as compared to reports by, Yoseph et al. (2005), Fikru et al. (2005) and Getachew et al. (2010) might reflect the seasonality of orbited mite intermediate hosts and differences in study period and locations. The negative value of confidence interval for *Anoplocephala* spp. indicates that they are rare parasites in the study area that indicate cross sectional study which is not a better study method. The prevalence of 8.1% for *G. aegypticus* recorded in the current study is in agreement with previous research done by Zerihun et al. (2009) reporting 5.7% in Sululta and Gefersa districts of central Oromia.

O. equi with prevalence rate of 6.5% was lower when compared with the work of Yoseph et al. (2001) in Wonchi who reported 32.4% and relatively similar to Alemayehu and Etaferahun (2013) who have reported 4% in south wollo zone. The low prevalence in this study might be the effect of deworming by the woreda veterinary clinic, variation in management system and relatively dry season during sample collection time in the present study area which desiccates the highly susceptible *O. equi* eggs. The parasite is ubiquitous but greater prevalence in areas of high rainfall (Radostitis et al., 2007).

Lower prevalence (7.5%) of *D. arnfieldi* was recorded in the present study as compared to Ayele et al. (2006) who have reported 32% in Dugda Bora District and Bewketu and Endalkachew (2013) who have reported 22.17% in and around Bahir Dar town. This difference in prevalence might be due to the ecological and climatically differences among localities.

Analysis of the degree of infection by GI parasites as determined by epg of donkey showed that the greatest proportion of young donkeys were with mild degree (45.7%) followed by moderate degree (20.0%) whereas the majority of adult and old donkeys were with mild degree of infection 43.3 and 45.6%, respectively. This observation is lower than the previous research of Matthee et al. (2002) and Getachew et al. (2009). This might be due to the effect of deworming in the study area. The difference in parasite prevalence between sexes might be due to the fact that females are found to have higher infection rates as they might have lower immunity due to gestation and lactation as stated by Ram (2009). The co-infection pattern observed in this study showed that donkey has the high chance of concomitant exposure to different GI parasites. Similar findings were reported by Yoseph et al. (2001).

This study confirmed that there is significant difference in the prevalence of the parasite among the different body condition scores and it is shown that GI parasites are more prevalent in animals with poor body condition than well-conditioned animals which are in agreement with the results of Ayele et al. (2006), which implies that the body condition score is a good indicator of parasitic burden, which can be used by farmers to identify donkeys with immediate requirement of anthelmintic remedies.

This study result is in agreement with Ayele et al. (2006) that there was no statistically significant difference ($p>0.05$) between age groups for GI parasite infections except *P. equorum*. This might be due to increased land of cultivation which restricts donkeys on small communal grazing land which allows the animals for continuous larvae exposure.

Identification of infective larvae of GI parasites showed that *S. vulgaris* (29.7%) and *S. edentatus* (16.7%) were the major larvae encountered. The prevalence of *P. equorum* and *D. arnfieldi* were 11.2 and 7.5%, respectively. This finding disagrees with observations of Ayele et al. (2010) and Yoseph et al. (2001) who reported 100%. These differences in prevalence might be due to intervention with anthelminthic and the ecological and climatic differences among localities.

Conclusion

The current study showed a decrease in prevalence of helminthes of donkeys in both coproscopic and larvoscopic methods of examination in the study area. This suggests that the mass deworming given by Woreda Veterinary Clinic reduce the parasitic infection. This study revealed that the major GI parasites that occurred were *S. vulgaris, P. equorum, S. edentatus, O. equi, D. arnfiedi* and *Cythostomum* spp. In the light of the results, it is considered that the infections caused by GI parasites, especially the *S. vulgaris, S. edentatus* and *P. equorum* are common in the region of the study, so greater importance should be given to this situation. This research indicated that infection with one parasite was found to be very common in this study than concurrent infection with two and three parasites. This study confirmed that there is significant difference in the prevalence of the parasite among the different body condition scores and it is shown that GI parasites are more prevalent in animals with poor body condition than well-conditioned animals.

RECOMMENDATIONS

1. Owners should be trained to improve the management system, especially in terms of the level of nutrition so that the animal can have good body condition that confers some level of resistance against GI parasite infection.
2. The decrease in the prevalence of parasite due to mass deworming is not necessarily satisfactory, so strategic parasitic control program should be designed with broad spectrum anthelmintic drugs with regular

evaluation of efficiency of anthelmintic.

3. Donkey owners should be educated on the economic importance and methods of control of helminthes of donkey.

4. Government and non-governmental organization should work together to improve the health and welfare of donkeys in the study area.

5. Further research on the economic importance, epidemiology and time of treatment of GI parasites of donkey in the study area is recommended.

Abbreviations: BCS, Body condition score; **CI,** confidence interval; **epg,** egg per gram of faeces; **GI,** gastrointestinal; **MOARD,** Ministry of Agriculture Rural Development; **rpm,** revolution per minute.

ACKNOWLEDGEMENTS

The authors thank the staff members of Woreda Veterinary Laboratory for their cooperation in accomplishment of this work.

REFERENCES

Abayneh T, Gebreab B, Tadesse G (2002). The potential role of donkeys in land tillage in central Ethiopia. Bull. Anim. Health Prod. Afr. 50:172-178.

Alemayehu R, Etaferahu Y (2013). Gastrointestinal Parasites of Equine in South Wollo Zone, North Eastern Ethiopia. J.Glob.Vet. 11:824-830.

Alemu G, Azage T, Alemu Y (2004). Research need of donkey utilization in Ethiopia. J. Anim. tra. 77-81.

Ayele G, Dinka A (2010). Study on strongyles and parascaris parasites population in working donkeys of central Shoa, Ethiopia. J. Livest. Res. Rural Dev. 22:1-5.

Ayele G, Feseha G, Bojia E, Joe A (2006). Prevalence of gastro-intestinal parasites of donkeys in Dugda Bora District, Ethiopia. J. Livest. Res. Rural Dev.18:2-6.

Bewketu T, Endalkachew N (2013). Prevalence of gastrointestinal helminthes of donkeys and mules in and around Bahir Dar, Ethiopia. Vet. J. 17:13-30.

LD (2011). Transplacental transmission of *Babessia equi (Theileria equi)* from carrier mares to foals. J. Parasit. Dis. 36: 31-33.

Crane M, Sevendesen A (1997). The professional Hand Books of the donkey. 3rd ed. Whittet Books Limitted, London. pp. 29-31.

Elisabeth D, Sevendesen M (1997). Professional donkey hand book.Anley road, London W14 OBY. pp. 61- 9.

Fikru R, Teshale S, Bizuneh M (2005).Prevalence of Equine gastrointestinal parasites in Western highlands of Oromia, Ethiopia. Bull. Anim. Health Prod. Afr. 53:161-166.

Food and Agricultural Organization FAO (2013). Food and Agriculture Organization Stat Database Available at http://faost at.fao.org/faostat/ form.

Gebrewold A, Tegegn A, Yami A (2004). Research needs of Donkey utilization in Ethiopia. A Resource Book of the Animal Traction Network for Eastern and Southern Africa (ATNESA), Technical
Center for Agriculture and rural cooperation (CTA), Wageningen pp.77-81.

Getachew M, Feseha G, Trawford A, Reid S (2009). A survey of seasonal patterns in strongylefaecal worm egg counts of working equids of the central midlands and lowlands, Ethiopia. J. Trop. Anim. Health Prod. 40:637-642.

Getachew M, Innocent G, Trawford F, Reid S, Love S (2010). Epidemiological features of fasciolosis in working donkeys in Ethiopia. J. Vet. Parasitol. 169:335-339.

Gulima D (2006). Epidemiological study of helminthosis in traction horses in Awi Zone, NorthWestern, Ethiopia. Vet. J. 10:37-54.

Gupta SK, Singla LD (2012) Diagnostic trends in parasitic diseases of animals. In: *Veterinary Diagnostics: Current Trends.* Gupta RP, Garg SR, Nehra V and Lather D (Eds), Satish Serial Publishing House, Delhi. pp. 81-112.

Ibrahim N, Berhanu T, Deressa B, Tolosa T (2011). Survey of Prevalence of Helminth Parasites of Donkeys in and Around Hawassa Town, Southern Ethiopia, J.Glob. Vet. 6:223-227.

Kaufmann J (1997). Parasitic Infection of Domestic Animals, a Diagnostic Manual, BirhavsenVerleg, Germany. pp. 5-21, 224-227.

Marshall K, Ali Z (2004). Donkeys, People and Development. A resource book of the animal traction network for eastern and Southern Africa (ATNESA). Technical center for agriculture and rural cooperation (CTA). pp. 77-81.

Matthee S, Krecek R, Milne S, Boshoff M, Guthrie A (2002). Impact of management interventions on helminth levels and body and blood measurements in working donkeys in South Africa. J. Vet. Parasitol. 107: 103-113.

Mezgebu T, Tafess K, Tamiru F (2013.). Prevalence of Gastrointestinal Parasites of Horses .and Donkeys in and around Gondar Town, Ethiopia. Open J. Vet. Med. 3:267-272.

Ministry of Agriculture and Rural evelopment (MOARD) (2012). Agriculture and Rural Development bulletin (Amharic version), 2 year. P 4.

Muleta B (2005). Preliminary study on helminthosis in equines in South and North Wollo zones. Ethiopia. J. Vet. 9:25-37.

Mushi E, Binta M, Chabo R, Monnafela L (2003).Seasonal fluctuation of parasitic infestation in donkeys (*Equusasinus*) in Oodi village, Kgatleng District, Botswana. J. South Afr. Vet. Assoc. 74:24-26.

Pearson R, Krecek R (2006).Delivery of health and husbandry improvements to working animals in Africa. J. Trop. Anim. Health Prod. 38:93-101.

Pereira JR, Vianna SS (2006).Gastrointestinal parasitic worms in equines in the Paraiba Valley, State of Sao Paulo, Brazil. J. Vet. Parasitol. 140:289-295.

Radostits O, Gay C, Hinchcliff K, Constable P (2007). Veterinary Medicine, Atextbook of the diseases of cattle, sheep, goats, pigs and horses.10th edition. Saunders-Elsevier. pp.1311-1315.

Ram C (2009). Prevalence of helminthes parasites in mules of Brick kiln of lalitpur District, Napal.

Saul C, Siefert L, Opuda-Asibo J (1997). Disease and health problems of donkeys: a case study from eastern Uganda. Paper presented at the international Animal Traction Network for Eastern and Southern Africa (ATNESA) workshop held 5-9 May 1997. DebreZeit, Ethiopia.

Sotiraki S, Badouvas A, Himonas C (1997). A survey on the prevalence of internal parasites of equines in macedonia and Thessalia-Greece. J. Equi. Vet. Sci. 17:550-552.

Starkey P, Starkey M (2013). Regional and world trends in donkey populations and Animal Traction Network for Eastern and Southern Africa Improving Donkey Utilization and Management; Debre Zeit, Ethiopia: ATENSA. pp. 230-237.

Sumbria D, Singla LD, Sharma A (2016). *Theileria equi* and *Babesia caballi* infection of equids in Punjab, India: a serological and molecular survey. Trop. Anim. Health Prod. 48:45-52.

Sumbria D, Singla LD, Sharma A, Bal MS, Kumar S (2015b). Multiplex PCR for detection of *Trypanosoma evansi* and *Theileria equi* in equids of Punjab, India. Vet. Parasitol. 211:293-299.

Sumbria D, Singla LD, Sharma A, Moudgil AD, Bal MS (2014). Equine trypanosomosis in central and western Punjab: Prevalence, haemato-biochemical response and associated risk factors. Acta Trop. 138:44-50.

Svendsen E (1997). Parasites Abroad in: The professional hand book of the donkey. Svendsen, E.D. (Ed.). 3rd Edition, Whittet Books, London. 227-238.

Thrusfield M. (2007). Veterinary Epidemiology. rd Ed. Blackwell Science Ltd, Oxford, UK. pp. 233-261.
Urquhart G, Aremour J, Duncan A, Dunn F, Jennis F (1996).Veterinary parasitology 2 edition. The University of Glasgw, Black Well Science, Scotland. pp. 3-137.
Uslu U, Guclu F (2007). Prevalence of endoparasites in horses and donkeys in Turkey. Bull. J. Vet. Inst. Pulawy 51:237-240.
Wells D, Krecek R, Wells M, Guthrie A, Lourens J (1998).Helminth levels of working donkeys kept under different management systems in the Moretele 1 district of the North-West Province, South Africa. J. Vet. Parasitol. 77:163-177.
Yilma JM, Feseha GA, Svendsen ED, Mohammed A (1991). Health problems of working donkeys in Debre-Zeit and Menagesha regions of Ethiopia. In: Donkeys, mules & horses in tropical agricultural development. Proc. Colloquium Organ. Edinburgh School Agric. Cent. Trop. Vet. Med. Univ. Edinburgh held in Edinburgh, Scotland, 3rd-6th Sept 1990. Centre Trop. Vet. Med. 336:151-155.
Yoseph S, Feseha G, Abebaw W (2001).Survey on helmenthiosis of equines in Wonchi, Ethiopia.J. Ethiopia Veterinary Association. 5:47-61.
Zerihun A, Bersissa k, Bojia E, Ayele G, Tesfaye M, Etana D (2009). Endoparasites of Donkeys in Sululta and Gefersa Districts of Central Oromia, Ethiopia. J. Anim. Vet. Adv. 10:1850-1854
Zerihun M (2008). The status of strongyle and Parascaris population in working donkeys in Central Ethiopia. DVM Thesis, FVM, AAU, DebreZeit, Ethiopia

Eukaryotic expression and characterization of BHV-1 glycoprotein D (gD) as a potential diagnostic antigen

M. Sylvestre*, Ramneek Verma, Ravi Kant Agrawal and Dipak Deka

School of Animal Biotechnology, Guru Angad Dev Veterinary and Animal Sciences University
Ludhiana-141004, Punjab, India.

Bovine herpesvirus-1 (BHV-1) causes Infectious bovine rhinotracheitis/Pustular vulvovaginitis in cattle. Glycoprotein D (gD) of BHV-1 represents a major component of the viral envelope and is a dominant immunogen. gD encoding gene was expressed in baculovirus-insect cell system. Viral genomic DNA extracted from BHV-1 grown on Madin-Darby Bovine Kidney (MDBK) cell monolayer was used as a template for PCR amplification of gD gene (1255 bp). Gel purified gD gene was used for directional cloning into pENTR/SD/D Directional TOPO vector to produce entry clone. Recombinant plasmids were screened by PCR and restriction enzyme (RE) digestion for gD gene insert. Endotoxin free purified plasmids were then subjected to LR recombination reaction with baculovirus linear DNA. LR recombination mix was transfected into Sf-9 cells and observed for appearance of cytopathic effects (CPE). Recombinant virus was serially passaged for 3 more generations and the 4th passage viral stock was used to infect fresh Sf-9 cells for gene expression study. Recombinant gD protein was immunoprecipitated and when subjected to SDS-PAGE and western blot analysis protein band of ~70 kDa was detected consistently. The recombinant gD protein was further weakly confirmed by dot-ELISA indicating its limited potential as a coating antigen in gD-based diagnostic ELISA.

Key words: Bovine herpesvirus-1 (BHV-1), Madin-Darby Bovine Kidney (MDBK) cells, Sf-9 cells, pENTR TOPO vector, Baculovirus mediated gene expression, glycoprotein D, eukaryotic expression,

INTRODUCTION

Bovine herpesvirus type-1 (BHV-1) causes various diseases worldwide (Biswas et al., 2013; Levings and Roth, 2013). It is the most common viral agent found in the semen of bovines (Saminathan et al., 2016) and can be transmitted through natural or artificial insemination (Godhardt-Copper et al., 2009). Infectious bovine rhinotracheitis (IBR) and infectious pustular vulvovaginitis (IPV) (Davis et al., 2014; Majumder et al., 2014) are few of the most important diseases which cause huge economic loss to dairy industry due to abortion and drop in milk production (Saminathan et al., 2016). BHV-1, large double stranded DNA virus (Guo et al., 2015; Kirchhoff et al., 2014), is one of three viruses responsible for the bovine respiratory disease complex (BRDC) associated with reduced immunity (Kirchhoff et al., 2014). It causes a latent infection in sensory neurons but can reactivate following an increase in corticosteroid level (da Silva et al., 2013). Apart from IBR and IPV, BHV-1 is

*Corresponding author. E-mail: smutayomba@gmail.com.

also responsible for many other clinical manifestations namely abortion, endometritis, infertility, mastitis, rhinotracheitis, encephalitis (Davis et al., 2014) conjunctivitis (Levings, 2012), balanoposthitis (Kaur et al., 2013; Muylkens et al., 2007; Saminathan et al., 2016) and is fatal to newborn calves (Engels and Ackermann, 1996). 12 envelope glycoproteins have been identified and seven among them, namely gB, gC, gD, gE, gH, gK and gL are known to be involved in viral attachment (Drummer et al., 2014; Biswas et al., 2013). gD gene is contiguous with gI gene with 141 bp region separating their two open reading frames (Chowdhury and Sharma, 2012). gB, gC, and gD are reported to be the major envelope glycoproteins recognized by both cellular and humoral immunity (Blanc et al., 2012) and consequently major BHV-1 immunogens (Collins et al., 1985).

All three glycoproteins are used in vaccine production and induce higher titer neutralizing antibodies with gD producing the highest titer (Dummer et al., 2014; Blanc et al., 2012). gD is reported to be potential candidate for production of subunit vaccines (Majumder et al., 2014) and its expression is limited to the alpha herpesvirus, the largest subfamily of herpesvirus (Connolly et al., 2001; Grauwet et al., 2014). Glycoproteins gB and gD participate in viral replication (Tikoo et al., 1995). gD abundance in the viral envelope and its role in initial stage of replication define it as a good target of the host immune response (Drummer et al., 2014) making it immunodominant and a good candidate for vaccine (Blanc et al., 2012; Majumder et al., 2014). These biological properties make the three glycoproteins powerful antigens in the study of BHV-1 immune response (Abdelmagid et al., 1998).

BHV-1 infection in India is endemic in nature and ELISA based diagnostic tests are being used commonly for seroprevalence studies in large population against several diseases including BHV-1. Most of these assays require viral antigen in bulk and recently diagnostic ELISAs based on recombinant protein are being developed as large scale production of recombinant viral protein is possible in safe and cost effective manner. With the recent development of marker viral vaccines, individual viral protein antigens will become a powerful tool for diagnostic evaluation of immune response as well as to differentiate infected animals from vaccinated ones (Kit and Kit, 1991; Drummer et al., 2014; Muylkens et al., 2007). Various expression system including insect cells have been developed for expression of different proteins of pathogens (Saminathan et al., 2016).

Keeping these points in view, this study was aimed at cloning for eukaryotic expression of BHV-1 gD and characterization of the expressed recombinant protein.

MATERIALS AND METHODS

Cell, virus and antibodies

MDBK cells were propagated in Dulbecco's minimum essential medium (DMEM) supplemented with 10% fetal bovine serum (FBS) and containing sodium bicarbonate, 2 mM L-glutamine, 10 mM HEPES. Sf-9 (*Spodoptera frugiperda*) cells were propagated in Grace's Insect Medium supplemented with 10% FBS (Invitrogen). Sf-900™ II Serum Free Media (Invitrogen) also supplemented with 10% FBS was used in later stage for protein expression study. A solution having both antibiotic and antimycotic activity (100×, HIMEDIA) containing amphotericin B, penicillin and streptomycin was added to the medium.

25 cm^2 cell culture flasks each containing (85-90%) monolayer of MDBK cells were used to propagate BHV-1 isolate IBR 216 II (available in the laboratory) at multiplicity of infection (m.o.i.) 0.1 and the virus was serially passaged 4 to 5 times.

Anti-sera against BHV-1 and Anti-gD mouse monoclonal antibody were used in this study; the first was available in animal biotechnology department and the second was procured from Biodot laboratory, New Delhi.

DNA extraction of BHV-1 and PCR

AuPrep GEN DNA Extraction kit (Life Technologies) was used to extract genomic DNA from Bovine herpesvirus-1 passaged in MDBK cell line. gD gene was amplified from 5 µl of template DNA by PCR. CACC overhang immediately preceding initiation codon sequence (ATG) and kozak sequence were two important features of the forward primer while the reverse primer was designed simply to amplify the gD gene from the codon immediately preceding the stop codon. The gD Forward primer was: 5' CACCATGGAAGGGCCGACATTG 3' and the reverse primer was 5' CCCGGGCAGCGCGCTGTAGTTG 3'. The actual size of gD gene is 1251 bp but addition of 4 bp, CACC, overhang increased the size of amplified product to 1255 bp.

PCR was carried in 50 µl volume made of 150 ng of DNA, 1 µl of each of primers at 25 pmol concentration, 6 µl of deoxynucleoside triphosphates (dNTPs) mix at 2.5 mM, 1.5 µl of magnesium sulphate at 50 mM concentration, 3 µl of dimethyl sulfoxide, 5 µl of enhancer solution, Pfx platinum buffer 1X and Pfx platinum DNA polymerase at 1.5 U. The conditions of PCR were: 94°C for 2 min, then 35 cycles of 94°C for 30 s, 50°C for 40 s, 72°C for 2 min and lastly the final extension at 72°C for 10 min in thermal cycler (Eppendorf). PCR product was visualized using ethidium bromide post stained agarose gel (1.5%) and its molecular weight was determined by comparing it to the 100 bp ladder (Fermentas).

Cloning of BHV-1 gD gene

A QIA Quick gel extraction kit (Qiagen) was used to purify the PCR product followed by directional cloning of the PCR product in pENTR™/SD/D-TOPO® vector (Invitrogen) as per the manufacturer's guideline. 2 µl of the cloning reaction were used to transform chemically competent *E. coli* host strain TOP10 cells and LB agar plates with 100 µg/ml of kanamycin were used for selection of transformed colonies. Selected clones (5 to 6 numbers) were grown overnight in LB broth at 37°C in a shaker incubator in presence of kanamycin (100 µg/ml). Recombinant plasmids were extracted from the broth culture by alkaline lysis method (Sambrook et al, 1990). The presence of BHV-1 gD gene and its correct orientation in the expression vector was confirmed by Touchdown/Colony PCR followed by PCR from extracted plasmids and the recombinant plasmid digestion with *Asc* I and *Not* I restriction enzymes. Gen Elute Endotoxin-free Plasmid Midiprep kit (SIGMA-ALDRICH) was used to prepare the plasmid DNA (free from endotoxin) which was then used as entry clone for recombination with baculovirus genomic DNA before transfection of the insect cells.

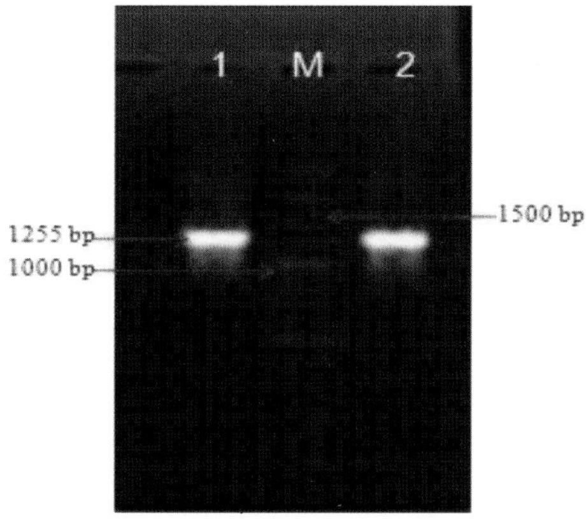

Figure 1. PCR amplified BHV-1 complete gD gene from genomic DNA. Lane 1, 2, Amplified gD gene positive samples; Lane M, 100 bp plus DNA ladder.

Transfection in Sf-9 cell line

The transfer of the gene of interest (gD) into the BaculoDirect^{TM} Linear DNA (Invitrogen) was mediated by LR recombination reaction. A transfection mixture was prepared using Cellfectin reagent and LR recombination mixture. Sf-9 cells in log phase with the viability greater than 95% were used for each transfection. Approximately 8×10^5 Sf-9 cells in 2 ml of complete growth medium were seeded per well in a six well plate followed by incubation at 27°C for one hour. Subsequently, in each well of Sf-9 cells, LR recombination mixture was added and again incubated. Selection of recombinant baculovirus encoding gD gene was done by adding 100 µM ganciclovir to the transfected Sf-9 cells. After 96 h of incubation at 27°C, cells were harvested upon observation of cytopathic effect. The P1 viral stock was used for 2 more passages up to P3. Sf-9 cells in 75 cm^2 cell culture flasks were infected with this P3 viral stock for gene expression study.

Ni-NTA column chromatography and immunoprecipitation

Ni-NTA Column chromatography which uses Ni-NTA superflow columns (Qiagen) and immunoprecipitation which uses Protein G Immunoprecipitaion kit (SIGMA) as recommended by the manufacturer (cell lysate (60 µl), Monoclonal antibody (5 µl) and 1X immunoprecipitation buffer "IP buffer" (535µl) were added to one spin column and cell lysate (60µl), Polyclonal antibody (15µl) and 1X IP buffer (525 µl) were added to another spin column to make the final volume 600 µl in each column. Both spin columns were incubated for 1 h at 4°C after which 30 µl of Protein-G-Agarose beads washed twice with 1X IP buffer and finally mixed with 50 µl of fresh 1X IP buffer were transferred into each spin column. Spin columns were then centrifuged at 12,000 rpm for 20 s at 4°C and the effluent were discarded. Beads were again washed twice with 1X IP buffer and 0.5 M NaCl by centrifugation at 12,000 rpm for 20 s followed by 4 times washing with 1X IP buffer. The last washing was performer with 0.1X IP buffer) were used to purify the recombinant gD protein from the P3 virus infected Sf-9 cells. Purified protein samples thus obtained were subjected to SDS-PAGE and western blot analysis.

SDS-PAGE and Western blot analysis

Sf-9 cells infected by recombinant baculovirus and non-infected ones, were harvested and prepared for SDS-PAGE by the method of sonication where centrifugation at 5000 rpm produced the pellet which was resuspended in 500 µl PBS and 5 µl protease inhibitor followed by sonication thrice at 5 microns for 10 s with a gap of 20 s each. Samples were then centrifuged again at 5000 rpm for 10 min and the supernatants were collected into new tubes for SDS-PAGE analysis. Samples along with the protein marker were run on 10% SDS-PAGE gel followed by staining with Coomassie Brilliant Blue (Sambrook et al., 1989). An unstained gel was blotted onto a PVDF membrane for Western blot and a SNAPid system (Millipore) was used for development. A solution of PBS with 0.1% Tween-20 and 1% BSA was used to block the membrane for 10 min at room temperature. The membrane was respectively incubated at room temperature with monoclonal antibody against BHV-1 gD and Goat anti-mouse HRP conjugate, the first at 1:300 dilution for 10 min followed by washing thrice with (PBS + 0.1% Tween 20) buffer but the second at 1:100 dilution for 10 min also followed by washing thrice with PBS. To develop the blot, DAB solution made of 1mg/ml diamino benzidine and 10 µl/ml hydrogen peroxide in PBS was used.

Dot ELISA

The following were used for Dot-ELISA: partially concentrated BHV-1, MDBK cell lysate, immunoprecipitated gD, Sf-9 infected cell lysate, non-infected Sf-9 cell lysate, PBS and blank. On dot-ELISA strip, 2 µl of each sample was spotted and it was kept for drying at 37°C for 1 h. 1% BSA was used for blocking for 30 min followed by 5 times washing with a solution of PBS containing 0.01% Tween-20, incubation with polyclonal antibody as primary antibody at 1:200 dilution and again washing once. The last incubation for 1 h at 37°C was done with secondary antibody, goat anti-rabbit HRP conjugate, diluted at 1:500 followed by washing once. DAB and hydrogen peroxide were used to develop the blot as described previously.

RESULTS

Cloning of gD gene and screening of the recombinant plasmids for presence of the insert

Genomic DNA of BHV-1 was isolated from partially purified virus and the complete gD gene (1255 bp) was amplified by PCR using specific primers to obtain gD gene fragments containing CACC base sequence at 5'end just preceding the initiation codon (Figure 1). Blunt end PCR amplified gene products were gel purified and directly used for cloning into PENTR/SD/D-directional TOPO cloning vector. Screening clones for gD gene insert was done by touch down PCR for presence of gD gene insert where PCR product of 1255 bp could successfully be amplified from recombinant plasmids. Clones having gD gene insert were grown for plasmids isolation and again the presence of gD gene insert from the purified recombinant plasmids was confirmed by amplification of 1255 bp product (Figure 2). The confirmation of complete gD gene's presence was also possible by digesting plasmids with *Asc* I and *Nco* I restriction enzymes which released 1297 bp fragment having additional 42 bp from multiple cloning site region of the plasmid (Figure 3).

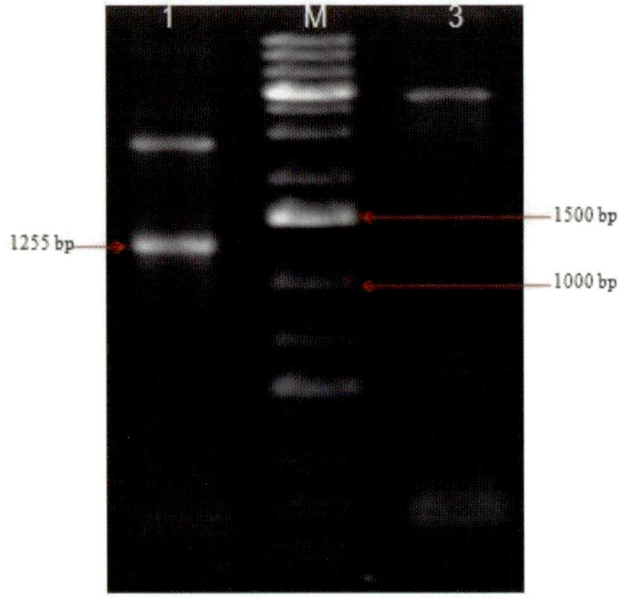

Figure 2. PCR amplification of gD gene (1255 bp) with gD gene specific F & R primers from pENTR-TOPO gD clones. Lane M, 1Kb DNA ladder;Lane 1, 3, pENTR-TOPO clones; Lane 1, positive clone.

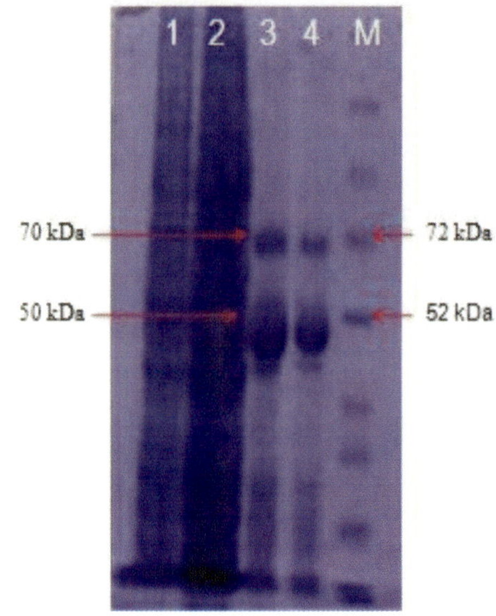

Figure 4. SDS-PAGE analysis of immunoprecipitated recombinant gD protein and partially purified BHV-1. Lane 1, Non infected Sf-9 cell lysate; Lane 2, Sf-9 infected cell lysate; Lane 3, Immunoprecipitated BHV-1; Lane 4, Immunoprecipitated gD; Lane M, Protein ladder.

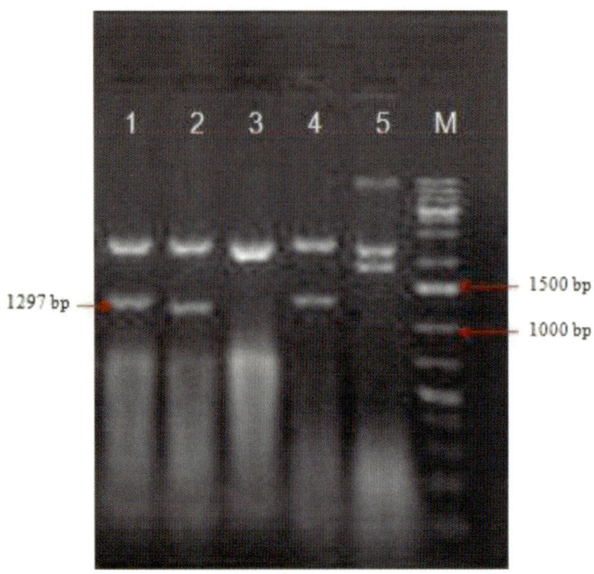

Figure 3. Release of gD gene insert by *Asc* I and *Nco* I RE digestion of the recombinant plasmids. Lane M, 1 kb DNA Ladder plus; Lane 1-5, Recombinant plasmids; Lane 1, 2, 4: Plasmids carrying gD gene insert.

Analysis of recombinant protein

The optimum duration for maximum protein expression was 72 h post infection as revealed by Western blot analysis. Immunoprecipitated expressed protein (from 72 h post infected cell lysate) was analyzed by SDS-PAGE where two bands of ~70 kDa and ~50kDa were observed (Figure 4). On western blot analysis with polyclonal anti BHV-1 serum, strong reaction of protein was observed with band of ~70 and 50 kDa (Figure 5). On SDS-PAGE together with western blot analysis (Figure 6a), gD protein was detected from 24 to 144 h post infection from Sf-9 cells, however the maximum expression being observed at 72 h (Figure 6b).

When expressed protein purified by immunoprecipitation was run on SDS-PAGE, a band of ~70 kDa and an additional band of ~50 kDa were observed. On western blot analysis using polyclonal anti BHV-1 serum, strong reaction of protein was observed with these bands (Figure 5 and 7), however the reaction being intense with polyclonal anti-BHV-1 compared to monoclonal.

The recombinant gD protein which appeared to be of a molecular mass of ~70 kDa was absent from uninfected cells. On western blot analysis, authentic gD (~70 kDa) and a polypeptide with an apparent molecular mass of ~70kDa were recognized by polyclonal antibody respectively in MDBK cells infected with BHV-1 and Sf-9 cells infected with recombinant baculovirus. This suggests that the recombinant gD is equivalent to the authentic gD.

Dot ELISA

The reaction of both immunoprecipitated gD protein and

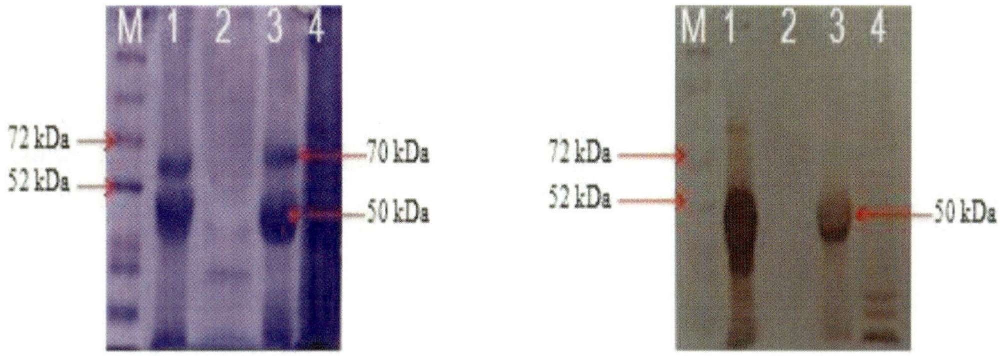

Figure 5. SDS-PAGE (left) and Western blot with Polyclonal antibody (right) analysis of the recombinant gD after 72 h of infection. Lane M, Protein ladder; Lane 1, Immunoprecipitated gD; Lane 2, Semi purified BHV-1; Lane 3, Immunoprecipitated gD; Lane 4, Non infected Sf-9 cell lysate.

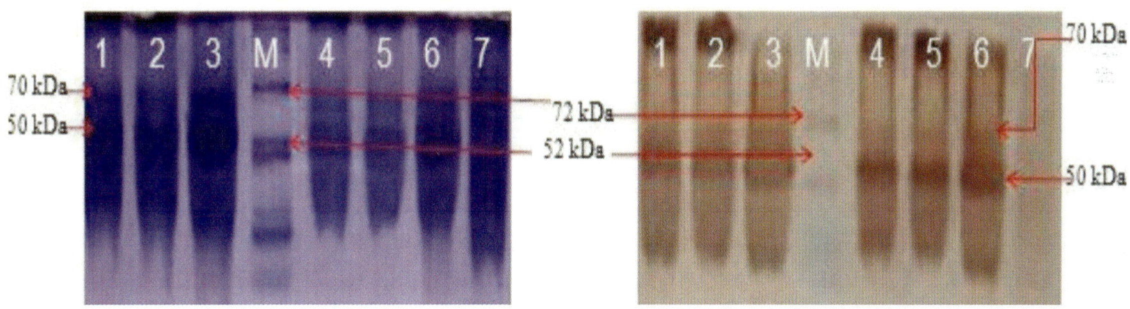

Figure 6. SDS-PAGE (left) (a) and Western blot with polyclonal antibody (right) (b) analysis of immunoprecipitated recombinant gD at different intervals of time after infection. Lane 1, Immunoprecipitated gD 24 h post infection; Lane 2, Immunoprecipitated gD 48 h post infection; Lane 3, Immunoprecipitated gD 72 h post infection; Lane M, Protein ladder; Lane 4, Immunoprecipitated gD 96 h post infection; Lane 5, Immunoprecipitated gD 120 h post infection; Lane 6, Immunoprecipitated gD 144 h post infection; Lane 7, Noninfected Sf-9 cell lysate.

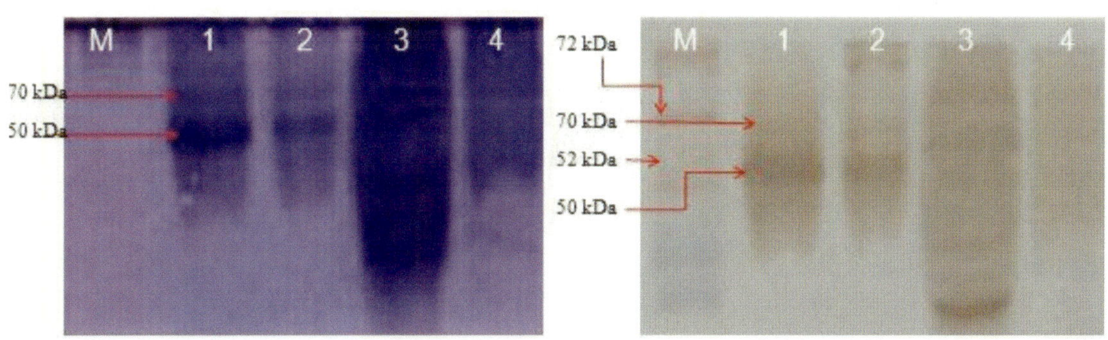

Figure 7. SDS-PAGE (left) (a) and Western blot (right) (b) analysis of the recombinant gD with monoclonal antibody. Lane 1: protein ladder; Lane 2, Immunoprecipitated gD; Lane 3, Immunoprecipitated BHV-1; Lane 4, Sf-9 infected cell lysate; Lane 5, Non infected Sf-9 cell.

gD protein recovered from infected Sf-9 cell lysate as shown in Figure 8, was also detected in Dot ELISA. As revealed by dark brown spots, the native protein gD recovered from both partially purified BHV-1 and BHV-1 infected cell lysate appeared to have fair reactivity with polyclonal antibody.

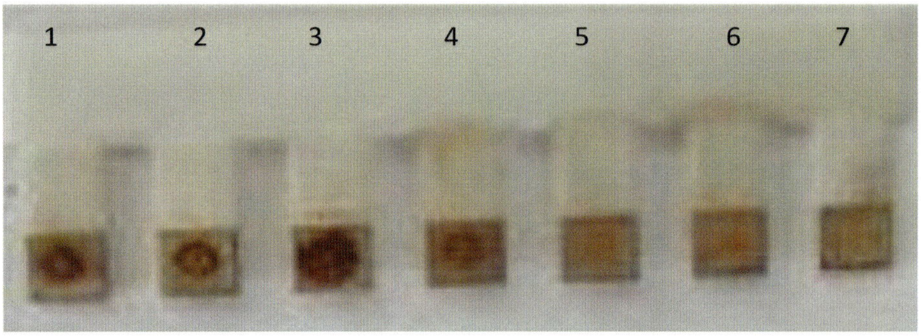

Figure 8. Dot ELISA (with polyclonal antibody) for detection of reactivity of the expressed gD recombinant protein. 1, Partially purified BHV-1; 2, MDBK infected cell lysate; 3,Immunoprecipitated gD; 4, Sf-9 infected cell lysate; 5, Non infected Sf-9 cell lysate; 6, PBS; 7, Blank.

DISCUSSION

As Abdelmagid et al. (1998) reported earlier, 72 h post infection was the optimum period for protein expression. Two bands of 70 and 50 kDa for the recombinant gD proteins were observed as revealed by SDS-PAGE and western blot analysis. Parker et al. (1991) reported to have expressed BHV-1 gp IV (D) of an apparent molecular mass of 63 kDa by recombinant baculovirus and its lower apparent molecular mass compared to the native protein indicated the incomplete glycosylation. The expressed protein appeared to be antigenically intact in this study as its reaction with polyclonal and monoclonal antibodies specific to gD was comparable to that of gD from BHV-1. These findings are in accordance with the work of Parker et al. (1991) and supported by the fact that Sf-9 cell are higher eukaryote and therefore having proper posttranslational modification (Hu, 2005).

The reactivity of anti gD monoclonal antibody with recombinant gD protein was found to be lower as compared to polyclonal antibody suggesting that the expressed protein is not being recognized properly by monoclonal antibody used as revealed by both dot ELISA and Western blot. This may result from modification or loss of epitope conformation due to protein denaturation during sample preparation together with or improper glycosylation as baculovirus infected cell display inability to correctly process some proteins (Hu, 2005) due to the fundamental nature of insect glycoprotein processing pathways (Jarvis, 2003). The poor reactivity of monoclonal antibody with a recombinant protein due to loss of native conformation of baculovirus expressed protein was also reported by Abdelmagid et al (1998) in the case of glycoprotein B (gB).

With both monoclonal and polyclonal antibodies, protein bands of 70 and 50 KDa were consistently detected in SDS-PAGE and western blot analysis. Blanc et al (2012) reported to have expressed glycoprotein D (gD) of 71 kDa and according to Van Donkersgoed et al. (1994) glycoprotein D (gD) of 71 kDa containing both N-linked and O-linked Oligosaccharides is synthesized first as a partially glycosylated precursor of 63 KDa.

Conclusion

BHV-1 gD could be successfully expressed using baculovirus based vector and insect cell system which was visualized as protein bands of 70 and 50 KDA in SDS-PAGE and Western blot assays. The expressed gD is equivalent to the authentic gD and has fair potential to be used as a diagnostic antigen for detection of BHV-1 specific antibodies.

REFERENCES

Abdelmagid OY, Mansour MM, Minocha HC, van Drunen Littel-van den Hurk S (1998). Evaluation of baculovirus-expressed bovine herpesvirus-1 (BHV-1) glycoproteins for detection and analysis of BHV-1-specific antibody responses. Vet. Microbiol. 61:249-259.

Biswas S, Bandyopadhyay S, Dimri U, Patra HP (2013). Bovine herpesvirus-1 (BHV-1)–a re-emerging concern in livestock: a revisit to its biology, epidemiology, diagnosis, and prophylaxis. Vet. Q. 33(2):68-81.

Blanc AM, Berois MB, Tomé LM, Alberto L, Epstein AL, Arbiza JR (2012). Induction of humoral responses to BHV-1 glycoprotein D expressed by HSV-1 amplicon vectors. J. Vet. Sci. 13(1):59-65.

Connolly SA, Whitbeck JC, Rux AH, Krummenacher C, Cohen GH, Eisenberg RJ (2001). Glycoprotein D homologs in herpes simplex virus type 1, pseudorabies virus, and bovine herpes virus type 1 bind directly to human HveC (nectin-1) with different affinities. Virol. 280(1):7-18.

Chowdhury S, Sharma B (2012). Transcription of gD and gI genes in BHV1-infected cells. J. Biosci. 37:971-977.

Collins JK, Butcher AC, Riegel CA (1985). Immune response to Bovine herpesvirus type 1 infections: Virus-specific antibodies in sera from infected animals. J. Clin. Microbiol .21:456-552.

da Silva LF, Kook I, Doster A, Jones C (2013). Bovine herpesvirus 1 regulatory proteins bICP0 and VP16 are readily detected in trigeminal ganglionic neurons expressing the glucocorticoid receptor during the early stages of reactivation from latency. J. Virol. 11214-11222.

Davis KJ, Syam RS, Chauhan RS (2014). Epidemiological studies on infectious bovine rhinotracheitis (IBR) in different parts of India. Int. J. Live. Res. 4(5).

Dummer LA, Leite FBL, van Drunen Littel-van den Hurk S (2014). Bovine herpesvirus glycoprotein D: a review of its structural characteristics and applications in vaccinology. Vet. Res. pp. 45:111.

Engels M, Ackermann M, (1996). Pathogenesis of ruminant herpesvirus infections. Vet. Microbiol. 53:3-15.

Godhardt-Cooper JA, Zoromski J, Toohey-Kurth K (2009). Evaluation of a blocking enzyme-linked immunosorbent assay for serological diagnosis of Bovine herpesvirus1. J. Vet. Diagn Invest.. 21:523-526.

Grauwet K, Cantoni C, Parodi M, Andrea de Maria, Devriendt B, Pende D Moretta L, Vitale M, Favoreel HW (2014). Modulation of CD112 by the Alphaherpesvirus gD protein suppresses DNAM-1–dependent NK cell-mediated lysis of infected cells. Proc. Natl. Sci. Acad.111(45):16118-16123.

Guo L, Yanling Yang Y, Liu L, Liao P, Wen Y, Wu H, Cheng S (2015). A proteomic study of the differential protein expression in MDBK cells after bovine herpesvirus type 1 infection (BHV-1) strain treatment. Int. J. Clin. Exp. Med. 8(3):4204-4211.

HU Y (2005). Baculovirus as a highly efficient expression vector in insect and mammalian cells. Acta Pharmacol. Sin. 26 (4):405-416.

Jarvis DL (2003). Developing baculovirus-insect cell expression systems for humanized recombinant glycoprotein production.Virology 310:1-7.

Kaur G, Dwivedi P N, Verma R, Sharma NS (2013). Prevalence of Bovine herpesvirus-1 in cattle and buffaloes in Punjab. Vet. World 6(6):343-345.

Kirchhoff J, Uhlenbruck S, Goris K, Keil GM, Herrler G (2014). Three viruses of the bovine respiratory disease complex apply different strategies to initiate infection. Vet. Res. pp.45:20.

Kit M, Kit S (1991). Sensitive glycoprotein gIII blocking ELISA to distinguish between pseudorabies (Aujeszky's disease)-infected and vaccinated pigs. Vet. Microbiol. 28:141-155.

Levings RL (2012). "Generation and characterization of virus-neutralizing bovine monoclonal antibodies to bovine herpesvirus 1 glycoproteins gB, gC, and gD" Graduate theses and dissertations. Paper 12862.

Levings RL, Roth JA (2013). Immunity to Bovine herpesvirus 1: II. Adaptive immunity and vaccinology. Anim. Health Res. Rev. 14(1):103-123.

Majumder S, Pandey AB, Ramakrishnan MA (2014). Cloning and sequence analysis of glycoprotein D gene of bovine herpesvirus 1. Adv. Anim. Vet. Sci. 2(2S):19-22.

Muylkens B, Thiry J, Kirten P. Schynts F,Thiry E (2007). Bovine herpesvirus 1 infection and infectious bovine rhinotracheitis Vet. Res. 38:181-209.

Sambrook J, Fritsch E, Maniatis T (1989). Molecular cloning (Vol. 2, pp. 14-9). New York: Cold spring harbor laboratory press.

Sambrook J, Fritsch EF, Maniatis T (1990). Molecular cloning: a laboratory manual, Ed 2nd.

Saminathan M, Rana R, Ramakrishnan MA, Karthik K, Malik YS, Dhama K (2016). Prevalence, diagnosis, management and control of important diseases of ruminants with special reference to Indian scenario. J. Exp. Bio. Agri. Sci. 4(3S).

Tikoo S, Campos M, Babiuk L (1995). Bovine herpesvirus 1 (BHV-1): Biology, pathogenesis, and control. Adv. Virus Res. 45:191-232.

Parker MD, Fitzpatrick DR, Zamb TJ, van den Hurk JV, Campos M, Harland R, Babiuk LA (1991). Expression of Bovine herpesvirus 1 glycoprotein IV by recombinant Baculovirus and analysis of its immunogenic propeerties. J. Virol. 65:263-71.

Van Donkersgoed J, Kowalski J, Van den Hurk JV, Harland R, Babiuk LA, Zamb TJ (1994). A subunit gIV vaccine, produced by transfected mammalian cells in culture induces mucosal immunity against bovine herpesvirus-1 in cattle. Vaccine 12:1295-302

Incidence and the history of *Echinococcus granulosus* infection in dogs within the past few decades in Libya

Mohamed, M. Ibrahem[1*], Wafa, M. Ibrahem[2], Kawther, M. Ibrahem[3], Badereddin, B. Annajar[4]

[1]Department of Zoology, Faculty of Sciences, University of Zawia, P. O. Box 16418, Zawia, Libya.
[2]Department of Parasitology, Faculty of Medicine, University of Zawia, P. O. Box 16418, Zawia, Libya.
[3]Department of Medicinal Chemistry, Faculty of Pharmacy, University of Zawia, P. O. Box 16418, Zawia, Libya.
[4]National Centre for Disease Control, Ain Zara, P. O. Box 71171, Tripoli, Libya.

***Echinococcus granulosus* is a tiny tapeworm that parasitizes the small intestine of canids, mainly dogs, which act as definitive hosts for the parasite. Infected dogs are the main source of infection to humans and livestock which act as intermediate hosts resulting in hydatid disease condition. *E. granulosus* is widely distributed in many parts of the world, and is very common in North African countries. In Libya, the rate of infection with echinococcosis in dogs was reported to be lower than 7 to 80% in stray dogs, 34.8 to 60% in sheep/guard dogs and 7.7 to 21.6% in farm/house dogs. This data fulfills the world health organization (WHO) criteria and suggests that the incidence of infection with echinococcosis/ hydatidosis in some parts of the country can be reaching the level of hyper endemic. Diagnosis of echinococcosis in infected dogs can be performed by isolating the parasite from their faeces or from the contents of their small intestine after necropsy. Recent developments in immunodiagnostic assays for echinococcosis in dogs have been described. Public health and risk factors as well as ways of hydatid disease treatment and various control strategies, including the use of veterinary vaccines, have also been discussed.**

Key words: Dogs, *Echinococcus granulosus*, prevalence, diagnosis, treatment, risk factors

INTRODUCTION

Echinococcus granulosus is a tapeworm that causes a condition known as echinococcosis in dogs, and hydatid disease or hydatidosis in humans and other ruminant animals (Chhabra and Singla, 2009). The parasite has been reported to occur in many parts of the world, and is very common in some agricultural regions, particularly, Northern Africa, Southern South America, Europe, the Middle East, South-Western Asia, and Australia (Figure 1), (Eckert and Deplazes, 2004). In these areas, the infection rate with *E. granulosus* in dogs was reported to be between endemic and hyper endemic (Dakak, 2010). The parasite requires two mammalian hosts for

*Corresponding author. E-mail: masoudibrahem@gmail.com.

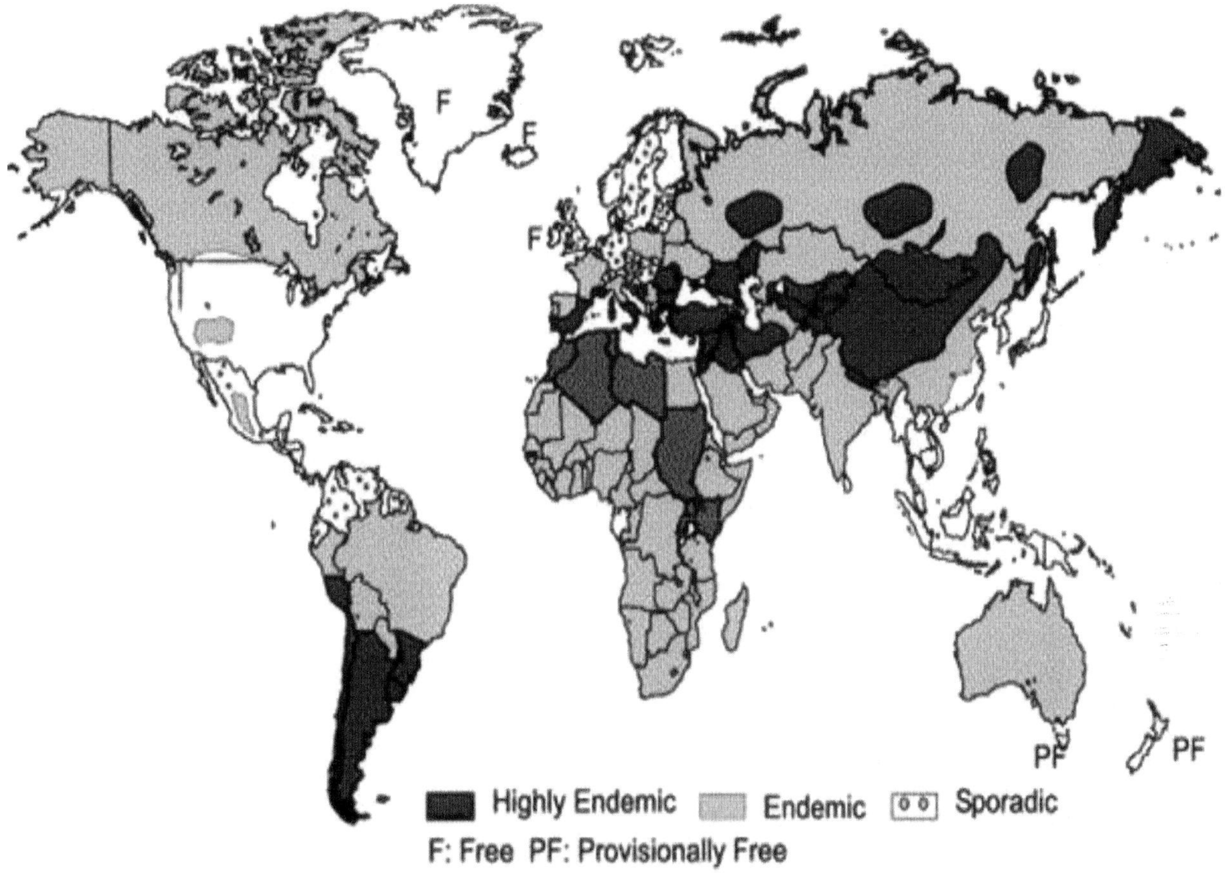

Figure 1. Worldwide distribution of *E. granulosus*. As seen from the map, echinococcosis infection in Libya in North Africa is highly endemic (adapted from Eckert and Deplazes, 2004).

completion of its life cycle; a definitive host, which is mainly carnivore for the adult stage and an intermediate host, which is mainly ungulates for the larval (hydatid cyst) stage (Figure 2). The life cycle of *E. granulosus* in Libya has a pastoral or domestic cycle in which dogs acquire the infection by eating the internal organs of infected sheep, goats, camels and cattle.

However, dogs in Libya are considered to be the main source of infection with cystic echinococcosis (CE) to various species of livestock as well as human. This cycle is potentially very important especially in areas where sheep farming is more common (Maureen, 2008). The adult form of the parasite is a minute white tapeworm, few millimeters long (3-7 mm) with three proglottids (segments) and some other features which help in species diagnosis morphologically (Thompson, 1995).

Due to the size of the parasite, dogs can carry hundreds or even thousands of them without showing any signs of illness at all. The parasites attach themselves to the wall of the small intestine of the definitive host using their hooks and in this place; they deposit a large number of eggs which are intermittently passed out in the host faeces. When the eggs are in the environment, they are dispersed by different means including wind, water, birds as well as through the fur of the infected dogs which is likely to become contaminated with the parasite eggs.

Eggs can also be found on the bodies of other animals sharing the same living environment, making them a source of transmission and distribution of the infection to humans and other ruminant animals. The intermediate hosts become infected with hydatid disease when they ingest the parasite eggs in their contaminated food or water. Once the eggs are ingested, they hatch in the duodenum releasing their embryos (the oncospheres) which subsequently penetrate the intestinal wall of the host entering the mesenteric vessels. They are then carried by the blood to the major filtering organs, mainly liver and lungs, but other sites may become involved, including the abdominal wall, brain, kidneys, bones, muscles and orbits (Polat et al., 2003; Bal et al., 2008).

The oncospheres requires about one year to transform and develop into full larval hydatid cysts with numerous tiny protoscoleces which are formed via asexual reproduction. Humans act as an intermediate hosts for *E. granulosus* and are infected when they accidentally ingest the parasite eggs from the definitive host by any way.

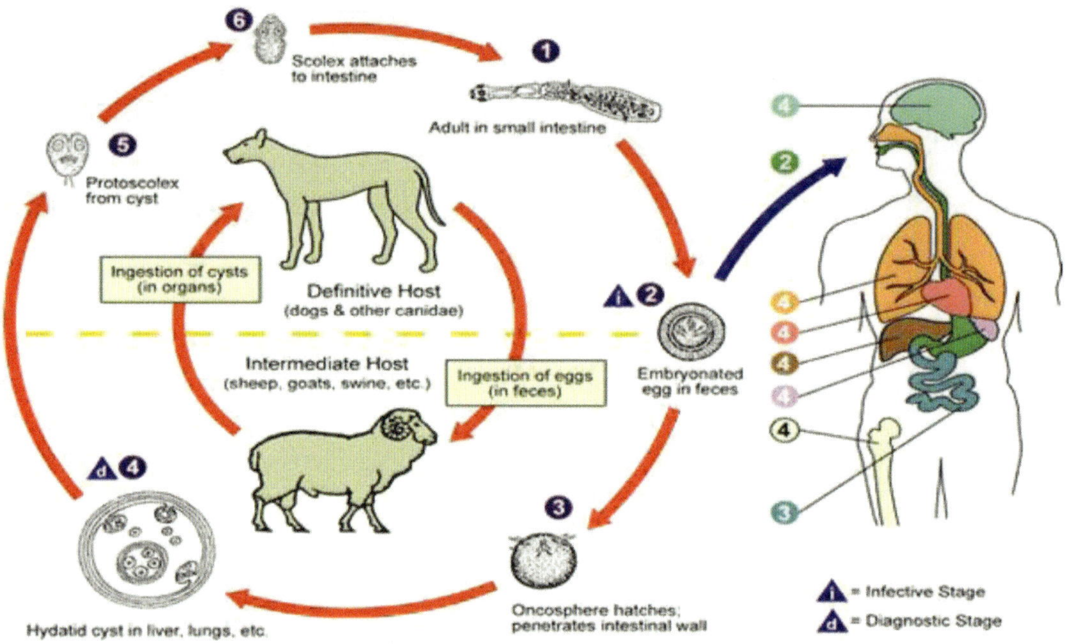

Figure 2. Illustration showing the life cycle of *E.granulosus* in both animals and humans. The life cycle of the parasite in animals involves six stages: 1) The adult worms resides attached to the bowel of the dogs. 2) Gravid segments release eggs that are passed out in the dog faeces. 3) The eggs are ingested by the ruminant animals and hatch in their bowels releasing oncospheres that invade the intestinal wall and travel through the circulating system to various organs of the host. 4). In the site, oncospheres develop into hydatid cysts producing protoscoleces and daughter cysts. 5) The ruminant infected organs ingested by dogs. 6) The protoscoleces attach to the intestinal wall of the dogs and start to develop gradually into adults in 32 to 80 days. The life cycle in humans: 2) Humans infected by eating food contaminated with the parasite eggs. 3) The ingested eggs hatch to release oncospheres in the small intestine. 4) Oncospheres migrate through the circulating system to different sites where they develop and produce hydatid cysts. (The image adapted from www.dpd.cdc.gov/dpdx).

The life cycle of the parasite is complete when dogs ingest hydatid cysts containing fully developed protoscoleces, which are subsequently released and attach themselves to the intestinal lining of the host. The protoscoleces start to develop into mature adult tapeworms within32- 80 days, depending on the species and the parasite strain. Humans are described as 'dead-end' hosts for the parasite, since the life cycle is usually completed when carnivores eat infected herbivores (McManus et al., 2003; Zhang et al., 2003).

However, it is mentioned in literature that, infected dead human bodies may contribute to complete the life cycle of the disease in some African villages where burial is not properly practiced and dogs can get access to those dead bodies (Macpherson et al., 1983). The research methodology consists of over 200 published articles on *E. granulosus* from different sources. The most appropriate publications covering the different sections in this paper were selected. This paper focuses mainly on the prevalence of *E. granulosus* infections in dogs in Libya since its discovery in 1961 to date and summarises the prospects of diagnosis, risk factors, treatment and the control and prevention strategies of the disease.

This study intends to provide base line epidemiological information on the incidence and the status of echinococcosis in dogs in Libya, and can be a source of information for the future studies.

Prevalence and the history of *Echinococcus granulosus* infection in dogs

According to scientists, the close relationship between humans and dogs started several thousands of years ago; this relationship facilitates the transmission of so many diseases including cystic hydatid disease.

Dogs in Libya, like any other country, can be classified into three groups, based on the type of their relationship to humans and other livestock: stray dogs, herding/sheep dogs and farm/house dogs. Stray dogs are the largest group in all urban and rural areas and they normally wonder freely during the night to scavenge on household waste materials, from which they may become infected with *E. granulosus* through eating dead animals and discarded offal contaminated with fertile hydatid cysts. These dogs are considered to be the main source of hydatid disease to human and livestock due to their ability to spread the parasite eggs over a wide range of areas, especially where the suitable herbivores are grazing.

The second group is the herding/sheep dogs which are used for shepherding and guarding sheep. These dogs may become infected with *E. granulosus* as a result of eating offal contaminated with fertile hydatid cysts provided by their owners or discarded by other people. Herding/sheep dogs are considered to be a source of infection to livestock by contaminating grazing pastures and water pools used for grazing and drinking respectively by the animal flocks. The third group is the farm/house dogs which are used for guarding the farm belongings including animals and the house contents from thieves.These dogs become infected with *E. granulosus* through contaminated meat or offal provided mostly by their owners.

Echinococcosis was discovered in Libya for the first time in 1961, when heavy infections with *E. granulosus* were detected in 60% of shepherd dogs and 10% of town dogs (Cicogna, 1961). Data available on the prevalence of echinococcosis in dogs is scattered and inadequate. Three different studies have been conducted on the prevalence of echinococcosis in stray dogs between 1986 and 1990, and the obtained results after necropsy were 11.8, 40.3, and 36.8% (Packer and Ali, 1986; Gusbi, 1987a; Awan et al., 1990) respectively. In sheep and house dogs, the infection rate with echinococcosis was reported to be 34.8 and 7.7% respectively (Gusbi, 1987a).

The low rate of infection with *E. granulosus* in house dogs compared to the other two groups of dogs is probably due to the fact that these dogs are kept within premises and under control most of the time and they rarely get access to contaminated offal. Another study on the incidence of echinococcosis in dogs was carried out by Buishi et al. (2005), who reported that 25.8% of stray dogs and 21.6% of farm/house dogs were found to be harbouring the parasite. Using Kato thick smear technique, Ben-Musa and Sadek (2007) investigated 50 samples of faeces from street dogs and found that 58% of the examined specimens were positive for *E. granulosus*.

Moreover, a recent study was conducted by Gusbi (2010) examining 151 stray dogs at post mortem from 14 localities distributed all over the country. The obtained results showed that 27.8% of the examined dogs were infected with *E. granulosus*. This study also elucidated that, the infection rate was generally greater in the coastal areas of the country which was between 26 and 80%, and was even worse in Zawia, El-Khumes, Misrata, Sirt and Tubruk, where more than 50% of stray dogs were found to be harbouring the parasite.

In contrast, a previous study showed that in southern regions such as Sebha and El-Kufra, the infection rate in stray dogs was less than 7% (Gusbi, 1987a). This could simply be explained by the fact that huge numbers of abattoirs exist in the highly populated northern areas and are unfortunately lacking proper disposal of offal. Also moderate temperatures and the relatively high humidity in the northern areas may contribute significantly in prolonging the survival rate of *E. granulosus* eggs, thus allowing for an increased chance of disease transmission and vice versa in the southern areas (Wachira et al., 1991).

Furthermore, the differences in local traditions of slaughtering animals in houses during social occasions and celebrations, which involves the disposal of unwanted offal and remains by feeding it to domestic dogs, may contribute to the indicated variations.

Public health risks associated with *E. granulosus* infection in dogs

Despite the establishment of comprehensive and successful control programmes for CE, *E. granulosus* still continues to have a wide geographical distribution. This may lead to the re-emergence of the disease in many endemic regions worldwide, which would easily spread from endemic to non-endemic areas, causing severe public health problems and considerable economic losses (Craig et al., 2003; McManus et al., 2003).

Echinococcosis is a serious zoonosis in certain rural populations where there is close contact with domestic dogs and where human infection with CE is reported to be between > 1 and < 200 cases per 100,000 populations (OIE, 2008). In most endemic areas, where domestic dogs act as a definitive host for *E. granulosus*, identification of risk factors for canine infection can provide useful information on potential human risk and can be useful for designing and monitoring the parasite control schemes based on treatment of infection in dogs. Agricultural or stock-raising lifestyle, low socio-economic status, climate, bad hygiene, illegal or uncontrolled slaughter, as well as uncontrolled dog populations have all been reported to be risk factors (Cetinkaya et al., 2005; King and Fairley, 2010).

Laboratory workers, animal handlers, veterinarians, dog owners are more prone to infection with hydatid disease due to their direct contact with the parasite eggs. On the other hand, Muslim families who have the religious practice of keeping dogs away from homes and avoiding direct contact are reported to be at low risk of being infected with CE (Akalin et al., 2014). Eggs are usually shed to the environment and may therefore, contaminate vegetables, fruits, water, or stick to animals' fur and human hands. Great hygienic care is essential, especially careful hand washing practices which constitute an important preventive measure. In humans, hydatid cysts of *E. granulosus* are usually developed in organs such as liver and lungs, so the symptoms of infection with the disease will be liver or lungs deficiency, however, X-ray, ultrasound investigation and blood tests should be undertaken regularly for those who are in contact with possible infected dogs. Significant risk factors for copro-positive owned dogs were found to be associated with non-restraint of dogs, in addition, people who do not de-worm their dogs, slaughter animals at home without proper veterinary inspection and have poor knowledge about the parasite transmission were also at high risk of acquiring human CE (Buishi et al., 2005).

Diagnosis of *E. granulosus* in dogs

Systematic diagnosis of *Echinococcus* infection in definitive hosts had always been an important component for establishing epidemiological parameters of echinococcosis and preventing human and livestock infection with CE (Sakai et al., 1995).

The problem of diagnosing *E. granulosus* in dogs has only been partially resolved, even after the introduction of biotechnology. It is more difficult to know when a dog is infected with *Echinococcus* parasites compared to the other cestods. This is due to the size of the parasite as well as their eggs, which can be easily missed out during faecal examinations and can be hard to differentiate them from *Taenia* eggs; however, this process still remains the most efficient way to detect the infection and should be performed regularly. Two major diagnostic methods have been used in dogs extensively. These are purgation with arecoline compounds and necropsy (Unruh et al., 1973; Craig et al., 1995; Eckert et al., 2001).

The purgation technique has been used in many control programmes all over the world in recent decades. The technique showed 100% specificity, but has certain limitations due to its poor sensitivity, as not all infected dogs respond to the purge and eliminate parasites. In addition to this, the technique is bio-hazardous, time consuming and must be administered by trained personnel (Craig et al., 1995; Eckert et al., 2001). Moreover, most of the epidemiological data and models have been developed from the results of this method (Torgerson et al., 2003). On the contrary, necropsy is the method of choice and is considered to be the more reliable tool for the diagnosis of the disease in dogs, but unfortunately has many limitations (Jenkins et al., 2000; Lopera et al., 2003).

Alternatively, immunodiagnostic techniques were used to detect specific antibodies or antigens in dogs. The detection of *E. granulosus* specific antigens in canine faeces was first reported by Babos and Nemeth (1962). During the last three decades, considerable progress has been achieved in various fields of echinococcosis research when several immunological and serological tests have evolved for the diagnosis of *Echinococcus spp.* in definitive hosts. Copro-antigen detection enzyme linked immunosorbent assay (cop-Ag-ELISA) test has been developed using polyclonal antibodies to *E.* granulosus excretory/secretory (ES) antigens, and appears to be valuable in detecting the infection in dogs with high specificity (96.5%) and sensitivity (87.5%) (Allan et al.,1992). Sandwich ELISA reported to be highly specific and capable in detecting immature and mature stages of *Echinococcus spp.* and this high specificity was found to be correlated to the worm burden and the duration of the infection (Craig et al., 1995; Ahmad and Nizami, 1998).

Some sandwich ELISA systems have been assessed for their ability to detect *E. granulosus* copro-antigens using monoclonal antibody produced against somatic extract of *Echinococcus multilocularis*. Although the test was very sensitive (100%) in naturally and experimentally infected animals, there were cases of cross-reactivity with *Taenia hydatigena* (Sakai et al., 1995; Malgor et al., 1997).

Overall, however, the test was the best laboratory-based test for ante mortem diagnosis of canine echinococcosis (Eckert et al., 2001). Parasite copro-antigens have been defined as parasite specific products in the faeces of the host that are amenable to immunological detection and are associated with the parasite metabolism (Allan et al., 2003).

Using copro-antigen sandwich ELISA, the sensitivity was between 83.33 and 100%, and the specificity was between 96.94 and 100% (Prathiush et al., 2008; Dalimi et al., 2010). Copro-ELISA test can also detect heat-stable antigens and has been used in a number of studies in the Middle East, Wales, Southern and Eastern Europe, and South America (Deplazes et al., 1992; Sakashita et al., 1995; Eckert et al., 2001).

The high sensitivity of monoclonal antibodies (MAb) to parasite specific antigens could increase the reliability of copro-antigen detection. Monoclonal antibodies for *E. granulosus* copro-antigen detection were produced namely, IgM murine monoclonal antibodies, EgC1 and EgC3, against E/S products of *E. granulosus* adult worms (Casaravilla et al., 2005).

Different studies from many countries suggest that copro-antigen ELISA is a valid test for detecting *E. granulosus* infection in living dogs. Thus, it is appropriate to apply this test in epidemiological studies (Magnaval et al., 2004; Buishi et al., 2005; Stefania et al., 2006; Kamiya et al., 2007; Zare-Bidaki et al., 2009). It would be useful to develop more specific techniques in cases where the presence of the parasite in the dog population is relatively low (Christofi et al., 2002), as well as for discrimination between dogs with *Echinococcus spp.* and those with other taeniid infections.

Copro-DNA-polymerase chain reaction (Copro-DNA-PCR) technique has been developed, and is only available for a limited number of species or genotypes in particular *E. multilocularis* and *E. granulosus* sheep strain (Craig et al., 2003; Mathis and Deplazes, 2006). Bretagna et al. (1993) was the first who developed a species-specific Copro-DNA-PCR for *E. multilocularis* and the technique showed 100% for both specificity and sensitivity, but the later can vary depending on worms quantity and maturity (Mathis and Deplazes, 2006). Copro-DNA-PCR could be improved if the parasite eggs are concentrated by using a process called sequential sieving and zinc chloride flotation (Mathis et al., 1996).

A PCR test developed by Cabrera et al. (2002) showed high levels of specificity and sensitivity for the identification of *E. granulosus* eggs from a contaminated environment. However, it is clear that the test did not cross-react with *E. multilocularis* but shared similar genetic sequences to other *Echinococcus spp.* such as *Echinococcus oligarthrus* and *Echinococcus vogeli.* A Copro-DNA-PCR assay developed by Stefanic et al. (2004) for detection of *E. granulosus* sheep strain (G1) showed 100% specificity against other *Echinococcus spp.* including *E. multilocularis* and *E. vogeli.* The PCR test used by Abbasie et al. (2003) gave 100% sensitivity and specificity using DNA samples extracted from 0.3 ml of faeces from 34 infected and 18 non-infected dogs, and the test gave a positive result even with a small number of *E. granulosus* eggs in the sample. For field application, the cop-Ag-ELISA has the potential for replacing necropsy examinations. The cop-PCR is a valuable method for the confirmation of positive copro-antigen results and the diagnosis of individual animals (Deplazes and Eckert, 1996). It is indeed considered to be the most specific diagnostic technique (Mathis and Deplazes, 2006).

Furthermore, when using specific primer along with cop-PCR, the *Echinococcus* infection can be diagnosed up to species level, with a specificity of 100% (Stefanic et al., 2004; Dinkel et al., 2004).

Treatment of echinococcosis in dogs with reference to human cystic hydatidosis

Until recently, surgery was the only option for treatment of hydatid disease in humans. However, medication and other surgical techniques (aspiration) are currently widely in use and can replace the need for surgical removal of hydatid cysts (Polat et al., 2002).

Nevertheless, in some cases, a surgery may be necessary, along with medication, to prevent the cyst from growing back. It has been agreed that an image-based, stage-specific approach is helpful in determining the choice of human CE treatment, whether it be percutaneous treatment, surgery, and anti-infective drug treatment or watch and wait (Brunetti et al., 2010).

Puncture aspiration, re-aspiration, injection and chemotherapy are also available for treatment of CE (Pawłowski et al., 2001). Percutaneous drainage has been widely used as an alternative to surgery in the treatment of hydatid cysts. Unlike surgical procedures, which normally start with the inactivation of the cyst contents followed by removal of all cyst components (Yorganci and Sayek, 2002; Menezes da Silva, 2003), The percutaneous drainage method does not involve the removal of the cyst membrane which is composed of laminated and germinative layers (Yorganci and Sayek, 2002). Percutaneous drainage may include puncture, aspiration of cyst contents, injection of scolicidal agents and finally re-aspiration of the injected fluid, as described by Ben-Amor et al. (1986), or by catheterization, as described by Akhan and Özmen, (1999).

Chemotherapy became a treatment option for hydatid disease decades ago when new anti-helminthic drugs were introduced. Benzimidazole carbamates were shown to kill the entire larval stage of the parasite by inhibiting the formation of microtubules, and thus destructing the uptake of glucose and interfering with the homeostasis of the parasite (Lacey, 1990), whereas praziquantel was found to be effective on protoscoleces (Heath and Chevis, 1974; Schantz et al., 1982).

Continuous or irregular treatment with albendazole is recommended for a period of up to 6 months, and to increase the efficacy of the treatment, praziquantel should be used, particularly in the case of cyst spillage (Teggi et al., 1993). It has been reported that the infection caused by adult worms in dogs can be successfully treated with praziquantel and it is advisable to confine dogs and/or use purgatives to facilitate the collection and disposal of infected faeces.

Most studies indicate that the effectiveness of albendazole as measured by the disappearance of the cysts, is generally less than 30% under ideal circumstances. However, 40 to 50% of cysts showed some response during the course of therapy such as shrinkage in their size or detachment of their components from the cyst wall. To increase its efficacy, albendazole must be taken daily for 4 to 6 weeks and should be repeated two or three times more. Additionally, using albendazole before and after operation was found to decrease the viability of cysts at the time of surgery, as well as significantly reducing the chances of cyst recurrence (Arif et al., 2008).

Oxfendazole is a benzimidazole drug which has been used in veterinary medicine to control nematode infections and was found to be effective against the intestinal stage of *E. granulosus,* as well as other cestodes in the gastrointestinal tract, thus could be used to treat infections in dogs, the principal reservoir for human infection (Gemmell et al., 1979).

Gonzales et al. (1996) examined the effect of the drug on the tissue stage of tapeworm infections and found that a single dose of 30 mg/kg of body weight of oxfendazole in pigs completely eliminated all tissue cysts of *Taenia solium*, a medically important human tapeworm. Nevertheless, hydatid cysts are much larger than and structurally different from the cysts of cysticercosis, suggesting the possible use of oxfendazole for the treatment of hydatid disease. Further studies carried out by Blanton et al., (1998) and Njoroge et al., (2005) used the same dose of oxfendazole on other animal species.

The results obtained after post mortem investigation showed that 97% of cysts from sheep and 93.3% of cysts from goats contained dead or absent protoscoleces, compared to 28 and 27.3% of cysts from untreated control sheep and goats respectively. In addition, 53% of cysts from treated animals were found to be heavily degenerated and even with the potentially viable cysts, there was evidence of severe damage to the wall, severe disorganization of the adventitial layer with invasion of inflammatory cells and in some cases frank necrosis with no apparent adventitial layer (Blanton et al., 1998).

More evaluation on oxfendazole was carried out against CE in sheep and the obtained results showed that, the number of fertile cysts decreased, the number of degenerated cysts increased and it was more efficacious against lungs and liver cysts at 49.6 to 61.2% and 91.8 to 100% respectively (Gavidia et al., 2009).

Based on the reported results, oxfendazole appears to be a promising alternative drug for the treatment of CE and may potentially become the drug of choice for the treatment of human hydatid disease in the near future. However, with poor response to most chemotherapeutic agents, cystic hydatidosis remains a primarily surgical disease and the importance of using chemotherapy lies in the prophylaxis against spillage during surgery, treatment of none operated cases and for use in areas where adequate surgical facilities are unavailable.

Control and prevention of echinococcosis transmission

Cystic hydatidosis continues to be a strong cause of morbidity and mortality in many parts of the world, however, complete eradication of CE is difficult to obtain and by using current control options to achieve such a goal will take several years of continuing attempts (Craig et al., 2007).

Control of unilocular hydatidosis is based on breaking the cycle of infection, either by preventing dogs from consuming infected organs of intermediate hosts or by preventing intermediate hosts from ingesting eggs present in dogs' faeces and treating infected dogs with effective cestocides, especially in urban environments. Cystic hydatid disease in humans was found to be caused by different genotypes of *E. granulosus* subspecies. Such genotypes include *for example, sensu stricto* (G1-G3), *equinus* (G4), *ortleppi* (G5) and *canadensis* (G6-G10) (Thompson, 2008).

In Libya, most human cases of CE are caused by sheep strain G1, cattle strain G5 and camel strain G6. These intermediate hosts are the most common reared animals in the country (Abushhiwa et al., 2010). Dogs are the most essential part for hydatid disease transmission to humans and other ruminant animals; however, vaccination of dogs provides a very practical and cost-effective Prevention strategy. A study by Zhang et al. (2006) indicated that vaccination of these animals with soluble native proteins obtained from protoscoleces of *E. granulosus* promotes significant suppression of worm growth and eggs production. In addition, control strategies need to focus on careful analysis of the local situations such as the cycle, ecology, and ethology of the animal hosts, as well as behavioural characteristics of the population at risk. It is most important to use newly developed tools such as imaging, molecular biology and immunology in both human and animals in any successful control programme. Moreover, anti-parasitic treatment, control of the definitive hosts, control of slaughtering, vaccination of the intermediate hosts, health education are also considered to be essential elements in any control programme (Ito et al., 2003).

As it is difficult to completely prevent the exposure to *Echinococcus* eggs from wild animals, food safety precautions combined with good hygiene can be helpful. All fruits and vegetables, especially those picked up from the wild, should be cleaned thoroughly with water to ensure the removal of the parasite eggs, if any. People who handle pets, or are involved in farming, gardening or preparing food, should wash their hands carefully before eating.

Furthermore, fences should be built around vegetable and fruit gardens to keep dogs and other canids away. Untreated water from sources such as lakes may also contain *Echinococcus* eggs and should therefore, be avoided. Unfortunately, over the past decades, there has been no CE control programme in Libya, but the high incidence of the disease in humans (1.4 to 2%) (Shambesh et al., 1999), and the high prevalence of hydatidosis in livestock, which has been reported to be 1.6 to 40% in sheep, 5.6 to 70% in goats, 2.7 to 56% in cattle, and 2.7 to 48% in camels (Ibrahem et al., 2016), suggests the need for an extensive control programme.

A control programme is most effective when implemented on a community or county-wide basis and must include the de-worming of all dogs, especially those with possible access to livestock offal, and this must be repeated at any time after any possible exposure. In endemic areas, where echinococcosis is considered to be a public health concern, dogs should be dosed with praziquantel every 6 weeks. The correct disposal of dead animals or animal viscera, elimination of stray dogs, keeping dogs away from children play grounds, personal hygiene (hand washing) are all essential tools in reducing the chances of the disease endemicity.

Despite the available epidemiological information on echinococcosis/hydatidosis in Libya, indicating that the disease is a public health concern, no effective control programme is currently in place. There is evidence suggesting that the incidence of echinococcosis and hydatidosis may have increased in the country during the last few years, due to the major social and political changes that affected veterinary and public health services following the collapse of the country government. Conducting screening surveys, using serological tests, may help in detecting early infections particularly in high risk groups.

CONCLUSION

Echinococcosis is a prevalent disease in all dog groups in Libya, with variable rates of infection (< 7 to 80% in stray dogs, 34.8 to 60% in sheep or guard dogs and 7.7 to 21.6% in farm or house dogs). Attempts to develop techniques with high specificity and sensitivity for the diagnosis of echinococcosis and hydatidosis are important in understanding the disease's epidemiology, especially in areas where CE is recently discovered. Control of hydatidosis is less effective without the support of dog-owners and this can only be achieved through increasing education and raising community awareness of the disease (Heath et al., 2006). High precautions should be taken in consideration regarding the risk factors influencing the transmission and spread of the disease in areas where the disease is recognised. In areas where home slaughter is practiced, dosing of dogs with a suitable taeniacide will be an important component in the hydatid control programme (Watson-Jones and Macpherson, 1988). In developing countries like Libya, imposing strict measures on offal disposal in abattoirs will certainly reduce disease transmission (Ito et al., 2003).

ACKNOWLEDGEMENTS

The authors would like to acknowledge people from UK, Elham M Ibrahem, BSc (Hon) and MSc-Distinction (Computer Sciences), Manchester University and Sarra M. Ibrahem, BSc (Hon), Accounting and Finance, Manchester Metropolitan University and MSc-Merit, Islamic Banking, Salford University for their important revision of the article linguistically.

REFERENCES

Abbasi I, Branzburg A, Campos-Ponce M, Abdel Hafez SK, Raoul F, Craig PS, Hamburger J (2003). Copro-diagnosis of *Echinococcus granulosus* infection in dogs by amplification of a newly identified repeated DNA sequence. Am. J. Trop. Med. Hyg. 69:324-30.

Abushhiwa MH, Nolan MJ, Jex AR, Campbell BE, Jabbar A, Gasser RB (2010). Genetic classification of *E. granulosus* cysts from human, cattle and camels in Libya using mutation scanning-based analysis of mitochondrial loci. Mol. Cell Probes 24:346-351.

Ahmad G, Nizami WA (1998). Copro-antigens: Early detection and suitability of an immunodiagnostic method for echinococcosis in dogs Vet. Parasitol. 77:237-244.

Akalin S, Kutlu SS, Caylak SD, Onal O, Kaya S, Bozkurt AI (2014). Seroprevalence of human cystic echinococcosis and risk factors in animal breeders in rural communities in Denizli, Turkey. J. Infect. Dev. Count. 8: 1188-1194.

Akhan O, Özmen MN (1999). Percutaneous treatment of liver hydatid cysts. Eur. J. Radiol. 32:76-85.

Allan JC, Craig PS, Garcia Noval J, Mencos F, Liu D, Wang Y, Wen H, Zhou P, Stringer R, Rogan MT, Zeyhle E (1992). Copro-antigen detection for immunodiagnosis of echinococcosis and taeniasis in dogs and humans. Parasitol. 104:347-356.

Allan JC, Wilkins PP, Tsang VC, Craig PS (2003). Immunodiagnostic tools for taeniasis. Acta Trop. 87:87-93.

Arif SH, Shams-ul-Bari, Wani NA, Zargar SA, Wani MA, Tabassum R, Hussain Z, Baba AA, Lone RA (2008). Albendazole as an adjuvant to the standard surgical management of liver hydatid cyst. Int J. Surg. 6:448-451.

Awan MAQ, Gusbi AM, Beesley WN (1990). *Echinococcus* in Libya. III. Further studies of *E. granulosus* in dogs. Ann. Trop. Med. Parasitol. 48:473-475.

Babos S, Nemeth I (1962). Az echinococcis szerodiagnoztikajanak kerderehez. Mag. Allat. Lap. 17:58-60.

Bal N, Nazim EK, Rabia A, Ali E, Fazilet K (2008). Uncommon locations of hydatid cysts. Saudi Med. J. 29:1004-1008.

Ben-Amor N, Gargouri M, Gharbi HA, Golvan YJ, Ayachi K, Kchouck H (1986). Treatment of hepatic hydatid cyst in sheep by echographic puncture. Tunis. Med. 64:325-331.

Ben-Musa NA, Sadek GS (2007). Prevalence of echinococcosis in street dogs in Tripoli district, Libya. J. Egypt Soc. Parasitol. 37:793-800.

Blanton R, Wachira TM, Zeyhle E, Njoroge EM, Magabo J, Schantz PM (1998). Oxfendazole treatment for cystic hydatid disease in naturally infected animals. Am. Soc. Microbiol. 42:601-605.

Bretagna S., Guilloun JP, Morand M, Houin R (1993). Detection of *Echinococcus multilocularis* DNA in fox faeces using DNA hybridisation. Parasitol. 106:193-199.

Brunetti E, Kern P, Vuitton DA (2010). Expert consensus for the diagnosis and treatment of cystic and alveolar echinococcosis in humans. Acta Trop. 114:1-16.

Buishi IE, Njoroge EM, Bouamra O, Craig PS (2005). Canine echinococcosis in northwest Libya: Assessment of coproantigen ELISA, and a survey of infection with analysis of risk-factors. Vet. Parasitol. 130: 223-232.

Cabrera M, Canova S, Rosenzvit M, Guarnera E (2002). Identification of *Echinococcus granulosus* eggs. Diagn. Microbiol. Infect. Dis. 44:29-34.

Casaravilla C, Malgor R, Rossi A, Sakai H, Nonaka N, Kamiya M, Carmona C (2005). Production and characterisation of monoclonal antibodies against excretory/secretory products of adult *Echinococcus granulosus*, and their application to coproantigen detection. Parasitol. Int. 54:43-49.

Cetinkaya Z, Ciftci IH, Demirel R, Altindis M, Ayaz E (2005). A seroepidemiologic study on cystic echinococcosis in Midwestern region of Turkey. Saudi Med. J. 26:350.

Chhabra MB and Singla LD (2009). Food-borne parasitic zoonoses in India: Review of recent reports of human infection. J. Vet. Parastol. 23:103-110.

Christofi G, Deplazes P, Christofi N, Tanner I, Economides P, Eckert J (2002). Screening of dogs for *E. granulosus* coproantigen in a low endemic situation in Cyprus. Vet. Parasitol. 104:299-306.

Cicogna D (1961). L'echinociccosi in Tripolitania. Boll. San. Del. Trip. pp. 2:3.

Craig PS, Gasser RB, Parada L, Caprera P, Parietti S, Brgues C, Acuttis A, Agulla J, Snowden K, Paolillo E (1995). Diagnosis of canine echinococcosis: comparison of coproantigen and serum antibody test with arecoline purgation in Uruguay. Vet. Parasitol. 56:293-301.

Craig PS, McManus DP, Lightwolers MW, Chabalgoity JA, Garcia HH, Gavidia CM, Gilman RH, Gonzalez AE, Lorca M, Naquira C, NietoA, Schantz PM (2007). Prevention and control of cystic echinococcosis. Latent Infect. Dis. 7:385-394.

Craig PS, Rogan MT, Campos-Ponce M (2003). Echinococcosis: disease, detection and transmission. Parasitol. 127:Suppl S5-20.

Dakak A (2010). Echinococcosis/hydatidosis: A severe threat in Mediterranean countries. Vet. Parasitol. 174:2-11.
Dalimi A, Motamedi GHR, Syavashi M, Paykari H, Hablolvarid MH (2010). Detection of *Echinococcus granulosus* infection in dogs using coproantigen enzyme linked immunosorbent assay. Arch. Razi. Inst. 65:9-14.
Deplazes P, Eckert J (1996). Diagnosis of the *Echinococcus multilocularis* infection in final hosts. Appl. Parasitol. 37:245-252.
Deplazes P, Gottstein B, Eckert J, Jenkins DJ, Ewald D, Jimenez-Palacios S (1992). Detection of *Echinococcus* coproantigens by enzyme linked immunosorbent assay in dogs, dingoes and foxes. Parasitol. Res. 78:303-308.
Dinkel A, Njoroge EM, Zimmermann A, Walz M, Zeyhle E, Elmahdi EI, Mackenstedt U, Romig T (2004). A PCR system for detection of species and genotypes of the *Echinococcus granulosus*-complex, with reference to the epidemiological situation in eastern Africa, Int. J. Parasitol. 34:645-653.
Eckert J, Deplazes P (2004). Biological, epidemiological and clinical aspects of echinococcosis, a zoonosis of increasing concern. Clin. Microbiol. Rev. 17:107-135.
Eckert J, Deplazes P, Craig PS, Gemmell MA, Gottstein B, Heath D, Jenkins DJ, Kamiya M, Lightowlers M, Meslin FX, Pawłowski ZS (2001). Echinococcosis in animals: clinical aspects, diagnosis and treatment. WHO/OIE Manual on echinococcosis in humans and animals: a public health problem of global concern. pp. 72-99.
Gavidia CM, Gonzalez AE, Lopera L, Jayashi C, Angelats R, Barron EA, Ninaquispe B, Villarrea L, Garcia HH, Verastegui MR, Gilman RH (2009). Evaluation of nitazoxanide and oxfendazole efficacy against cystic echinococcosis in naturally infected sheep. Am. J. Trop. Med. Hyg. 80: 367-372.
Gemmell MA, Johnstone PD, Oudemans G (1979). The effect of oxfendazole on *Echinococcus granulosus* and *Taenia hydatigena* infections in dogs. Res. Vet. Sci. 26:389-390.
Gonzales AE, Garcia HH, Gilman RH, Gavidia CM, Tsang VCW, Bernal T, Falcon N, Romero M, Lopez-Urbina MT (1996). Effective, single-dose treatment of porcine cysticercosis with oxfendazole. Am. J. Trop. Med. Hyg. 54:391-394.
Gusbi AM (1987a). Echinococcosis in Libya. I. Prevalence of *Echinococcus granulosus* in dogs with particular reference to the role of the dogs in Libyan Society. Ann. Trop. Med. Parasitol. 81:29-34.
Gusbi AM (2010). The prevalence of *E. granulosus* infection in dogs and the parasitic risk in Libya. 4th Sci. Congr. Egypt. Soc. Anim. Manag. 112-119.
Heath D1, Yang W, Li T, Xiao Y, Chen X, Huang Y, Yang Y, Wang Q, Qiu J (2006). Control of hydatidosis. Parasitol. Int. 55:247-252.
Heath DD, Chevis RAF (1974). Mebendazole and hydatid cysts. Lanc. 2:218-219.
Ibrahem, MM, Ibrahem WM, Abdorrahem MM, Ibrahem KM (2016). Livestock Hydatid Disease (Cystic Hydatidosis) in Libya: A review. Am. J. Anim. Vet. Sci. 11:70-84.
Ito A, Urbani C, Jiamin Q, Vuitton DA, Dongchuan Q, Heath DD, Craig PS, Zheng F, Schantz PM (2003). Control of echinococcosis and cysticercosis: A public health challenge to international cooperation in China. Acta Trop. 86:3-17.
Jenkins D J, Fraser A, Bradshaw H, Craig PS (2000). Detection of *Echinococcus granulosus* coproantigens in Australian canids with natural or experimental infection. J. Parasitol. 86:140-145.
Kamiya M, Lagapa JT, Ganzorig S, Kobayashi F, Nonaka N, Yuzaburo O (2007). Echinococcosis risk among domestic definitive hosts, Jap. Emerg. Infect. Dis. 13:346-47.
King CH, Fairley JK (2010). Cestodes (Tapeworms). In. Mandell GL, Bennett JE, Dolin R (Eds). Principles and Practice of Infectious Diseases. 7th edition. Philadelphia, Churchill Livingstone. pp. 3607-3616.
Lacey E (1990). Mode of action of benzimidazole. Parasitol. Tod. 6:112-115.
Lopera L, Moro P, Chavez A, Montes G, Gonzales A Gilman R (2003). Field evaluation of a coproantigen enzyme linked immunosorbent assay for diagnosis of canine echinococcosis in a rural Andean village in Peru. Vet. Parasitol. 117:37-42.
Macpherson CNL, Karstad L, Stevenson P, Arundel JH (1983). Hydatid disease in the Turkana District of Kenya. III. The Significance of Wild Animals in the Transmission of *Echinococcus granulosus*, with particular reference to Turkana and Masailand in Kenya. Ann. Trop. Med. Parasitol. 77:66-73.
Magnaval JF, Boucher C, Morassin B, Raoul F, Duranton C, Jacquiet P, Giraudoux P, Vuitton DA, Piarroux R (2004). Epidemiology of alveolar echinococcosis in southern Cantal, Auvergne region, France. J. Helminthol. 78:237-242.
Malgor R, Nonaka N, Basmadjian I, Sakai H, Carambula B, Oku Y, Carmona C, Kamiya M (1997). Coproantigen detection in dogs experimentally and naturally infected with *Echinococcus granulosus* by a monoclonal antibody-based enzyme linked immunosorbent assay. Int. J. Parasitol. 27:1605-1612.
Mathis A, Deplazes P (2006). Copro-DNA tests for diagnosis of animal taeniid cestodes. Parasitol. Int. 55:87-90.
Mathis A, Deplazes P, Eckert J (1996). An improved test system for PCR-based specific detection of *Echinococcus multilocularis* eggs. J. Helminthol. 70:219-22.
Maureen A (2008). More about *Echinococcus* tape worm in dogs. Worms & Germs Blog, Ont. Vet. Coll., Centre for Public Health and Zoonosis.
McManus DP, Zhang W, Li J, Bartley PB (2003). Echinococcosis. Lanc. 362:1295-1304.
Menezes da Silva A (2003). Hydatid cyst of the liver: Criteria for the selection of appropriate treatment. Acta Trop. 85: 237-242.
Njoroge E, Mbithi P, Wachira T, Gathuma J, Gathura P, Maitho TE, Magambo J, Zeyhle MSE (2005). Comparative study of albendazole and oxfendazole in the treatment of cystic echinococcosis in sheep and goats. Int. J. Appl. Res. Vet. Med. 3:97-101.
Office International des Epizootics (OIE) (2008). Echinococcosis/ hydatidosis. Terrestrial manual.
Packer DE, Ali TM (1986). *Echinococcus granulosus* in dogs in Libya. Ann. Trop. Med. Parasitol. 80:137-139.
Pawloeski ZS, Eckert J, Vuiton DA, Ammann RW, Kern P, Craig PS, Dar KF, Rosa F, de Filice C, Gottesein B, Grimm F, Macpherson CNL, Sato N, Todorov T, Uchino J, Sinner W, von Wen H (2001). Echinococcosis in humans: clinical aspects, diagnosis and treatment. In. Eckert J, Gemmell MA, Pawloeski ZS, (Eds). Manual on echinococcosis in humans and animals: A public health problem of global concern. WHO/OIE. pp: 20-66.
Polat KY, Balik AA, Oren D (2002). Percutaneous drainage of hydatid cyst of the liver: long-term results. HPB. 4:163-166.
Polat P, Mecit K, Fatih F, Selami S, Melike BK, Adnan O (2003). Hydatid Disease from Head to Toe 1. Radiographics 23(2):475-494
Prathiush PR, Placid ED, Ananda KJG (2008). Diagnosis of *Echinococcus granulosus* infection in dogs by a coproantigen sandwich ELISA. Vet. Arch. 78:297-305.
Sakai H, Malgor R, Basmadjian I, Gallardo R, Carmona C, Sato H, Oku Y, Kamiya M (1995). An enzyme linked immunosorbent assay (ELISA) for the detection of *Echinococcus granulosus* coproantigen in dogs. Japan J. Parasitol. 44:453-461.
Sakashita M, Sakai H, Kohno H, Ooi V, Oku V, Vagì K, Ito M, Kamiya M (1995). Detection of *Echinococcus multilocularis* coproantigens in experimentally infected dogs using murine monoclonal antibody against adult worms. Jap. J. Parasitol. 44:413-420.
Schantz PM, Van den Bossche H, Eckert J (1982). Chemotherapy for larval echinococcosis in animals and humans: Report of a workshop. Z. Parasit. 53:5-26.
Shambesh MK, Craig PS, Macpherson CNL, Rogan MT, Gusbi AM, Eechtuish FE (1999). An extensive ultrasound and serologic study to investigate the prevalence of human cystic echinococcosis in northern Libya. Am. J. Trop. Med. Hyg. 60:462-468.
Stefania S, Avram E, Cozma V (2006). Detection of *Echinococcus* coproantigens by enzyme linked immunosorbant assay in dogs from the northwest of Romania. Bull. USAMV-CN 63:395-398.
Stefanic S, Shaikenov BS, Deplazes P, Dinkel A, Torgerson PR, Mathis A (2004). Polymerase chain reaction for detection of patent infections of *Echinococcus granulosus* (sheep strain) in naturally infected dogs. Parasitol. Res. 92: 347-351.
Teggi A, Lastilla MG, De Rosa F (1993). Therapy of human hydatid disease with mebendazole and albendazole. Antimicrob. Agents Chemother. 37:1679-1684.
Thompson RCA (2008). The taxonomy, phylogeny and transmission of

Echinococcus. Exp. Parasitol. 119:439-446.

Thompson RCA (1995). Biology and systematics of *Echinococcus*. In: Thompson RCA, Lymbery AJ (Eds.). The biology of Echinococcus and hydatid disease. Cab International. pp. 1-50.

Torgerson PR, Shaikenov BS, Rysmukhambetova AT, Abdybekova AM, Usenbayev AE, Baitursi nov KK (2003). Modelling the transmission dynamics of *Echinococcus granulosus* in rural Kazakhstan. Vet. Parasitol. 114:143-153.

Unruh DHA, King JE, Eaton RDP, Allen JR (1973). Parasites of dogs from Indian settlements in northwestern Canada: A survey with public health implications. Can. J. Comp. Med. 37:25-32.

Wachira TM, Macpherson CNL, Gathuma JM (1991). Release and survival of *Echinococcus* eggs in different environments in Turkana, and their possible impact on the incidence of hydatidosis in man and livestock. J. Helminthol. 65:55-61.

Watson-Jones DL, Macpherson CNL (1988). Hydatid disease in the Turkana district of Kenya. VI. Man-dog contact and its role in the transmission and control of hydatidosis amongst the Turkana. Ann. Trop. Med. Parasitol. 82:343-356.

Yorganci K, Sayek I (2002). Surgical treatment of hydatid cysts of the liver in the era of percutaneous treatment. Am. J. Surg. 184:63-69.

Zare-Bidaki M, Mobedi I, Naddaf SR, Kia EB, Mahmoudi M, Piazak N, Nekouie H, Sadeghieh Ah ari S, Habibzadeh Sh, Siavashi M (2009). Prevalence of *Echinococcus spp.* infection using coproantigen ELISA among canids of Moghan plain, Iran. Iran J. Public Health 38:112-118.

Zhang W, Li J, McManus PD (2003). Concepts in immunology and diagnosis of hydatid disease. Clin. Microbiol. Rev. 16:18-36.

Zhang W., Zhang Z., Shi B, Li J, You H, Tulson G, Dang X, Song Y, Yimiti T, Wang J, Jones MK, McManus DP. (2006). Vaccination of dogs against *Echinococcus granulosus* the cause of cystic hydatid disease in humans. J. Infect. Dis.194:966-974.

Prevalence of tick-borne haemoparasitic diseases (TBHDS) and haematological changes in sheep and goats in Maiduguri abattoir

Egbe-Nwiyi T. N.[1], Sherrif G. A.[1] and Paul B. T.[2*]

[1]Department of Veterinary Pathology, University of Maiduguri, Maiduguri, Nigeria.
[2]Veterinary Teaching Hospital, University of Maiduguri, Maiduguri, Nigeria.

A preliminary survey was conducted to determine the prevalence of some tick-borne haemoparasitic diseases (TBHDs) and their effects on the haematological parameters of sheep and goats in Maiduguri abattoir. A total of 200 blood samples were collected from sheep (n = 100) and goats (n = 100) from November 2015 to May 2016. Giemsa stained blood smears were prepared and examined under light microscope, to screen for haemoparasites. Packed cell volume (PCV) was determined by microhaematocrit centrifugation technique while haemoglobin (Hb) concentration was determined by Sahli's method. The total white blood cell (WBC) and red blood cell (RBC) counts were estimated with Neubauer hemocytometer while erythrocyte indices were calculated. The results showed 13.5% overall prevalence of tick-borne haemoparasitic diseases in sheep 13 (6.5%) and goats 14 (7.0%). There was no significant ($p>0.05$) differences in prevalence of haemoparasites between sexes and age groups of sheep and goats. Anaplasma ovis and Babesia ovis were identified in the study of which A. ovis [23 (11.5%)] was higher ($p<0.05$) than B. ovis [2 (1.0%)]. A single co-infection of A. ovis and B. ovis was encountered in sheep. The mean values of PCV, Hb and RBC counts of infected sheep were lower ($p<0.05$) than the uninfected sheep. Similarly, the mean values of Hb and WBC of were significantly ($p<0.05$) lower in infected goats. This stud has reports important tick-borne haemoparasitic diseases in sheep and goats. We recommend tick control using suitable acaricides, periodic screening and treatment of small ruminants in Maiduguri.

Key words: Anaemia, *Anaplasma ovis*, *Babesia ovis*, haemoglobin, packed cell volume, white blood cell count.

INTRODUCTION

Sheep and goats are common household livestock in Nigeria. They are particularly important in the northern region, where a greater proportion can be found (Blench, 1999). Generally, three breeds of goats (Sahel, Sokoto red and West African dwarf) and four breeds of sheep (Balami, Ouda, Yankasa and West African dwarf) are recognized in Nigeria (Blench, 1999).The socio-economic importance of sheep and goats varies in different parts of

*Corresponding author. E-mail: bpaulgadzama@unimaid.edu.ng. Tel: +23480695940333.

the country, but they generally have agricultural, cultural and economic values (Lawal-Adebowale, 2012; Adamu and Balarabe, 2012). Most commonly, their flesh is recognized as sources of protein for human consumption, and their hides and skin also generates revenue (Lawal-Adebowale, 2012).

The productivity of sheep and goats in the Sahel zone of Nigeria is threatened by diseases and inclement weather conditions. Among parasitic diseases, sub-clinical gastrointestinal parasitism is responsible for great economic losses (Singla, 1995; Singh et al., 2017a, b). The incidence of parasitic infections with special reference to tick-borne intracellular haemoparasites of the genus *Anaplasma*, *Babesia* and *Theileria* has been linked with significant losses in productivity of small ruminants in the tropics and subtropical areas of the world (Soulsby, 1982; Jatau et al., 2011; Adamu and Balarabe, 2012; Demessie and Derso, 2015; Salih et al., 2015; Sumbria and Singla, 2017). Anaplasma species are mainly transmitted by various species of the genus *Amblyomma*, *Dermacentor*, *Ixodes* and *Rhipicephalus* (Soulsby, 1982) and occasionally by biting flies of the genus *Tabanus* (Radostits et al., 2007).

The disease is caused by *Anaplasma ovis* in small ruminants and is characterized by anaemia, high fever, weight loss, breathlesness, incoordination, abortion and death (Khan, 2005). *A. ovis* has a worldwide distribution and is responsible for huge losses in sheep and goats stock, with considerable impact on the economy of developing countries in tropics and subtropics, which rely heavily on small ruminant production (Rymaszewska and Grenda, 2008). Babesiosis in sheep and goats is caused by *Babesia motasi, Babesia foliata, Babesia taylori* and *Babesia ovis* (Soulsby, 1982). In sheep and goats, the disease is characterized by fever, anaemia, icterus, haemoglobinuria, anorexia, and death (Demessie and Derso, 2015). Other species of haemoparsites such as *Theileria hirci* (Metenawy, 1999), *Theileria ovis* (Okaiyeto et al., 2008), *Trypanosoma vivax, T. congolense* and *T. brucei* (Samdi et al., 2008) have also been reported in small ruminants in Nigeria.

Sheep and goats contribute significantly to food security and value chain of the Nigerian economy (Lawal-Adebowale, 2011), but their productivity is threatened by ticks and associated haemoparasitic diseases, especially Babesiosis and Anaplasmosis (Okaiyeto et al., 2008; Jatau et al., 2011). This study was therefore conducted to investigate the prevalence of tick-borne haemoparasites and the associated changes in haematological parameters of slaughtered sheep and goats in Maiduguri abattoir.

MATERIALS AND METHODS

Study area

This study was conducted in Maiduguri, the capital city of Borno state, located in the Sahel savannah zone of North-eastern Nigeria, between latitude 11°50′48″N and longitude 13°09′25″E of the equator. The climate of Maiduguri is characterized by a short period of rainfall from June to October, followed by a long period of dry season for the rest of the year (Hess et al., 1995). Sheep and goats are among the important household livestock in Maiduguri and its environs. They are mainly raised under traditional semi-intensive or free-range management systems in low income communities (Figure 1).

Sample collection

A total of 200 blood samples was randomly collected from sheep (n=100) and goats (n=100), consisting of 50 males and females. 5 mls of blood was collected immediately after slaughter from the severed jugular vein into vacutainer tubes, containing 1 mg of ethylene diaminetetra-acetic acid (EDTA).

The age, sex and specie of each animal were also identified based on morphometric characteristics and recorded in a case book. The samples were transported on icepacks at 4°C to the veterinary parasitology and clinical pathology laboratories, University of Maiduguri for parasitological and haematological examinations.

Laboratory examination

In the laboratory, thin and thick blood smears were prepared on clean glass slides and stained with Giemsa according to standard protocol described by Soulsby (1982), to screen for the presence of haemoparasites. The stained blood films were examined with oil immersion objective (×100) of a compound microscope (Gupta and Singla, 2012). Identification of haemoparasites was performed using morphologic characteristics (Soulsby, 1982).

The packed cell volume (PCV) was determined by microhaematocrit method; haemoglobin (Hb) by Sahli's method; the total white blood cell (WBC) and red blood cell (RBC) counts by Neubauer hemocytometer while erythrocyte indices, mean corpuscular volume (MCV), mean corpuscular haemoglobin(MCH) and mean corpuscular haemoglobin concentration (MCHC) were calculated using standard formula (Brar et al., 2000).

Statistical analysis

Chi Square test was computed with statistical package for social sciences (SPSS) version 22, to determine the prevalence of haemoparasites and its associations with age and sex of sheep and goats. The student's t-test was performed to determine the difference between mean haematological parameters of infected and uninfected sheep and goats. Significant differences were declared at $P<0.05$.

RESULTS

The results obtained from this study has shown that out of 200 blood samples of sheep and goats examined, 27(13.5%) were positive for various tick-borne haemoparasites. The results further revealed 13(6.5%) and 14(7.0%) of infected animals were sheep and goats, respectively. There was no significant difference ($p>0.05$) in prevalence of tick-borne haemoparasites among the different sexes and age groups of sheep and goats

Table 1. Prevalence of tick-borne haemoparasitic diseases in sheep and goats.

Variable	No. examined		No. (%) infected		×2 (1df)	p-value	95% CI
	Sheep	Goats	Sheep	Goats			
Age							
Young	32	38	5 (5.0)	3 (3.0)	0.9379	0.3328	0.3174 – 1.430
Adult	68	62	8 (8.0)	11 (11.0)	-	-	-
Sex							
Male	50	50	5 (5.0)	6 (6.0)	0.05395	0.8163	0.4036 – 2.048
Female	50	50	8 (8.0)	8 (8.0)	-	-	-
Total	100	100	13 (6.5)	14 (7.0)	0.03263	0.8566	0.9169 – 1.110

N= 200.

Table 2. Distribution of tick-borne haemoparasites in sheep and goats in Maiduguri.

Animal species	No. Examined	Haemoparasites		
		Anaplasma ovis	*Babesia ovis*	Mixed infection
Sheep	100	10 (5.0)	1 (0.5)	2 (1.0)
Goats	100	13 (6.5)	1 (0.5)	0 (0.0)
Total	200	23 (11.5)	2 (1.0)	2 (1.0)

Table 3. Mean (±SE) haematological parameters of uninfected and infected sheep.

Parameter	Uninfected(n=87)	Infected(n=13)	Normal (Khan, 2005)
PCV (%)	30.99 ± 0.31*	25.54 ± 0.69*	27-45
Hbg (g/dL)	10.69 ± 0.15*	8.72 ± 0.29*	9-15
WBC ($x10^3/\mu L$)	10.17 ± 0.12	10.45 ± 0.76	4-12
RBC ($x10^6/\mu L$)	12.62 ± 0.15*	9.39 ± 0.63*	9-15
MCV (fL)	24.64 ± 0.22	24.25 ± 1.27	28-40
MCH (pg)	8.48 ± 0.83	8.16 ±0.44	8-12
MCHC (mg/dL)	35.06 ±0.52	32.95 ± 0.93	31-34

*p<0.05 denotes significant difference between infected and uninfected group.

(Table 1).

The two species of haemoparasites identified in this study were tick-borne *A. ovis* and *B. ovis*. There was no significant difference (p>0.05) in prevalence of infection with haemoparasites in sheep and goats. However, the prevalence of *A. ovis* (11.5%) in both sheep and goats was significantly (p<0.05) higher than *B. ovis* (1.0%). Furthermore, 2(1.0%) sheep had co-infection with *A. ovis* and *B. ovis* (Table 2).

The mean values of PCV, Hb and RBC counts of infected and uninfected sheep were significantly (p<0.05) different. Furthermore, the mean PCV (25.54 ± 0.69) was below normal range (27 to 45) of values for sheep (Table 3). Similarly, the mean Hb concentration and WBC counts of infected and uninfected goats were significantly (p<0.05) different but fell within normal range of values for goats (Table 4). Other haematological parameters of infected and uninfected sheep and goats were comparable (p>0.05).

DISCUSSION

The results obtained from our present study revealed that tick-borne haemoparasites are prevalent in both sheep and goats examined at slaughter in Maiduguri. The study further revealed a numerically higher prevalence in female adult sheep and goats than their counterparts. The occurrence of haemoparasites in both sheep and goats in this study may be associated with previous

Table 4. Mean (±SE) haematological parameters of uninfected and infected goats.

Parameter	Uninfected (n=87)	Infected (n=13)	Normal (Khan, 2005)
PCV (%)	27.35 ± 0.36	25.64 ± 1.03	22-38
Hbg (g/dL)	9.53 ± 0.13*	8.81 ± 0.40*	8-12
WBC (x10^3/μL)	9.88 ± 0.11*	8.97 ± 0.33*	4-13
RBC (x10^6/μL)	12.94 ± 0.30	11.91 ± 0.89	8-18
MCV (fL)	21.83 ± 0.37	23.59 ± 1.04	16-25
MCH (pg)	7.58 ± 0.14	7.52 ± 0.33	5.2-8.0
MCHC (mg/dL)	35.41 ± 0.56	33.99 ± 0.97	30-36

*p<0.05 denotes significant difference between infected and uninfected group.

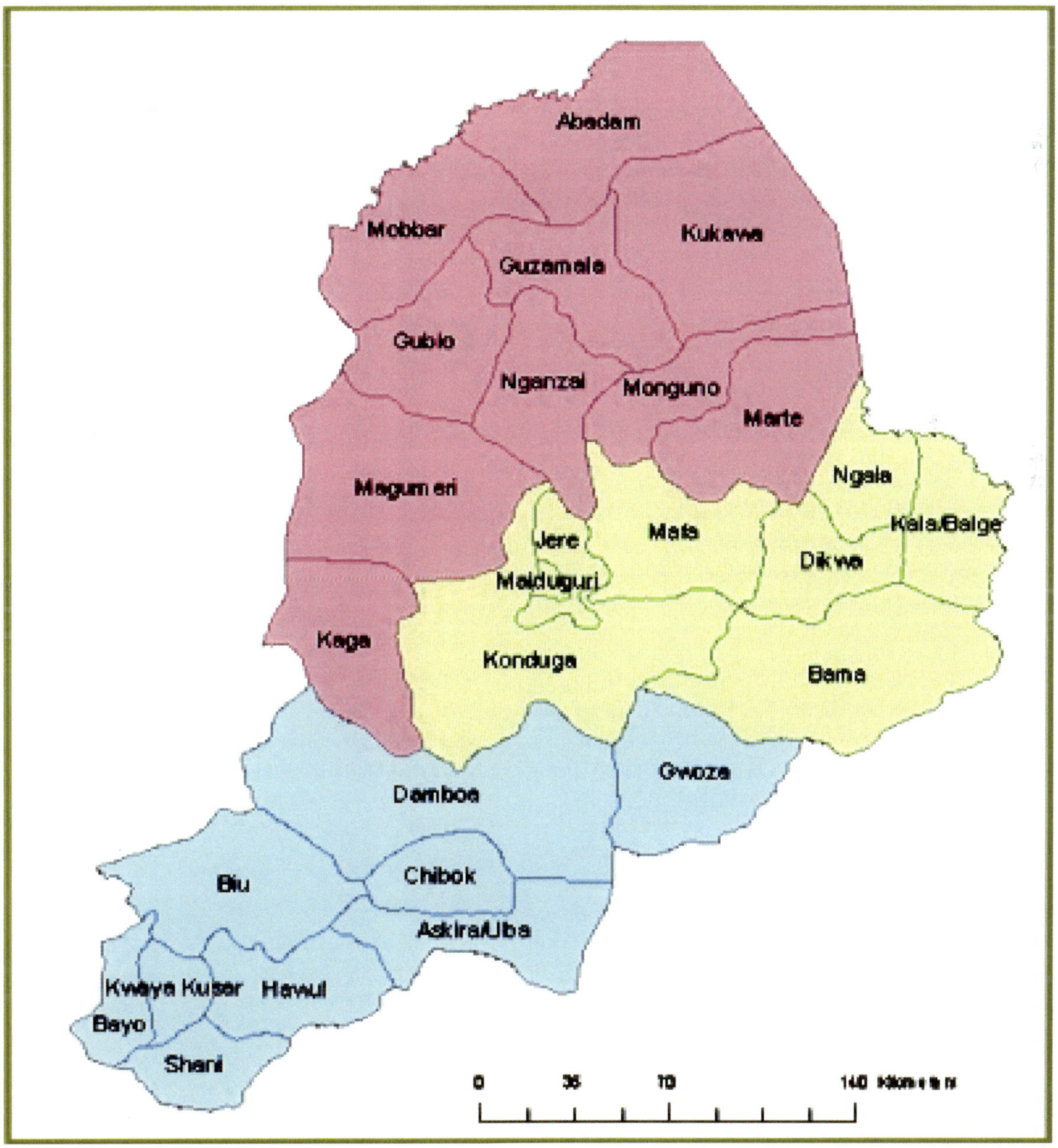

Figure 1. Map of Borno state showing Maiduguri, the study area.

reports on high prevalence of ixodid ticks in livestock in Maiduguri and environs (James-Rugu and Jidayi, 2004; Oparah and Ezeh, 2011; Musa et al., 2014; Paul et al., 2017). Ticks of the genus *Amblyomma*, *Rhipicephalus* including subgenus *Boophilus*, *Hyalomma* and *Dermacentor*, which are potential vectors of *Anaplasma* and *Babesia* species in sheep and goats were previously reported in Borno state (James-Rugu and Jidayi, 2004; Oparah and Ezeh, 2011; Musa et al., 2014; Paul et al., 2017). Furthermore, the sheep and goats slaughtered in Maiduguri are raised under extensive and semi-intensive management systems in outdoor environments graze alongside with cattle. These increase their exposure to the arthropod vectors.

Both *A. ovis* and *B. ovis* were identified in this study. *A. ovis* was the most prevalent species in both sheep and goats. This finding agrees with previous reports (Okaiyeto et al., 2008; Jatau et al., 2011; Adamu and Balarabe, 2012). The prevalence of these parasites elsewhere in Nigeria was linked with suitable microclimate favouring the propagation of their arthropod vectors (Jatau et al., 2011). Similarly, the prevalence of haemoparasites in slaughtered cattle in Maiduguri was linked with conditions favouring the bionomics of ixodid ticks (Paul et al., 2016).

Moreover, *A. ovis* is a ubiquitous organism that has been reported in all the six continents (Rymaszewska and Grenda, 2008) and especially in the tropics and subtropics, due to the abundance of its tick vectors (Jongejan and Uilenberg, 2004). The low prevalence of *B. ovis* recorded in both sheep and goats in this study agreed with previous reports (Bell-Sakyi et al., 2004; Jatau et al., 2011). This finding could be attributed to the enzootic occurrence of babesiosis in indigenous animals in Nigeria. Sheep and goats usually develop strong immunity in early life and resist subsequent challenges favourably by preventing establishment of the parasite (Soulsby, 1982).

This study revealed that, infection with haemoparasites in sheep caused a significant ($p<0.05$) reduction in PCV, Hb and total RBC counts. Furthermore, our results show a significant ($p<0.05$) reduction in the Hb concentration and total WBC count of goats. The anaemia observed in this study characterized by a reduction in PCV and Hb concentration of infected sheep and goats, is consistent with previous reports. Anosa (1988) reported that, anaemia is a predominant feature that often serves as a reliable indicator for severity of haemoparasitic infections. Rymaszewska and Grenda (2008) observed that progressive anaemia usually develops during anaplasmosis and babesiosis.

Furthermore, Anumol et al. (2011) reported that haemoparasites are responsible for most cases of anaemia in goats. The pathogenesis of anemia in haemoparasitic infections is multifactorial in nature; emergence of parasites from RBC, mechanical rupture of RBC, spontaneous lysis of RBC due to increased osmotic fragility, direct removal of non-infected erythrocytes by phagocytosis and adsorption of circulating antigen-antibody complexes to the surface of RBC, leading to their removal by phagocytosis as described by Soulsby (1982).

The observed reduction in WBC counts of infected goats in this study has been previously reported. A significant reduction in total WBC counts of dromedary camels infected with babesiosis in Saudi Arabia was described by Swelum et al. (2014). This finding could be linked with concurrent infections and stress which may lead to immune suppression. Helminthosis and bacterial infections are usually encountered concurrently with haemoparasitic infections under field conditions in Nigeria (Okaiyeto et al., 2008; Jatau et al., 2011), which may complicate the clinical course of haemoparasitic infections.

Conclusion

This study has revealed the presence of important tick-borne haemoprotozoan parasites in slaughtered sheep and goat in Maiduguri. The prevalence of *A. ovis* and *B. ovis* was accompanied by anaemia in sheep and goats. This finding suggests that *A. ovis* and *B. ovis* are common causes of anaemia leading to decreased productivity of sheep and goats in Maiduguri and environs.

RECOMMENDATION

Molecular studies used to characterize *Anaplasma* and *Babesia* genotypes and specific tick vectors responsible for the transmission of these parasites in Maiduguri, in other to aid proper planning of effective control measures is recommended.

Meanwhile, vector control with effective acaricides and the periodic screening and treatment of sheep and goats in Maiduguri with suitable antiprotozoal drugs will reduce the impact of tick-borne haemoparasitic diseases which enhance their productivity.

ACKNOWLEDGEMENT

This work was made possible with the full support received from the Veterinary officer in charge of Maiduguri central abattoir, to which we are very grateful. We are especially grateful to Mallam Ismaila Gadaka in the Veterinary Clinical Pathology Laboratory and Mallam Ya'uba Mohammed in the Parasitology and Entomology

Laboratory, both in the Faculty of Veterinary Medicine, for their technical support in the laboratory analysis of the samples.

REFERENCES

Adamu BS, Balarabe LM (2012). Prevalence of haemoparasites of sheep and goats slaughtered in Bauchi Abattoir. Int. J. Appl. Biol. Res. 4(1&2):128-133.

Anosa VO (1988). Haematological and biochemical changes in human and animal Trypanosomosis. Part 1 Revue d'Elevage Medicine Veterinarie des pays Tropicaux 41:65-78.

Anumol J, Tresamol PV, Saranya MG, Vijayakumar K, Saseendranath MR (2011). A study on aetiology of anemia in goats. J. Vet. Anim. Sci. 42:61-63.

Bell-Sakyi L, Koney EBM, Dogbey O, Walker AR (2004). *Ehrlichia ruminantum* seroprevalence in domestic ruminants in Ghana. I. Longitudinal survey in the greater Accra region. Vet. Microbiol. 100:308-313.

Blench R (1999). Traditional Livestock Breeds: Geographical distribution and dynamics in relation to the ecology of West Africa: Overseas Development Institute Portland House Stag Place London. 122:7-21.

Brar RS, Sandhu HS, Singh A (2000). Veterinary Clinical Diagnosis by Laboratory Methods (1st Ed) India: Kaylani Publishers. pp. 29-150.

Demessie Y, Derso S (2015). Tick Born Diseases of Ruminants: A review. Adv. Biol. Res. 9(4):210-224.

Gupta SK, Singla LD (2012). Diagnostic trends in parasitic diseases of animals. In: Veterinary Diagnostics: Current Trends. Gupta RP, Garg SR, Nehra V and Lather D (Eds), Satish Serial Publishing House, Delhi. pp. 81-112.

Hess TM, Stephens W, Maryah UM (1995) Rainfall trends in the North East Arid Zone of Nigeria 1961-1990. Agric. For. Meteorol. 74:87-97.

James-Rugu NN, Jidayi S (2004). A survey on the ectoparasites of some livestock from some areas of Borno and Yobe States. Niger. Vet. J. 25 (2):48-55.

Jatau ID, Abdulganiyu A, Lawal AI, Okubanjo OO, Yusuf HK (2011). Gastrointestinal and haemoparasites of sheep and goats at slaughter in Kano, Northern Nigeria. Sokoto J. Vet. Sci. 9(1):7-11.

Jongejan F, Uilenberg G (2004). The global importance of ticks. Parasitology 129: 129(S1):S3-S14.

Khan CM (2005). The Merck veterinary Manual. 9th ed. USA: Merck and Company Incorporated: pp.18-32.

Lawal-Adebowale AO (2012). Dynamics of ruminant livestock management in the context of Nigerian Agricultural System. InTech. pp. 61-80.

Metenawy TM (1999). Blood parasites of sheep and goats. Parkistan Vet. J. 19(1):43-45.

Musa HI, Jajere SM, Adamu NB, Atsanda NN, Lawal JR, Adamu SG, Lawal EK (2014). Prevalence of tick infestation in different breeds of cattle in Maiduguri, North-eastern Nigeria. Bangladesh J. Vet. Med. 12(2):161-166.

Okaiyeto SO, Tekdek LB, Sackey AKB, Ajanusi, OJ (2008). Prevalence of haemo and Gastrointestinal parasites in sheep kept by the Nomadic Fulanis in some Northern states of Nigeria. Res. J. Anim. Sci. 2(2):31-35.

Opara MN, Ezeh NO (2011). Ixodid ticks of cattle in Borno and Yobe States of Northeastern Nigeria: breed and coat colour preference. Anim. Res. Int. 8(1):1359-1365.

Paul BT, Bello AM, Haruna NM, Dauda J, Ojo TD, Gadzama MA (2017). Infestation of Zebu cattle (*Bos indicus* Linnaeus) by hard ticks (Acari: Ixodidae) in Maiduguri, North eastern Nigeria. Persian J. Acarol. 6(3):213-224.

Paul BT, Bello AM, Ngari O, Mana HP, Gadzama MA, Abba A, Malgwi KD, Balami SY, Dauda J, Abdullahi AM (2016). Risk factors of haemoparasites and some haematological parameters of slaughtered trade cattle in Maiduguri, Nigeria. J. Vet. Med. Anim. Health 8(8):83-88.

Radostits OM, Gay GC, Hinchiff KW, Constable PO (2007). Veterinary Medicine: A text book of the disease of cattle, sheep, goat, pigs and horses. 10th ed. Saunders Elsevier London, New York pp. 2047-1533.

Rymaszewska A, Grenda S (2008). Bacteria of the genus *Anaplasma*-characteristics of Anaplasma and their vectors: A Review. Vet. Med. 53(11):573-584.

Salih DA, Hussein AM El, Singla LD (2015) Diagnostic approaches for tick-borne haemoparasitic diseases in livestock. J. Vet. Med. Anim. Health 7(2):45-56.

Samdi S, Abenga JN, Fajinmi A, Kalgo A, Idowu T, Lawani F (2008). Seasonal variation in Trypanosomosis Rates in small Ruminants at the Kaduna Abattoir, Nigeria. Afr. J. Biomed. Res. 11:229-232.

Singh E, Kaur P, Singla LD, Bal MS (2017a). Prevalence of gastrointestinal parasitism in small ruminants in western zone of Punjab, India. Vet. World 10(1):61-66.

Singh R, Bal MS, Singla LD, Kaur P (2017b). Detection of anthelmintic resistance in sheep and goat against fenbendazole by faecal egg count reduction test. J. Parasitic Dis. 41(2):463-466.

Singla LD (1995). A note on sub-clinical gastro-intestinal parasitism in sheep and goats in Ludhiana and Faridkot districts of Punjab. Indian Vet. Med. J.19:61-62.

Sumbria D, Singla LD (2017). Thwack of Worldwide Weather Transformation on Vector and Vector-Borne Parasitic Infections. ARC J. Anim. Vet. Sci. 3(2):1-10.

Soulsby EJL (1982). Helminths Arthropods and Protozoa of Domesticated Animals 7th ed. London, U.K: Bailliere Tindall. P 809.

Swelum AA, Ismael AB, Khalaf AF, Abouheif MA (2014. Clinical and laboratory findings associated with naturally occurring babesiosis in dromedary camels. Bull. Vet. Institute Pulawy. 58(2):229-233.

A cross-sectional study on bovine Schistosomiasis in and around Kemissie, Dawa Cheffa District

Alemu Aylate[2]*, Mohammed Hussen[1], Alebachew Tilahun[2] and Ashenafi Kiros[3]

[1]School of Veterinary Medicine, Wollo University, Dessie, Ethiopia.
[2]School of Veterinary Medicine, Wolaita Sodo University, Sodo, Ethiopia.
[3]Ministry of Livestock and Fisheries, National Animal Health Diagnostic and Investigation Center

A cross sectional study was conducted in and around Kemissie, Dawa Cheffa District to estimate the prevalence and identify possible risk factors for the disease in the study area. Animal identification based on age, sex, breed and body condition score and management system of the study animals were taken into account followed by coprological examination for the presence of the developmental stages of parasites or parasite in naturally infected cattle. For this purpose, four hundred and five randomly selected animals were examined during the study period out of which 75 (18.5%) were found positive for schistosomiasis based on fecal examination. Variation together with age and sex of animals did not show statistical significance (P>0.05) in the disease occurrence. However, the prevalence of the disease was highest in young animals (23.14%), followed by adults (17.61%) and least in old animals (15.49%). On the other hand, statistical significant association (P<0.05) was seen with the variation of breeds, body condition score and management systems in the disease occurrence. In conclusion, relatively moderate prevalence (18.5%) was recorded in and around Kemissie and based on the results obtained, recommendations were forwarded.

Key words: Cattle, coproscopy, Kemissie, prevalence, Schistosomiasis.

INTRODUCTION

Animal production has been considered as the main component of agricultural development in most parts of sub-Saharan Africa. Like in many developing countries of the region, domestic animals play a crucial role in Ethiopia. They provide food in the form of meat and milk, and non-food items such as draft power, manure and transport services as inputs into food crop production, and fuel for cooking. Livestock are also a source of cash income through sales of the above items, animal hides determine social status within the community. Ethiopia is known for its high livestock population, being the first in Africa and tenth in the world (Gebrecherkos and Berihun, 2012). The recent livestock population estimate shows that the country has about 52.1 million heads of cattle, 24.2 million sheep, 22.6 million goats and 44.9 million poultry (MoARD, 2013).

Trematode parasitism is one of the biggest problems reducing ruminant productivity around the world and

*Corresponding author. E-mail: wsusvm2014@gmail.com.

skins. Furthermore, they act as a store of wealth and (Vercruysse and Claerebout, 2001). In Ethiopia, the potential of livestock sector is not efficiently and fully exploited due to several constraints like malnutrition,traditional management practice, poor genetic makeup and prevailing diseases. Among the prevailing diseases in the country, trematodes are one of the main parasitic problems of cattle and other ruminants (Fromsa et al., 2011).

These parasitic diseases are found in vast water lodged and marshy grazing field, a condition anticipated to be ideal for the propagation and maintenance of the intermediate host snails and hence the high prevalence of trematode infection (Solomon and Abebe, 2007).

Among these trematode infections, Schistosomiasis (also known as Bilharzias) is economically important worldwide. It is a chronic and debilitating tropical disease caused by adult blood flukes (parasitic trematode worms) of the genus, *Schistosoma* that deposit eggs in blood vessels surrounding the bladder or gut of infected mammalian hosts (McManus et al., 2009).

It is an endemic disease of cattle in Africa and Asia while at least 165 million cattle are infected with bovine Schistosomiasis worldwide. Animal Schistomes are mainly restricted to tropical and sub tropical areas (Upadhayay, 2005). It has a restricted distribution, which is found commonly in northern, eastern, southwestern and central parts of Ethiopia (Habtamu and Mariam, 2011). Routine diagnosis of visceral Schistosomiasis relies heavily on observation of clinical signs and fecal examination for eggs of the parasite. It is a zoonotic disease affecting both humans and livestock. The growing interest in organic, outdoor and aquaculture farming are likely to present higher risk of infection (Chhabra and Singla 2009).

The blood flukes are grouped under the genus *Schistosoma* (McCauley et al., 1984) and the family Schistosomatidae. Schistosomes under this group are elongate, unisexual and dimorphic trematodes, which inhabit the blood vessels of their hosts. Members of Schistosomatidae show morphological and physiological peculiarities which set them apart from all other trematodes. Firstly, they are dioecious, the male bearing the female in a ventral canal, gynaecophoric canal and secondly they live in the blood stream of warn-blooded hosts, being the only trematodes to do so (Smyth, 2005). One of the most important in animals is *Schistosoma bovis* which occurs in the portal and mesenteric veins of cattle, sheep and goats in Central, East and West Africa, the Mediterranean area and in the Middle East (Soulsby, 2006).There are three main species of Schisotomes infecting humans, *Schistosoma mansoni*, *Schistosoma japonicum* which inhabit the mesenteries around the intestine and *S. haematobium*, which are found in the venules surrounding the bladder (Upadhayay, 2005).

Although, little or no overt clinical signs may be seen over a short period, frequent Schistosome infections, in the long term, cause significant losses to the herd (Ravindran et al., 2007).The disease is characterized by its chronic nature and affects the productivity and reproduction performances; and predisposes animals to other diseases (McCauley et al., 1984). Within the last five years, no work has been done indicating the current situation of bovine schistosomosis in the study area. Therefore, the aims of this study were to estimate the current prevalence of bovine schistosomosis and to identify major risk factors associated with the disease in the study area.

MATERIALS AND METHODS

Study area

The study was conducted to determine the prevalence of bovine Schistosomosis in and around Kemissie, Dawa Cheffa District from September 5, 2011 to May 10, 2012, Oromo Nations Zone of the Amhara Regional state, Northeastern Ethiopia. It is located at 325 km North of Addis Ababa. The approximate geographical location of the area is between 10°01' to 11° 25' N and 39° 41' to 40° 24' E. The altitude of the area ranges from 1000 to 2500 m above sea level and the maximum temperature is 33°C and the minimum temperature of the area is about 12°C. The mean annual rainfall of the area ranges from 600 to 900 mm. The area has a long heavy rainy season from June to September and short rainy season from March to May (OZARD, 2006).

Study population

The study was conducted in local Zebu and cross breeds between exotic and local breeds of cattle in the study area that was managed under extensive and semi-intensive management systems in the study area. The study population comprises of cattle at different age (De launta and Habel, 1986) and sex category. Four peasant associations (PAs) were selected purposively for their accessibility (convenience) of transportation and nearness to towns. These PAs were Kemissie, Shekla, Woledi and Tuche, all of which are under the same climatic and geographical features (OZARD, 2006). All the local breeds were often kept out-doors grazing on a marshy land and watered on natural rivers whereas most of the crossbreeds were kept in-door especially during milking periods where there is sufficiently gathered feed resources but watering is usually out-door especially during the dry season where it is difficult to fetch from a distant area for animals to drink. During sampling, deworming history of individual animals was obtained from the owners and recently dewormed animals were excluded from being sampled.

Study design

The study design for this particular study was cross sectional. The sampling method used was simple random sampling. To determine the sample size, an expected prevalence of 50% was taken into consideration since there was no previous study conducted recently within the last five years in the study area. The desired sample size for the study was calculated by the formula given by Thursfield (2005) with 95% confidence interval and 5% absolute precision and it was 384. However, to increase the precision level, 405 animals were selected randomly from the selected PAs of the study area.

Study methodology

Sample collection and transportation

About 10 g (Foreyt, 2001) of fresh fecal samples were collected per rectum from each cattle using sterile rectal plastic gloves and placed in a clean plastic container and each sample was clearly labeled with animal identifications, such as body condition score (Nicholson and Butterworth, 1986), sex, age (De launta and Habel, 1986), breed and management systems for each animal on a data recording format.

Coprological examination

Coproscopy was used to determine positivity of the animals for the disease. Fecal samples collected from the study animals directly from the rectum were stored in a clean universal bottle containing 10% formalin and labeled separately. A modified simple sedimentation technique (Gupta and Singla, 2012) was employed. Each sample was repeatedly examined more than four times recommended by Habtamu and Mariam (2011) to observe the eggs of the parasites by using a light microscope.

Data analysis

Data were entered and stored in a Microsoft Excel spread sheet program and were coded for analysis. SPSS version17.0 software, data were analyzed. Chi-square ($\chi 2$) test was used to determine the variation in the infection and prevalence among ages, sexes, breeds, body condition score and management systems. Statistical significance was set at $P<0.05$ to determine whether there are significant differences between the parameters measured between the groups.

RESULTS

Out of 405 fecal samples examined, an overall prevalence of 18.5% was observed as 75 samples were found positive for schistosomiasis in the study area. Slightly higher prevalence of the disease was seen in young cattle (23.14%) followed by adults (17.61%) and least in old age (15.49%) as shown in Table 1. However, the prevalence of schistosomiasis iid not vary significantly ($p>0.05$) among the age groups.

Prevalence of Schistosomiasis in female and male animals was 18.66 and 18.37%, respectively. However, no significant difference ($P>0.05$) was observed between sexes (Table 2).

Prevalence of the disease in the cross breeds (48.61%) was higher, which showed higher variation from local breeds (11.41%). The result of statistical analysis revealed a significant difference ($P<0.05$) between breeds of animals (Table 3).

Prevalence of schistosomiasis in poor body condition animals (31.16%) was found to be highest. However, the prevalence in animals with medium and good body condition was 9.38 and 1.28%, respectively. A significant difference ($P<0.05$) in prevalence was observed in body condition of the study animals (Table 4).

The prevalence of the disease in animals under semi-intensive management system (59.26%) was higher. However, the prevalence of the disease in animals under extensive management was only 12.25%. The result of statistical analysis revealed a significant difference ($P<0.05$) in each management system (Table 5).

DISCUSSION

An overall prevalence of 18.5% bovine schistosomiasis was recorded based on coprological investigation. This result agrees with previous reports of Getachew et al. (2006) in Kemissie who reported similar prevalence of 17.2% as in the present case. This may be because both studies were conducted in the same study area. However, the result of the present study was not in agreement with the previous reports by Ameni et al. (2001) who reported higher prevalence (28%) in Kemissie. This may be due to climatic changes such as repeated draught leading to drying of natural habitats of the intermediate host, snail and the larval stages of the parasite may not be reached by infective stages and may decrease their population leading to decrease in the prevalence of the disease in the area. Hansen and Perry (1993) reported that schistosomiasis is closely associated with large permanent water bodies such as ponds, lakes and marshy pastures; and according to Urquhart et al. (1996), it may be due to development of resistance for the disease when animals are repeatedly exposed to the infection in the study area. The prevalence of the disease was also not in agreement with the previous reports in different areas by different authors; Habtamu and Mariam (2011), 37.3% in Bahir Dar; 43% in Bati (Getachew et al., 2006), 57.3% in India (Ravindran et al., 2007). This might be due to the differences in temperature, moisture, humidity, availability of large permanent water bodies and soil that might favor multiplication and survival of the intermediate host, snails. Hansen and Perry (1993) reported that a key determinant in the epidemiology of bovine schistosomiasis is the relative abundance of the intermediate hosts and their ability to develop and survive in the environment and associated with large permanent water bodies. It was also reported by Urqhart et al. (1996) that *Schistosoma* species are totally dependent on water as a medium for infection in both the intermediate host and final host.

Prevalence of the disease in different age groups has values of 23.14% in young, 17.61% in adults and 15.49% in old animals with a non-statistical difference ($P > 0.05$). However, the result of the study indicates that the prevalence of the disease decreases as age increases. This may be because young animals have lower immunity when compared with adult and older cattle. According to the reports by Habtamu and Mariam (2011), calves are traditionally weaned at about 1.5-2 years and then allowed to graze with adult cattle. In addition to this, adult and old group of cattle are left to graze on the field where cercaria infection is high, furthermore in this group

Table 1. Prevalence of bovine schistosomiasis in different age groups.

Age	Animals examined	Animals affected	Prevalence (%)	χ2	P value
Young	121	28	23.14		
Adult	142	25	17.61	2.653	0.265
Old	142	22	15.49		

Table 2. Sex wise prevalence of bovine schistosomiasis.

Sex	Animals examined	Animals affected	Prevalence (%)	χ2	P value
Male	196	36	18.37	0 .006	0.940
Female	209	39	18.66		

Table 3. Breed wise prevalence of bovine schistosomiasis.

Breed	Animals examined	Animals affected	Prevalence (%)	χ2	P value
Local	333	38	11.41	62.703	0.00
Cross	72	35	48.61		

Table 4. Body condition score based prevalence of bovine schistosomiasis.

Body condition score	Animals examined	Animals affected	Prevalence (%)	χ2	P value
Poor	199	62	31.16		
Medium	128	12	9.38	43.511	0.00
Good	78	1	1.28		

Table 5. Prevalence of bovine Schistosomiasis based on management system.

Management	Animals examined	Animals affected	Prevalence (%)	χ2	P value
Extensive	351	43	12.25	68.538	0.00
Semi-intensive	54	32	59.26		

of animals, acquired immunity is not established, hence egg shed in these animals is high. There was statistically non-significant difference ($P > 0.05$) between the sexes categories indicating that it has no effect on the prevalence of the disease. This may be because exposure of both sex groups in similar pasture lands and watering points is the same and eventually developing the disease equally (Habtamu and Mariam, 2011).

A significant difference ($P < 0.05$) was observed between breeds in the study animals. High prevalence was recorded in cross breed cattle (48.61%) than in local breeds (11.41%). This wide gap may be due to local breeds acquired a high degree of immunity as a result of repeated natural exposure to the disease for a longer period. The main manifestation of immunity was suppression of worm fecundity (Cheng, 1986). It was also reported that local cattle that naturally acquired infections are capable of reducing egg production. Furthermore, there is difference in natural or innate immunity between indigenous and cross breed of cattle (Habtamu and Mariam, 2011).

The results of this study indicated that there is a significant difference in body condition scoring ($P<0.05$). Infection rates in poor body condition animals were significantly highest (31.16%), moderate in medium (9.38%) and least in animals having good body condition

(1.28%). Based on the reports of Urqhart et al. (1986) and Hansen and Perry (1993), the disease causes anorexia and emaciation which leads to weakening of the immune status of the animal that leads to low immune response to the parasite and predisposes animals to other diseases McCauley et al. (1984). This indicates the importance of the disease in causing poor body condition (emaciation).

An attempt was also made to analyze the prevalence of the management system of the animals. The prevalence of the disease in animals that were kept under semi-intensive management system was higher (59.26%) than animals kept under extensive management system (12.25%). The result of statistical analysis revealed that there is a significant difference ($P < 0.05$) in the management system. This may be because extensively managed animals acquired a high degree of immunity as a result of repeated natural exposure to the disease (Cheng, 1986). However, animals kept in semi-intensive management system become susceptible to the infection as they have no acquired immunity to withstand the disease.

CONCLUSION AND RECOMMENDATIONS

The result of this study indicated that schistosomiasis is a moderately prevalent bovine infection in the study area. Even though its prevalence seems lower, it has higher economic importance due to loss of productivity and mortality in animals and it is a zoonotic disease. However, it is evident that proper evaluation of the epidemiology of the disease is absent in the study area recently. The major risk factors associated with the disease on this finding were management system, body condition score and cattle breeds. However, sex and age were not that much significant in this study. However, the prevalence of the disease was highest in young cattle followed by adults and least in older age animals. The result of the present study showed that there is a reduction in its prevalence when compared with previous reports in the study area. However, micro dams constructed for irrigation purpose may be threatening factors to increase its prevalence again in the future in the area. In the area, no measures being taken to control the disease and no drugs available in veterinary clinics even though the disease is endemic.

Therefore, detailed studies should be conducted on the epidemiology of the disease to expand and implement disease investigation and control strategy. Young aged animals should be kept at home or the weaning time of calves should be extended until they become mature or until their immunity develops well. Fencing water bodies is supposed to be practiced to reduce water contamination with fluke eggs. Applications of molluscicide ought to be used to reduce snail population at seasons where the number of the population increases in the area.

ACKNOWLEDGEMENT

The authors thank Wollo University School of Veterinary Medicine for technical support and facility provision.

REFERENCES

Ameni G, Erko B, Bogale T (2001). Preliminary study on the major bovine trematode infection around Kemissie, Northeastern Ethiopia and treatment trial with praziquantel. Bull. Anim. Health. Prod. Afr. 49:62-67.

Cheng TC (1986).General Parasitology, 2nd edition, Academic Press, Medical University of South Carolina, Charlton. pp. 332-342.

Chhabra MB, Singla LD (2009). Food-borne parasitic zoonoses in India: Review of recent reports of human infections. J. Vet. Parasitol. 23(2):103-110.

De launta A, Habel RE (1986). Applied Veterinary Anatomy. W.B. Saunders Company. USA.

Foreyt WJ (2001). Veterinary Parasitology Reference Manual, 5th edition, Black well,Lowa State University Press, Washington DC, USA. P 3.

Fromsa A, Meharenet B, Mekibib B (2011). Major Trematode Infections of Cattle Slaughtered at Jimma Municipality Abattoir and the Occurrence of the IntermediateHosts in Selected Water Bodies of the Zone. J.Anim. Vet. Adv. 10(12):1592-1597.

Gebrecherkos, Berihun A (2012). Prevalence of bovine fascilosis in municipal Abattoir of Adigrat, Tigray, Ethiopia. Mekelle University College of Veterinary Medicine, Mekelle Ethiopia.

Getachew T, Tesfu K, Berhanu E, Legesse W, Ahmed A, Nega B, Girmay M (2006). Pilot control of fasciolosis and related animal fluke infections by the use of Endod and reduced morbidity: I pre-intervention studies. Ethiop. vet. J. 10(1):67-70.

Gupta SK, Singla LD (2012). Diagnostic trends in parasitic diseases of animals. In: *Veterinary Diagnostics: Current Trends.* Gupta RP, Garg SR, Nehra V and Lather D (Eds), Satish Serial Publishing House, Delhi. pp. 81-112.

Habtamu A, Mariam SW (2011). Repeated simple sedimentation technique and prevalence of bovine schistosomosis in selected sites of Bahir Dar woreda. Ethiop. Vet. J.15(1).

Hansen J, Perry B (1993). The Epidemiology, Diagnosis and Control of Helminth Parasites of Ruminants, 2nd edition, published by the ILRAD, Nairobi, Kenya. pp. 40-41.

McCauley EH, Majid AA, Tayeb A (1984). Economic evaluation of the production impact of bovine schistosomiasis and vaccination in the Sudan.Preven. Vet. Med. 2(6):735-754.

McManus DP, Li Y, Gray DJ, Ross AG. (2009). Conquering 'snail fever': schistosomiasis and its control in China. Exp. Rev.Anti-infect.Ther. 7(4): 473-485.

Ministry of Agriculture and Rural Development(MoARD)(2013).Major challenges and Achievements in Ethiopian Livestock production.

Nicholson MJ, Butterworth MH (1986). A Guide to Body Condition Scoring in Zebu Cattle. International Livestock Center for Africa (ILCA). Addis Ababa, Ethiopia.

OZARD (2006). Annual Report, Oromya Zone Agricultural and Rural Development Department, Amhara Regional State, Kemmisse. P 19.

Ravindran R, Lakshmanan B, Ravishankar C, Subramanian H (2007). Research note. Visceral schistosomiasis among domestic ruminants slaughtered in Wayanad, South India. Southeast Asian J. Trop.Med. Public Health 38(6):1008.

Smyth JD (2005). Animal Parasitology. Cambridge University Press.3rd edition. London. P 236.

Solomon W, Abebe W (2007). Effects of a strategy antehelmtic treatment intervention bovine fasciolosis. A conducted in facilities in endemic area in north western Ethiopia. Vet. J. 11(2):59-68.

Soulsby EJL (2006). Helminths, Arthropods, and Protozoas of Domestic Animals. 7th edition. London. P 72.

Thrusfield M (2005). Veterinary Epidemiology.2nd edition, UK, Blackwell Sci. pp. 228-247.

Upadahayay AKU (2005). Textbook of Preventive Veterinary Medicine. 1st edition. pp. 380-381.

Aerobic and anaerobic bacterial isolates from the respiratory tract of sheep slaughtered at Addis Ababa Abattoirs Enterprises, Central Ethiopia

Addisu Awukew Yegoraw[1*], Addis Kassahun Gebremeskel[2], Tesfaye Sisay Tesema[3] and Biruk Tesfaye Birhanu[4]

[1]School of Veterinary Medicine, Wolaita Sodo University, Wolaita, Ethiopia.
[2]School of Veterinary Medicine, Hawassa University, Hawassa, Ethiopia.
[3]Unit of Health Biotechnology, Institute of Biotechnology, College of Natural and Computational Sciences, Addis Ababa University, Ethiopia.
[4]College of Veterinary Medicine and Agriculture, Addis Ababa University, Debrezeit, Ethiopia.

The present study was an endeavor to isolate and identify the various bacteria localizing pneumonic lungs and the associated tracheas of sheep slaughtered at Addis Ababa Abattoirs Enterprise, Central Ethiopia, in both aerobic and anaerobic conditions. A total of 60 pneumonic lungs and 60 tracheal swabs were examined bacteriologically. From all the samples collected, a total of 440 bacterial isolates (239 from the aerobic culture and 201 from the anaerobic culture) were obtained. The result of aerobic isolates include: *Staphylococcus* species (31.38%), *Pasteurella hemolytica* (29.71%), *Bacillus* species (10.04%), *Bibersteinia trehalosi* (6.69%), *Micrococcus* (3.77%), *Escherichia coli* (3.35%), *Streptococcus* species (2.51%), *Rhodococcus equi* (2.93%), *Pseudomonas* species (2.09%), *Klebsiella pnuemonea* (0.84%), *Actinobacillus* species and *Bordetella* species (1, 29%); whereas *Staphylococcus* species (26.87%), *P. hemolytica* (37.81%), *Bacillus* species (3.98%), *B. trehalosi* (10.45%), *Micrococcus* (3.48), *E. coli* (6.97%), *Streptococcus* species (0.5%), *Rhodococcus equi* (0.5%), *Klebsiella pneumoniae* (2.99%) and *Actinobacillus* species (1.49%) were among anaerobic isolates. Thus, isolation of multiple bacterial species from the respiratory tracts of pneumonic sheep in this study signifies their possible role in the involvement of respiratory diseases. Appropriate prevention and control methods should be established along with identification of the most pathogenic species by future studies.

Key words: Bacteria, lung, pneumonia, sheep, trachea.

INTRODUCTION

Ethiopia is home to various indigenous sheep breeds. From the total livestock population of the country, sheep owns about 46%. Despite this huge resource, Ethiopian sheep productivity remains far lower than expected. The

*Corresponding author. E-mail: tiwoadd@gmail.com.

major biological constraints contributing to low productivity include bacterial and parasitic infections (Kaur et al., 2009; Leta and Meles, 2014; CSA, 2014-15; Fikru and Gebeyehu, 2015; Gebremeskel et al., 2017; Pawar et al., 2017; Singh et al., 2017).

The lungs are continuously exposed to air that contains dust, bacteria, fungi, viruses and various noxious agents and defense against these potentially harmful materials is controlled by a complex of protective mechanisms (Mohan et al., 2013). Stress factors such as inclement of weather, cold and stress of weaning, transportation, poorly ventilated housing and nutritional deficiencies have predisposing roles. In addition, concurrent infections with some viruses, bacteria or parasitic infestation degrade the potential of the host to combat infections (Gebremeskel et al., 2017; Gupta et al., 2009; Radostits et al., 2000).

The impact of respiratory disease is extensive and can be measured as the sum of the direct economic losses occurring due to mortality, morbidity, treatment and prevention costs. Loss of production (reduced animal performance and carcass quality) and the indirect costs such as labor, infrastructures and intangibles (Jim, 2009; Monot et al., 2015).

A number of bacterial, viral and parasitic agents participate in sheep respiratory diseases, however most important include: mycoplasma species such as Mycoplasma ovipneumoniae, Mycoplasma.arginini, Mycoplasma agalactiae (Lin et al., 2008), lung worms particularly (*Dictyocaulus filaria*) (Borji et al., 2012) and bacteria like *Pasteurella multocida, Manhemia haemolytica*, *Chlamydia psittaci*, *Histophilus somni,* which can suppress the animal's immune system, allowing opportunistic microorganisms to colonize the lung and cause the disease (Angen et al.,1998; Radostits et al., 2000; Tesfaye et al., 2013; Fulton, 2009; Alemneh and Tewodros, 2016).

Therefore, objectives this study is to identify most bacterial pathogens involved in pneumonic lung of sheep as well to compare and contrast the types of isolated bacterial species in different sites of the respiratory system both in aerobic and anaerobic environments.

MATERIALS AND METHODS

Study area

The study was conducted from October 2010 to April 2011 at Addis Ababa abattoir enterprises, central Ethiopia. Geographically Addis Ababa is located 9°2' N and 38° 42'E having elevation of 2400 above sea level (a.s.l) and mean annual rainfall of 1800 mm. The city has average minimum and maximum annual temperature of 10.7 and 23.6°C, respectively (NMSA, 2005; Jury and Chris, 2013).

Study animals and sampling strategy

The study was conducted on 60 randomly selected sheep lungs with pneumonic lesions and tracheal swabs slaughtered at Addis Ababa Abattoirs Enterprises. Samples were kept separately and transported to the School of Veterinary Medicine, Microbiology Laboratory of Addis Ababa University in a cool box containing ice pack at 4°C.

Sample collection

Tracheal swabs

Samples were taken with sterile cotton swabs moistened with tryptose soya broth from the trachea of sheep. Two swabs were introduced directly into the trachea of slaughtered sheep and rubbed smoothly against the mucosa in a circular motion. The swabs were allowed to remain in contact with the secretions for up to 1 min, and the two swabs collected from each sheep were kept in a tryptose soya broth transport medium and transported to the laboratory (Lees et al., 1990; OIE, 2008).

Pneumonic lung tissue

Samples of pneumonic lung tissue were collected at post mortem for microbial culture. Each piece of tissue was placed in a fully labeled separate sterile screw capped universal bottle. Containers were fully labeled with the date, tissue and sterile instruments (knife, scalple, forceps and scissors) were used for collecting specimens for microbiological cultures. After collection and transportation to the laboratory, the samples were processed immediately (Gebremeskel et al., 2017).

Bacteriological sample processing

Culturing the tracheal swabs

The broth culture samples were incubated overnight under aerobic and anaerobic conditions, respectively. After 24 h of incubation the samples were thoroughly agitated, mixed and a loop of broth cultures was taken and streaked over labeled Petri plates containing blood agar base supplemented with 7% sheep blood as described by Quinn et al. (1994).

Culturing the lung tissues

The outer surfaces of the lungs were first seared with a heated spatula, followed by cutting and mincing of the inner surface of the lungs using sterile scissors and forceps, and then transferred to sterile Petri dish. The minced interior part of the lungs were further incised with sterile scalpel blade, then printed on the blood agar and streaked with wire loop. All bacteriological procedures were conducted in a level two biological safety cabinet.

Cultural characterization and bacteriological examination

The growths of typical colonies on blood agar were characterized based on the presence or absence of hemolysis, the type of hemolysis and general appearance of the colonies (color, shape, size, consistency etc.). On MacConkey agar, the colonies were examined for the presence or absence of growth, general appearance and ability to ferment lactose (Sharma and Adlakha, 1996; Alemneh and Tewodros, 2016). All cultures were incubated under aerobic and anaerobic conditions at 37°C for 24 to 48 h.

Isolation and Identification

Single colony type from pure cultures on blood agar was transferred to nutrient agar for a series of primary and secondary biochemical tests. Primary tests such as Grams staining, motility, catalase, oxidase, and oxidative-fermentative (O-F) tests were conducted. In addition, secondary biochemical tests including indole, methyl red, and citrate utilization tests were performed for further confirmation of the isolates. General procedures for isolation and identification of Gram positive and Gram negative bacteria were as described by Carter (1984) and Quinn et al. (1994).

Data analysis

Descriptive statistics was performed to analyze the data obtained from the study. The number of each species/genera was expressed as a percentage in comparison to the total number of isolates.

Ethical approval

The study considered direct observation of slaughter animals in the abattoirs and took appropriate samples for further microbiological examination. As a result of this study, no animal was subjected to suffer. Nevertheless, ethical approval was conducted by Research Ethical Approval Committee of Addis Ababa University, School of Veterinary Medicine, Ethiopia.

RESULTS

The predominant species among the aerobic isolates were *Staphylococcus* species (31.38%), followed by *M. haemolytica* (29.71%), *Bacillus* species (10.04%), *B. trehalosi* (6.69%), *Micrococcus* species (3.77%), *E. coli* (3.35%), *Rhodococcus equi* (2.93%), and *Pseudomonas* species (2.09%). On the other hand *Streptococcus*, *Bordetella*, *Klebsiella* and *Actinobacillus* were among the least encountered bacterial genera as indicated by Figure 1.

The majority of the isolates (aerobic and anaerobic) colonize the two anatomical sites investigated with *Streptococcus*, *Rhodococcu equi*, *Pseudomonas*, and *Actinobacillus* as exceptions which were not seen in trachea. However, a general increase in the isolation rate was observed as one that goes down the respiratory tract. In a nutshell, Gram positive bacteria were the predominant species inhabiting the respiratory tract in aerobic condition, whereas Gram negative bacteria predominate in anaerobic conditions.

A total of 191 facultative bacteria were isolated in anaerobic condition with Gram negative bacteria as the dominant isolates. The isolated bacteria with their isolation rate include *M. haemolytica* (37.81%), *Staphylococcus* species (26.87%), *B. trehalosi* (10.45%), *E. coli* (6.97%), *Bacillus* species (3.98%), *Micrococcus* species (3.48%), *K. pneumonae* (2.99%), *Actinobacillus* species (1.49%), *Streptococcus* species (0.5%) and *Rhodococcus equi* (0.5%) as denoted by Figure 2.

DISCUSSION

The present study assessed the frequency and type of aerobic and facultative anaerobic bacteria isolated from ovine pneumonic lungs and their associated trachea at Addis Ababa Abattoir Enterprises, Central Ethiopia among which several of them were isolated. A number of workers such as Gebremeskel et al. (2017), Akloul and Mohammed (2016), Sarker et al. (2016), Porter et al. (1994), Al Sultan (1995), Barbour et al. (1997), Almeida et al. (1986), Okolo (1985), Esra et al. (2009) and Richard et al. (1986) have isolated similar bacteria from pneumonic lungs of domestic animals. The invariable isolation of those organisms from pneumonic lungs of various animal species may indicate their significance in various respiratory syndromes in different animal species (Megra et al., 2006).

Among 239 isolates, *Staphylococcus* species were the dominant bacteria having high proportion accounts (23.25 and 35.95%) of the trachea and lung isolates, respectively. In agreement to this study *Staphylococcus* species were isolated and reported in high proportion by few studies such as Alley (1975) and Queen et al. (1994). Other investigations includes that by Esra et al. (2009) who isolated *Staphylococcus* spp. from unhealthy *Holstein* cattle nasal cavities with high frequency and percentage, and Asaduzzaman et al. (2013) who reported on *Staphylococcus* species from Black Bengal goat in Bangladesh. These indicate that there is a probability of association between these bacteria and pneumonic syndrome of lung. The bacteria are commensally living in the mucous membrane of the upper respiratory tract of animals and are opportunistic pathogens (Rashid et al., 2014; Quinn et al., 1994).

Bacillus species has been described as ubiquitous microbes found in nature as normal micro-flora. Thus, their role in the pathogenesis of respiratory infections is thought to be insignificant (Carter et al., 1995; Garedew et al., 2010). A high proportion of *Bacillus* species was obtained mainly from the lungs in this study. Other studies reported similar data such as Asaduzzaman et al. (2013), Garedew et al. (2010), Rajiv et al. (2000) and Shigidi (1973) from various domestic animals.

Micrococcus species is known primarily to be a normal flora of the respiratory tract. However, in most of the infections along with other pathogens, it may flare up and act as a secondary invader (Akloul and Mohammed, 2016; Carter, 1984). Our finding indicated that only 3.77% of *Micrococcus* species were isolated from ovine pneumonic lungs, with similar studies found to have agreed with present results such as Marru et al. (2013) and Esra et al. (2009).

Streptococcal are resident flora of the upper respiratory tract mucous membrane and commonly associated with suppuration and abscess formation (Quinn et al., 1994; Obasi et al., 2001). Although streptococci have not been associated with respiratory problems in ruminants, they are well known pathogens in humans, equine and camels. In this study, isolation of these bacteria might be an indication of its involvements as opportunistic

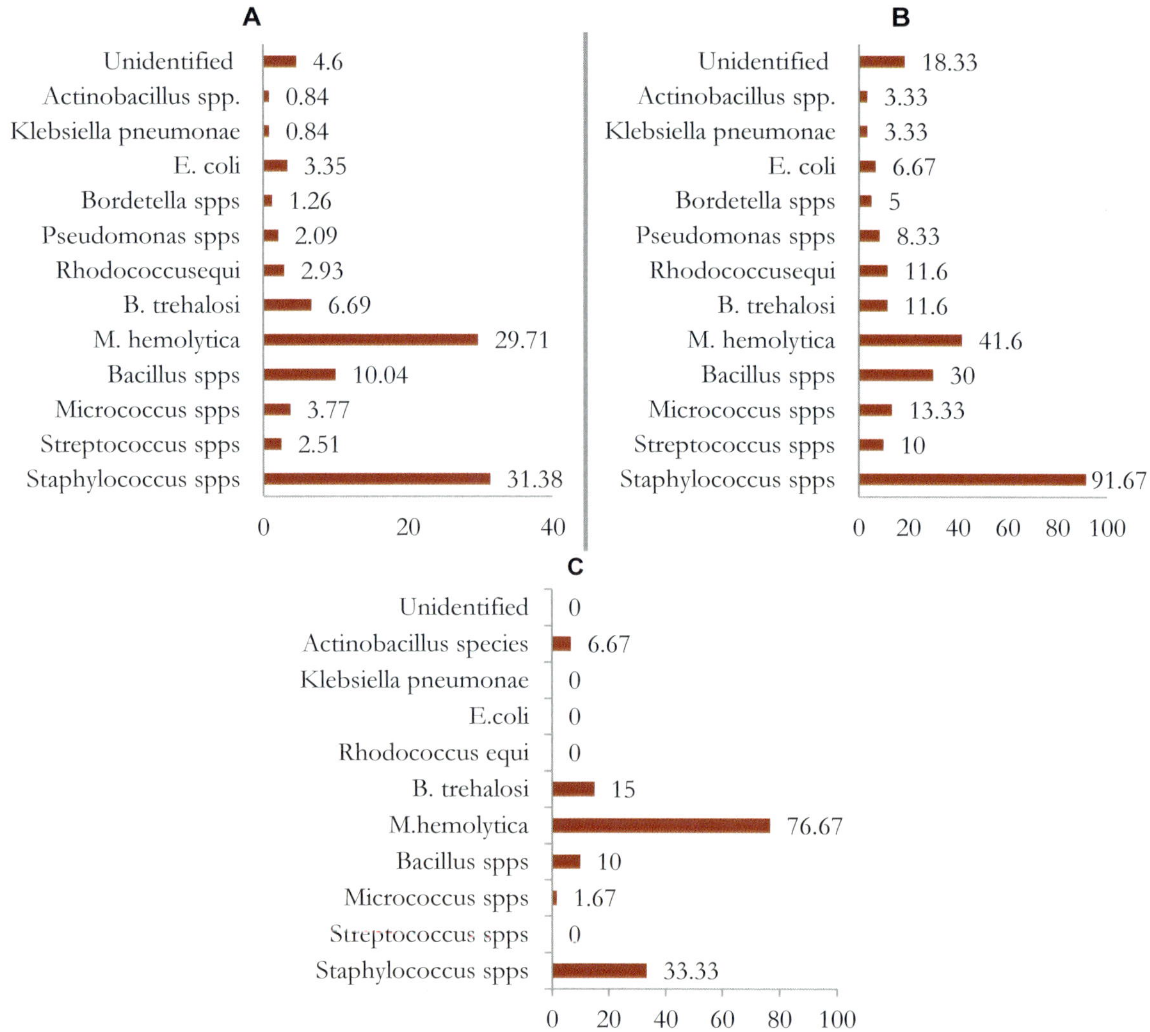

Figure 1. Bacterial isolates (%) under aerobic condition from respiratory tract of sheep slaughtered at Addis Ababa Abattoirs Enterprises. (A) Overall proportion of bacterial isolates; (B) Bacterial Isolates from lung; (C) Bacterial isolates from trachea.

pathogens in sheep pneumonia. *M. haemolytica*, is a normal flora of the upper respiratory tract and may play a secondary role after the primary initiating agent suppressed the host's defense mechanisms, and favors the multiplication of *Pasteurella* species leading to bronchopneumonia (Aiello and May, 1998; Buxton and Frazer, 1977). Stress factors with or without viral infections interact to suppress the host defense mechanisms which allow the proliferation of commensal bacteria in the respiratory tract of animals (Baker, 1998).

Conclusion

This study revealed that the isolation of multiple bacterial species from the respiratory tracts of pneumonic sheep signifies their possible role in the involvement of respiratory disease complex. However, viruses and mycoplasma species are expected to reside in the respiratory tract. Therefore, the extent of the impact of respiratory diseases on sheep production and a complete understanding of the respiratory microbial flora, both culturable and unculturable condition give future research warranty.

ACKNOWLEDGMENTS

The authors are indebted to Addis Ababa University for the support to conduct this study.

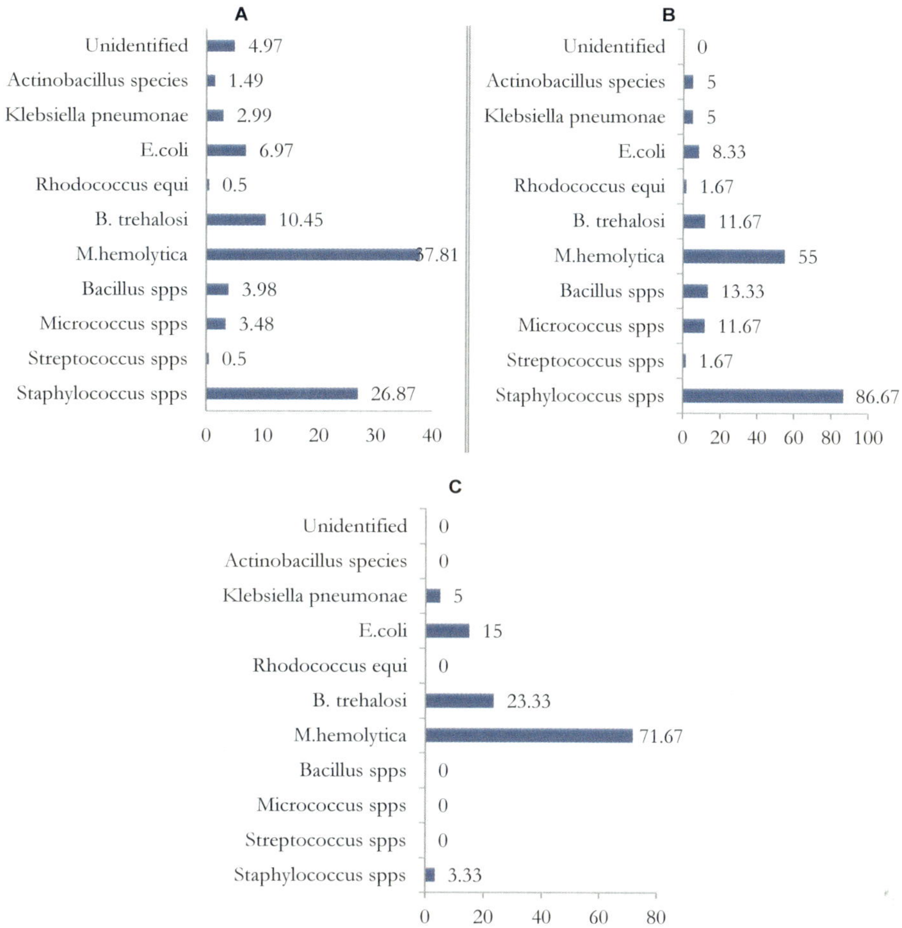

Figure 2. Bacterial isolates (%) under anaerobic condition from the respiratory tract of sheep slaughtered at Addis Ababa Abattoirs Enterprises. (A) Overall proportion of bacterial isolates; (B) Bacterial Isolates from lung; (C) Bacterial isolates from trachea.

REFERENCES

Aiello E, May A (1998). The Merck Veterinary Manual. 8th ed. Merck and Co., Inc.,NewJersey. USA, pp. 1053-1057.

Alley MR (1975). The bacterial flora of the respiratory tract of normal and pneumonic sheep. New Zealand Vet. J. 23(6):113-118.

Akloul K, Mohammed NM (2016). Pneumonia in Algerian OuledDjellal sheep: Bacteriological study and macroscopic aspect of lung lesions. Afr. J. Microbiol. Res. 10.40:1685-1693.

Alemneh T, Tewodros A (2016). Sheep and goats pasteurellosis: Isolation, identification, biochemical characterization and prevalence determination in FogeraWoreda, Ethiopia. J. Cell Anim. Biol. 10(4):22-29.

Al Sultan II (1995). Bacterial isolation from pneumonic lungs in sheep. Iraq J. Vet. Sci. 8(2):213-215.

Almeida PFJ, AlvesFS J, Santos LF, Posa JS, DE-Almeida PF (1986). Revista de Micro Biologica, Brazil 17(3):213-215.

Angen O, Aherns P, Teptimeicer C (1998). Development of a PCR test for identification of *Haemophilus somnus* in pure and mixed cultures. Vet. Microbiol. 63:39-48.

Asaduzzaman KHM, Nazmul HN, Mostafizur R, Khondokar SA (2013). Isolation and identification of bacteria from upper respiratory tract of Black Bengal goat in Bangladesh and investigation of some epidemiological parameters related to pneumonia. Sci. J. Microbiol. 2(11):207-213.

Baker JC (1998). Respiratory disease of cattle. In: Merck Veterinary Mannual. 8ed. Merck and Rhone-Poulence Company, pp. 1068-1069.

Barbour EKJ, Nabbut NH, Hamadeh SK, Al Nakhli HM (1997). Bacterial identity and characterstics in healthy and diseased respiratory tract of sheep and calves. Am. Vet. Res. Commun. 21(6):401-430.

Borji H, Azizzadeh M, Ebrahimi M, Asadpour M (2012). Study on small ruminant lungworms and associated risk factors in northeastern Iran. Asian Pacific J. Trop. Med. 5(11):853-856.

Buxton, Fraser G (1977). Animal Microbiology Volume 1. Black well Scientific Publications Edinburgh, London, pp. 151-163.

Carter GR (1984). Diagnostic procedures in veterinary bacteriology and mycology, 4th ed., pp.12-47.

CSA (Central Statistical Authority) (2014-15). Ethiopian agricultural sample survey. Vol. II Report on livestock and livestock characteristics. Statistical Bulletin 388. CSA, Addis Ababa, Ethiopia.

Esra S, Yhaya K, Selattin K (2009).Bacterial examination in the nasal cavity of apparently healthy and unhealthy Holstein cattle. J. Anim. Vet. Advan. 8:2355-2359

Fikru S, Gebeyew K (2015). Sheep and goat production systems in Degehabur Zone, Eastern Ethiopia: challenge and opportunities. J. Advan. Dairy Res. 3:134.

Fulton RW (2009). Bovine Respiratory disease research (1983-2009). Anim. Health Res. Rev. 10(2):131-139.

Garedew L, Gelagay A, Roman Y, Aschalew Z, Esayas G (2010). Isolation of diverse bacterial species associated with maedi-visnainfection of sheep in Ethiopia. Afr. J. Microbiol. Res 4(1):14-21.

Gupta MP, Kumar H, Singla LD (2009). Trypanosomosis concurrent to

tuberculosis in black bucks. Ind. Vet. J. 86:727-728.
Jim K (2009). Impact of Bovine Respiratory Disease (BRD) from the perspective of the Canadian beef producer. Anim. Health Res. Rev. 10(2):109 -110.
Jury MR, Funk C (2013).Climatic trends over Ethiopia: regional signals and drivers. Int. J. Climatol. 33(8):1924-1935.
Gebremeskel AK, Tesema TS, Yegoraw AA, Birhanu BT, Mekuria SA (2017). Isolation and Characterization of Bacterial Species from Respiratory Tracts of Cattle Slaughtered in Addis Ababa City, Central Ethiopia. World Vet. J. 7(1):14-20.
Kaur S, Singla LD, Hassan SS, Juyal PD (2009). Standardization and application of indirect plate ELISA for immunodiagnosis of paramphistomosis in ruminants. J. Parasitic Dis. 33(1-2):70-76.
Lees VW, Meek AH, Rosendal S (1990). Epidemiology of *Haemophilus somnus* in young rams. Can. J. Vet. Res. 54(3):331.
Leta S, Mesele F (2014). Spatial analysis of cattle and shoat population in Ethiopia: growth trend, distribution and market access. SpringerPlus 3(1):310.
Lin YC, Miles RJ, Nicholas RA, Kelly DP, Wood AP (2008). Isolation and immunological detection of Mycoplasma ovipneumoniae in sheep with atypical pneumonia, and lack of a role for Mycoplasma arginini. Res. Vet. Sci. 84(3):367-373.
Marru HD, Anijajo TT, Hassen AA (2013). Study on Ovine pneumonic pasteurellosis: Isolation and Identification of Pasteurellae and their antibiogram susceptibility pattern in Haramaya District, Eastern Hararghe, Ethiopia." BMC Vet. Res. 9(1):239.
Megra T, Sisay T, Asseged B (2006).The aerobic bacterial flora of the respiratory passageways of healthy goats in Dire Dawa Abattoir, Eastern Ethiopia. Revue de médecinevétérinaire 157:84-87.
Mohan M, Aprajita, Panwar NK (2013). Effect of Wood Dust on Respiratory Health Status of Carpenters. J. Clin. Diagn. Res. 7(8):1589-1591.
Monot M, Archer F, Gomes M, Mornex JF, Leroux C (2015). Advances in the study of transmissible respiratory tumours in small ruminants. Vet. Microbiol. 181(1-2):170-177.
NMSA (2005). National metrology service agency, Ethiopia.
Obasi OL, Ragi MA, Adogwa T, Natala AJ (2001). The effect of climaticfactors on the occurrence and gross pathological lesion in bacterial pneumonia of ovine and caprine hosts in Zaria, Nigeria. Glob. J. Pure Appl. Sci. 7:57-60.
Office International des Epizooties (OIE) (2008). Manual for terstitial animal disease. https://web.oie.int/eng/normes/MMANUAL/2008/pdf/2.04.15_MCF.p
Okolo MIO (1985). Pathological conditions found in Goat killed at Slaughter houses in Nusuku. Nig. J. Anim. Prod. 12(125):61-65.
Pawar PD, Khasnis MW, hong CD, Khole RP, Mhase PP, Singla LD (2017). Coproprevalence and successful management of parasitic infections in sheep in Pune district of Maharastra.. Proceedings of 25th National Congress of Veterinary Parasitology and International Symposium on Current Concepts in Diagnosis & Control of Parasitic Diseases to Combat Climat Change (15-17 February, 2017) at Veterinary College, Shimoga. P 56.
Porter JF, Connor K, Donachie W (1994). Isolation and characterization of Bordetellaparapertussis-like bacteria from ovine lungs. Microbiology 140(2):255-261.
Queen C, Ward AC, Hunter DL (1994). Bacteria isolated from nasal and tonsillar samples of clinically healthy Rocky Mountain bighorn and domestic sheep. J. Wildlife Dis. 30(1):1-7.
Quinn PJ, Carter ME, Markery B, Carter GR (1994). Clinical Veterinary Microbiology. London: Wolfe Publishing Company, pp. 178-182.
Radostits OM, Gar CC, Blood DC, Hinchcliff KW (2000). Veterinary Medicine.A text book of the Disease of Cattle, Sheep, Pigs, Goats and Horses.9th ed., Harcourt Publishers Limited, London Philadelphia, pp. 701-867.
Rajiv K, Katoch RC, Prasenjit D (2000). Bacteriological studies on pneumonic Gaddi sheep of Himachal Pradesh. Ind. Vet. J. 77:846-848.
Rashid MM, Ferdoush MJ, Dipti M, Roy P, Rahman MM, Hossain MI, Hossain MM (2014). Bacteriological and pathological investigation of goat lungs in Mymensingh and determination of antibiotic sensitivity. Bangladesh J. Vet. Med. 11(2):159 166.
Richard YJ, Menour NJ, Cuiguen FJ, Avier CJ, Borges E, Fontain, MJ,Audar J, Brunet J, Pailhac C (1986). Bacteriological study on sheep lungs from the abattoir. Reve De Medecine Veterinaire 137(10):671-680.
Sarker CK, Hossen A, Yousuf MA, Uddin MA, Akter MS, Rahman M, Rahman MB (2016). Isolation, identification and characterization of bacterial flora from the respiratory tract of apparently healthy sheep. Asian J. Med. Biol. Res. 1(3):677-685.
Sharma SN, Adlakha SC (1996). Text book of Veterinary Microbiology. New Delhi: Vikas Publishing House, pp. 63-55.
Shigidi AM (1973). Aerobic micro flora of respiratory tract of camels. Sudan J. Vet. Sci. Anim. Husband.14 (1):9-14.
Singh R, Bal MS, Singla LD, Kaur P (2017). Detection of anthelmintic resistance in sheep and goat against fenbendazole by faecal egg count reduction test. J. Parasitic Dis. 41(2):463-466.
Tesfaye B, Tessema TS, Tefera G (2013). Diversity of bacterial species in the nasal cavity of sheep in the highlands of Ethiopia and first report of Histophilus somni in the country. Trop. Anim. Health Prod. 45(5):1243-1249.

Prevalence of endo-parasites in donkeys and camels in Karamoja sub-region, North-eastern Uganda

Jesca Nakayima[1]*, William Kabasa[2], Daniel Aleper[1] and Duke Okidi[1]

[1]National Livestock Resources Research Institute (NaLIRRI), P.O Box 96 Tororo, Uganda.
[2]College of Veterinary Medicine, Animal Resources and Bio-security (CoVAB), P.O. Box 7062, Kampala, Uganda.

Donkeys (*Ass-Equus-assinus*) and camels (*Camelus dromedarius*) in Uganda are mainly owned by low income earners and peasant farmers, mainly in the semi-arid North-eastern Uganda in Karamoja and Sebei sub-regions. The animals however, seem to receive little or relatively no veterinary care. This study was carried out in Moroto and Amudat districts, Karamoja sub-region, Uganda in March 2016. Faecal samples of 110 randomly selected camels and donkeys of all age and sex were collected directly from their rectum. The faecal samples were examined by flotation method, sedimentation technique, McMaster egg counting technique and faecal culture to identify and determine the burden of parasites in different age groups. Lungworms ovaculture revealed *Dictyocaulus cameli* (29.3%) of camels and *Dictyocaulus arnfieldi* (15.4%) of donkeys. Cestode eggs detection revealed family *Anoplocephalidae* which includes seven species of cestodes identifiable as eggs in faeces or as adults in the gastro-intestinal tract of camels (18.3%) and donkeys (15.4%). Coccidia species included *Eimeria cameli* (11%) and *Eimeria Leuckarti* (3.85%) in camels and donkeys, respectively. Trematodes were detected in 5 camels as *Fasciola gigantica*. Overall, EPG count was observed for strongyles at 58.5% in camels and 42.3% in donkeys. The results of this study will provide insights into the health of donkeys and camels in Uganda and provide a way forward to their veterinary care and management for improved production and productivity.

Key words: Gastrointestinal parasites, donkey, camels, Karamoja, Uganda.

INTRODUCTION

Donkeys and camels are subject to severe work and in bondage, working in extremely strenuous conditions, over laden, underfed and ill-used especially for draught purposes. They are sore footed, constantly burdened by parasites (Atawalna et al., 2015; Tsegaye and Chala, 2015; Ismail et al., 2016; Anvari-Tafti et al., 2013), with little or no veterinary care. An attempt to study parasitism in these species has only been recent.

Parasitic helminthes are one of the most common factors that constrain the health and working performance of camels and donkeys worldwide. Parasites cause various degrees of damage depending on the species and number present, nutritional and the immune status of the animal (Sumbria et al., 2014; Sumbria and Singla,

*Corresponding author. Email: jescanl2001@yahoo.co.uk.

2015). Infection by endo-parasites in camels and donkeys are responsible for problems including poor body condition, reduced power output, diarrhea, colic, emaciation, impaired growth, poor reproductive performance, short lifespan and predisposition to other infectious diseases (Ayele, 2006; Fikru et al., 2005; Getachew et al., 2010; Yoseph et al., 2005).

The prevalence, species composition and epidemiology of helminthes affecting donkeys and camels have not been previously investigated in Uganda. Donkeys and camels are used in arid and mountain villages, both as saddle animals and for carriage. In camels and donkeys, nematodes are seen to be most prevalent, while cestodes and trematodes are less occurring (Arslan and Umur, 1998; Bakirci et al., 2004; Demir et al., 1995). *Eimeria* species can also be encountered (Arslan and Umur, 1998; Bakirci et al., 2004; Ozer and Küçükerden, 1992).

Nematode infection was the most prevalent challenge in these species. A heavy internal parasite burden can adversely affect the health of donkeys and camels particularly when called upon to work and as it is often the case, is undernourished and stressed (Sonja et al., 2000).

The present study was therefore designed to generate baseline data on the prevalence and species composition of helminth parasites of donkeys and camels in Uganda.

MATERIALS AND METHODS

Faecal samples were collected from Karamoja sub-region in two districts namely: Moroto: N 2° 31' 41.604", E 34° 39' 28.794" and Amudat: N 1° 47' 29.841", E 34° 54' 23.583" districts, Uganda. The study was conducted in March 2016. The camels and donkeys were classified as: infant, juvenile, sub-adult and adult. Male and female animals were sampled (Table 1).

Karamoja sub-region is a semi-arid region, the livelihoods of the people depend on pastoralism. Cattle, sheep and goat are kept in large numbers for meat, milk, blood, dowry, prestige. Donkeys and camels are kept for draught power, meat and milk. Faecal samples were collected directly from the rectum of the animal using a gloved hand, into polyethene bags, labeled using details such as source, age, sex, species and general condition of animal for easy identification, cold chain was maintained in the field and the samples were hurriedly taken to the parasitology laboratory for analysis to avoid larval development.

Samples were kept in refrigerator at 4°C if immediate processing was not possible, but it had been processed within 48 h or as soon as possible. Direct faecal smear, sedimentation and floatation techniques were the utilized parasitological techniques to identify the eggs in faeces and examined microscopically (10 and 40×) for presence of parasite ova following their procedures (Forety, 2001). Identification of the eggs was made on the basis of their morphology (Soulsby, 1982). Quantitative faecal examination was performed by using McMaster technique (Gordon and Whitlock, 1939) to determine the number of egg per gram of faeces (EPG) and performed according to the procedure described by Urquhart et al. (1996). Faecal culture using Baermann technique to determine lungworm larvae, *Dictyocaulus arnifieldi* and *Dictyocaulus cameli* was also undertaken. Level of infection was extrapolated from infection severity index (Soulsby, 1986) where animals are said to have mild, moderate and severe nematode infestation if their faecal egg counts are less than 500, 500-1000 and more than 1000, respectively.

Table 1. Physical characteristics of the animals.

Identity	Camel	Donkey	Total
Sex			
Male	36	1	37
Female	46	25	71
Age			
Infant	9	1	10
Juvenile	29	0	29
Sub-adult	7	1	8
Adult	37	24	61

Data management and analysis

The data collected from the study area was entered into Microsoft Excel spread sheet and the data was coded appropriately and analyzed using SPSS version 16 statistical software. Analysis Of variance (ANOVA) test was applied to test the statistical association existing among the risk factors such as species, sex, age and body condition scoring with the presence of the infection.

RESULTS

The total number of donkeys was 26, while camels were 82 giving a total of 108 animal samples analyzed. Number of positive cases for Strongyle EPG was 48 for camels and 11 for donkeys giving a prevalence of 58.5% for camels and 42.3% for donkeys. The mean EPG count was 1056 for camels and 323 for donkeys. The number of positive cases for *Anoplocephalidae* family of cestodes was 15 for camels and 4 for donkeys, giving a mean count of 74.4, prevalence of 18.3% in camels and 27, prevalence of 15.4% in donkeys (Table 2). Lung worm larvae reported *Dictyocaulus arnfieldi* in donkeys with 4 cases at a mean count of 0.4 and a prevalence of 15.4%. While *Dictyocaulus cameli* recorded 24 cases with a mean count of 1 at a prevalence of 29.3%.

Coccidia reported *Eimeria cameli* in camels with 9 cases in camel at a mean count of 34 at a prevalence of 11%, while *Eimeria leuckarti* in donkeys reported 1 case with a mean count of 11.5 at a prevalence of 3.85%.

Mixed infections were reported. Infections with one parasite species were 22 (26.8%) in camels and 8 (30.8%) in donkeys. Infections with 2 parasite species were 24 (29.3%) in camels and 6 (23%) in donkeys. Infections with 3 parasite species were 7 (8.5%) in camels and none in donkeys (Table 3).

Level of infection

Animals were said to have mild, moderate and severe

Table 2. Prevalence of endo parasites of donkeys and camels from Karamoja sub-region, Uganda.

Parasite/animal (mean EPG count)	No. positive camel/donkey	Camel (n = 82)	Donkey (n = 26)	Total
Strongyle eggs (EPG)	48/11	1056 (58.5%)	323 (42.3%)	1379
Dictyocaulus arnfieldi	0/4	N/A	0.4 (15.4%)	0.4
Dictyocaulus cameli	24/0	1 (29.3%)	N/A	1
Anoplocephalidae	15/4	74.4 (18.3%)	27 (15.4%)	101.4
Eimeria cameli	9/0	34 (11%)	N/A	34
Eimeria leuckarti	0/1	N/A	11.5 (3.85%)	11.5
Trematodes	5/0	12 (14.6%)	0	12

Table 3. Prevalence of various parasitic infections in camels and donkeys.

Infection status	Camels	Donkeys	Total
Infection with one species	22 (26.8%)	8 (30.8%)	30 (27.8%)
Infection with two species	24 (29.3%)	6 (23%)	30 (27.8)
Infection with three species	7 (8.5%)	0	7 (8.5%)
Infection with four species	0	0	0
General infection rate	51 (62.3%)	14 (53.8%)	65 (60.3%)

Table 4. Level of infection of strongyles in different age groups of donkeys and camels.

Age groups	Mild	Moderate	Severe	Total
Donkeys				
Infant	0	0	1 (3.85%)	1 (3.85%)
Juvenile	0	0	0	
Sub-adult	0	0	1 (3.85%)	1 (3.85%)
Adult	6 (23%)	2 (7.7%)	1 (3.85%)	9 (34.6%)
Camels				
Infant	0	0	4 (4.9%)	4 (4.9%)
Juvenile	5 (6%)	3 (3.7%)	4 (4.9%)	12 (14.6%)
Sub-adult	1 (1.2%)	1 (1.2%)	3 (3.7%)	5 (6%)
Adult	7 (8.5%)	4 (4.9%)	16 (19.5%)	27 (33%)

nematode infestation if their faecal egg counts are less than 500, 500-1000 and more than 1000, respectively (Table 4). Statistical analysis revealed a significant difference between the mean Strongyle EPG between the two districts, Moroto and Amudat (p=0.000), *Eimeria* EPG (p=0.018) and Trematode EPG (p=0.048), for the two districts; Mean Strongyle EPG Moroto (1281.8), Amudat (260); Mean *Eimeria* EPG Moroto (10.6), Amudat (60.0); Mean Trematode EPG Moroto (0.30), Amudat (0.25). The mean Strongyle EPG between species, camel and donkey was significant at p=0.020. Mean *Eimeria* EPG was statistically significant for location (p=0.018) and sex (p=0.017). Mean Trematode EPG was significant for location (p=0.048) and sex (p=0.006).

DISCUSSION

Lungworm infection characterized *D. cameli* of camels and *D. arnfieldi* as the parasite of horses and donkeys. *D. arnfieldi* has donkey as its normal host. While pathogenicity is limited in the donkey, the parasite may provoke severe clinical lungworm disease in the horse.

The family *Anoplocephalidae* comprises seven species of cestodes that inhabit the gastro-intestinal tract of camels and donkeys as adults or eggs found in the faeces. These include: *Moniezia expanza, Moniezia benedeni*, *Stilesia globipunctata*, *Stilesia vittata*, *Avitellina centripunctata, Avitellina woodland* and *Thysaniezia ovilla.*

Ugandan camels (*Camelus dromedaries*) were infected with *E. cameli* (11%) while 3.85% donkeys had *Eimeria leuckarti*. It is believed that the infection of coccidia is concern mainly with young horses and donkeys, especially foals. Although, it has been reported that *E. leuckarti* is more prevalent among young foals and only occasionally is it detected in adult animals (Souza et al., 2009). Watering devices should be protected from faecal contamination. Diagnosis is based on clinical signs and the demonstration of high numbers of oocysts in the diarrhoeic faeces. Cystic structures containing immature oocysts occur in the intestinal mucosa. In the present study, in all the cases, no clinical signs were documented in the animals excreting *E. leuckarti* oocysts, while there were some doubt about the pathogenicity of *E. leuckarti*, diarrhea of several days duration, and acute massive intestinal hemorrhage leading to rapid death have been described in foals (Radostits et al., 2006). However, the infection is rarely evidenced by clinical signs. Difficulties in the diagnosis of coccidia infection in camels, horses and donkeys cause the parasitosis not to be diagnosed in a routine coproscopical examination.

Trematodes were detected in 5 camels as *Fasciola gigantica*. Trematodes whose eggs may appear in the faeces including: *Fasciola hepatica* (liver flukes), *Fasciola gigantica* (giant liver fluke), *Dicrocoelium* spp. (liver flukes), *Eurytrema pancreaticum* (pancreas fluke), *Schistosoma bovis* and *Schistosoma mattheei* (blood flukes).

Strongyle eggs were quantified to determine egg per gram of faeces (EPG). Strongyles were taken as a group, speciation of the nematodes by ovaculture was not done. All the camels and donkeys were in good health and body condition except one sick donkey in Moroto which was in poor body condition. For this reason, autopsy was not done and hence adult worms were not studied. Therapy and prophylaxis for all the above mentioned helminth parasites is the same as for cattle.

Veterinary health care provision in Uganda does not cater for donkeys and camels at all. No veterinary intervention for these animals in Uganda is available at all. Yet these animals are kept in arid and mountainous areas of Karamoja and Sebei sub-region in North-eastern Uganda. They are kept for milk, meat, dowry, prestige and carriage.

Mixed infections were encountered comprising of double infections or triple infections of Strongyle, coccidian, cestode, trematode and lungworms. The challenge of mixed infections exacerbates the compromised health condition of the animal which could result in debilitation and death of the animal.

The number of eggs per gram can be calculated by counting the number of eggs within the grid of each of the 2 chambers, ignoring those outside the squares, then multipling the total by 50; this gives the eggs per gram of faeces (e.p.g.). Reading the count should not be delayed beyond the recommended time as the flotation fluid may distort or destroy delicate eggs. Therefore, it is advisable to only process a few samples at a time.

When interpreting McMaster results, it must be remembered that a number of factors can influence the occurrence, recognition or numbers of helminth eggs found in a faecal sample. In particular, the number of eggs is not necessarily indicative of the number of worms present. Reasons for this include: Eggs are produced only by fertile adult female (or hermaphrodite) worms and will, therefore, be absent in immature or single sex infections. The daily output of eggs by fertile females is influenced by host-physiological factors such as stress or lactation (increased) or immunity (decreased). Chemotherapy can also affect egg-production e.g. corticosteroids (increased) or sub-lethal anthelmintic doses (decreased). Some food-stuffs may have a similar effect e.g. tannin-rich forages (decreased). The concentration of eggs (per gram of faeces) is influenced by the daily volume of faeces being produced by the host, the rate of passage by the ingesta through the intestine, and the distribution of eggs throughout the faecal mass. Some types of eggs are heavier than others and may not float well in solutions of lower specific gravity (e.g. *Fasciola*). Some eggs from different species are indistinguishable (particularly trichostrongylids and strongylids). This complicates clinical interpretation as some species (e.g. *Haemonchus*) produce many more eggs per day than others (e.g. *Ostertagia*).

The mean EPG was statistically significant for male and female animals for *Eimeria* (p=0.017) and Trematodes (p=0.006). Although in this study, mean EPG *Eimeria* was higher in males (68.6) than females (12.1), and Trematodes male (0.34) and females (0). Female animals are ideally more prone to helminth infections physiologically because of stress, pregnancy and lactation conditions which compromise their immunity. The mean Strongyle EPG was 1056.1 in camels and 323.1 in donkeys. The mean Strongyle EPG between species, camel and donkey was significant at (p=0.020). It could be explained that donkey is a hardier animal, closer to wildlife species. Hence, it has a stronger resistance to infections naturally, more tendency as a reservoir host. However, fewer donkeys than camels were sampled in this study.

Conclusion

Helminthes infection is endemic in camels and donkeys in Uganda. A wide range of species of helminthes that plague donkeys and camels was detected in Karamoja sub-region, Uganda. The observation of multiple infections with high prevalence and high overall EPG suggest the presence of favorable environmental conditions for survival, infection and perpetuation of helminthes of camels and donkeys in Uganda. There is complete lack of veterinary service provision to these animals and lack of awareness of animal welfare. Information on the different aspects of parasitology of these animals is also limited. Production and productivity of camels and donkeys in Uganda is compromised by the little or no veterinary care and welfare of these animals.

ACKNOWLEDGEMENT

This study was financially supported by the Government of Uganda under National Agricultural Research Organization (NARO).

REFERENCES

Anvari-Tafti M, Sazmand A, Hekmatimoghaddam S, Moobedi I (2013). Gastrointestinal helminths of camels (*Camelus dromedarius*) in center of Iran. Trop. Biomed. 30(1):56-61.

Arslan MO, Umur S (1998). The helminth and Eimeria (Protozoa) species in horse and donkey in Kars. Acta. Parasitol. Turcica. 22:180-184.

Atawalna J, Emikpe BO, Sallah EK, Shaibu W, Folitse RD (2015). The Health Problems, Gastrointestinal and Blood Parasites Commonly Associated With Donkeys in the Upper East Region of Ghana. Afr. J. Biomed. Res. 18:37-41.

Ayele CF (2006). Principal health problems of donkeys in Dugda Bora district of Ethiopia. In: Proceedings of the 5th International Colloquium on Working Equines Thethe Future for Working Equines. Eds: Pearson AA, Muir CC, Farrow MM. The Donkey Sanctuary, Sidmouth. pp. 162-168.

Bakirci S, Çirak VY, Gülegen E, Karabacak A (2004). Parasites found by faecal examinations in horses in the Gemlik Military Stud Farm. Acta. Parasitol. Turcica. 28:35-37.

Demir S, Tinar R, Kaplan A (1995). Helminths obtained from a donkey. Acta. Parasitol. Turcica. 19:119-123.

Fikru R, Reta D, Teshale S, Bizunesh M (2005). Prevalence of equine gastrointestinal parasites in western highlands of Oromia, Ethiopia. Bull. Anim. Health Prod. Afr. 53:161-166.

Forety WJ (2001). Veterinary Parasitology. Reference Manual, Fifth Edition, Iowa State University Press.

Getachew AM, Trawford AF, Feseha G, Reid SWJ (2010). Gastrointestinal parasites of working donkeys in Ethiopia, Trop. Anim. Health Prod. 42:27-33.

Gordon HM, Whitlock HV (1939). A new technique for counting nematode eggs in sheep faeces. J. Counc. Sci. Ind. Res. 12:50-52.

Ismail AA, Seri HI, Ahmed NK, El Tigani-Asil El TA, Bashar AE, Abakar AD (2016). A Survey of Seasonal Gastrointestinal Parasitic Infections in Donkeys from a Semiarid Sub-Saharan Region, Sudan. Hindawi. J. Pathog. P 8.

Ozer E, Küçükerden N (1992). Helminth and *Eimeria sp.* found in equids in Elazig and region. Doga Tr. J. Vet. Anim. Sci. 17:217-221.

Radostits OM, Gay CC, Hinchcliff KW, Constable PD (2006). A text-book of the diseases of cattle, horses, sheep, pigs and goats. Veterinary Medicine E-Book, 10th Edition. Vet. med. Saunders.

Sonja M, Rosina CK, Susan AM (2000). Prevalence and Biodiversity of helminth parasites in donkey from South Africa. J. Parasitol. 86:756-762.

Soulsby E (1982). "Helminths, Arthropods and Protozoa of Domestic Animals," Bailliere TinDall, Toronto.

Soulsby EJL (1986). Helminthes, Arthropods and Protozoa of Domesticated Animals (7thedn) Bailliere Tindall London. 167-174

Souza PNBD, Bomfimb TCB, Huber F, Abboud LCS, Gomes RS (2009). Natural infection by Cryptosporidiumsp. Giardia sp. and Eimeria leuckarti in three groups of equines with different handlings in Rio de Janeiro. Brazil. Vet. Parasitol. 160:327-333.

Sumbria D, Moudgil AD, Singla LD (2014). Equine Piroplasmosis: Current status. Veterinaria 1(1):9-14.

Sumbria D, Singla LD (2015). Recent Diagnostic and control approaches in Equine piroplasmosis. Veterinaria 2(1):1-6

Tsegaye B, Chala A (2015). Prevalence of endoparasitic helminths of donkeys in and around Haramaya district, Eastern Ethiopia. JVMAH 7:221-224.

Yoseph S, Smith DG, Mengistu A, Teklu F, Firew T, Betere Y (2005). Seasonal variation in the parasite burden and body condition of working donkeys in East Shewa and West Shewa regions of Ethiopia. Trop. Anim. Health Prod. 37:35-45.

A study on sero prevalence of foot and mouth diseases in West and South West Shoa zones of Oromia regional state, central Ethiopia

Kebede Shanko Hordofa*, Tesfaye Rufael Chibsa and Enquibaher Kasaye

Mekelle University, Ethiopia

Cross-sectional study was conducted from December, 2008 to April, 2009 to determine the sero prevalence of foot and mouth disease (FMD) virus in West and South West Shoa zones of Oromia regional state, central Ethiopia. The samples were processed with the 3 ABC ELISA kits that can able to identify natural infected animal from vaccinated animals. From the total sera of 421 tested, the overall sero prevalence of FMD in cattle was 15.0% (63/421). The prevalence rate was higher (22%) in the South west shoa zone than West shoa zone (5.6%). The difference was statistically significant (ρ<0.05). At district level, the highest sero prevalence were recorded at Dawo (26.7%), Alemgana (26.2%), Kokir (24.4%) and Haramaya (21.4%) districts, which were located at south west shoa zone. The difference among districts were statistically significant (ρ<0.05). Statistically difference was also observed between different age groups (ρ<0.05); being higher in adult (19.3%) followed by calves (9.3%). The sero prevalence of male and female were 16.0 and 14.1%, respectively, and which was not statistically significant (ρ>0.05). The sero prevalence of FMD was found higher in mid highland (16.8%) than highland attitude (6.7%) which was statistically significant (ρ<0.05). The result of this study indicated that FMD is highly prevalent in the South West Shoa zone than West Shoa zone due to contact of different origin of animals, and free animals movement in search of feed and water in zone. Age and attitude were also found as an important risk factor for the diseases. Finally, it is recommended that, sero typing of the virus circulating in the study area should be undertaken for effective control of the disease.

Key words: Foot and mouth disease (FMD), Sero prevalence, West Shoa, South west shoa, 3 ABC ELSA.

INTRODUCTION

Ethiopia has the largest livestock inventories in Africa, possessing more than 31 million cattle, 48 million small ruminants, 1.5 million camels, 7 million equines and 52 million chickens (Desta, 1999). Livestock is an integral part of all farming system in it. They provide milk, meat, hides and skin, and the drought power required for tilling the farm land (Asseged, 2005). However, due to the higher prevalence of different diseases like foot and

*Corresponding author. E-mail: sh.kebeko@yahoo.com.

mouth diseases (FMD) and poor management system, the country is not utilizing this huge potential in livestock resource (Hussen, 2006).

FMD, which is also known as aphthous fever (Kahrs, 2001), is a major global animal health problem (Murphy et al., 1999). It is the most contagious transboundary animal disease (TAD) affecting cloven hoofed animals (FAO, 2007) characterized by the formation of vesicles in the mouth, at coronary band and skin of inter digital cleft (Radostits et al., 2000). The disease is an infection, worldwide in incidence, caused by an entero virus of the genus aphtho virus, family picornaviridae which occurs as seven major A, O, C, SATI, SAT2 , SAT3 and Asia 1 (Radostits et al., 2000). Each serotypes of FMD virus is antigentically district (Kitching, 1987). All the seven (7) serotype produce a disease that is clinically indistinguishable but immunologically district and infection with one serotypes does not confer immunity against the other (Richard, 1998).

According to the office of international des epizootics (OIE, 1990), FMD ranks first among the notifiable infection disease of animals (OIE, 2000). The disease is notoriously contagious that it can be spread as much as 50 (fifty) miles downwind from one out break area to another (Sainsbury, 2000). Introduction of the virus types or subtypes to regions where they were previously absent, lead to epidemics of varying magnitude (Gibbs, 1981). When the disease breaks out in susceptible cattle, it spreads very rapidly, and the morbidity rates approximate 100%. The disease is rarely fatal expect in young anima (Kahan and Scottlline, 2005).

The disease has an incubation period of 3 to 14 days, and excretion of the virus from infected animals in all secretion and excretion usually begins before the appearance of the visible clinical signs (kitching and Donaldson, 1987). Initial virus multiplication occurs mainly in the pre-pharyngeal area and the lungs (Burrows et al., 1981). Acutely infected cattle salivate profusely and develop a nasal discharge (mucoid and muco purulent). Following pyrexia (about 40°C) vesicles appears on the dorsum of the tongue, hard palate, dental pad, lips, gums, muzzle, coronary band and inter digital space with consequent lameness. The lesions are susceptible to secondary bacterial infection. At this stage, it also include linking, cannot eat and move. Other signs include licking of the feet or shifting weight from one leg to other, holding one hoof off the ground, lagging behind the herd, lying down and reluctance to rise (Woodbury, 1995). Vesicles may also be seen on the teats of lactating animals. Morbidity is high and young caves may die before the appearance of clinical signs due to virus infection of the developing heart muscle and the production of a severe myocarditis (Woodbury, 1995). However, most animal recover within 2 weeks.

FMD has a great potential for causing severe economic loss in susceptible cloven-hoofed animals (OIE, 2000). Greater losses can result from refusal of FMD free countries to import livestock and livestock products from infected regions (Kahrs, 2001). Adult mortality is not very high but causes heavy economic losses (losses of flesh, diminished milk production, mastitis and calf mortality and infertility etc). This combined with the time and money spent treating animals, and their long convalescence contributes to consider it as the most important animal disease in a world context (Solomon, 1980). The disease occasionally transmitted to humans causing a self limited, febrile illness, characterized by pain in the limps excessive salivation and the appearance of vesicular lesions on the buccal or lingual epithelium and on the skin of hand, feet and other parts of the body (Lennette et al., 1979). Very few cases have been reported even among people working with infected carcasses and laboratories. However, humans can also be vehicle for transmission of the disease to animals (Radostits et al., 2000).

No specific treatment exist for FMD; however, proper animal husbandry practice and treatment of secondary bacterial infection reduce losses (Hirsh and Zee, 1996), treatment with mild disinfectants and protective dressing to inflamed areas to prevent secondary bacterial infection is recommended in endemic countries where slaughter policy is not in force. If, however a disease outbreak occurs in suckling calves, no treatment will be possible (Seifert, 1990). Given the law absolute production of pastoral herds compared with commercial or semi commercial dairy with, some workers assume that FMD is relatively minor disease in pastoral. However, at certain time of years pastoralist rely heavily on milk for food and therefore, they often prioritize FMD due to its impact on milk supply. They also associate FMD with mortality in claves and "Chronic FMD" cases showing heat intolerance, reduced fertility and other signs (Rufael, 2006).

There is no reliable figure for the prevalence of FMD in different countries. The disease generally occurs in the form of an outbreak that rapidly spread from herd to herd before it is controlled (Radostits et al., 2000). The disease is endemic in Ethiopian, the main incidence to the stress of harvesting and trashing (Solomon, 1980). The occurrence of FMD in Ethiopia is increasing, and in 1999 almost 10% of cattle were under risk of infection, and in 2000 and 2001 a total of 27 and 88 disease outbreaks were reported, respectively (Esayas et al., 2005).

Four of the seven serotype of FMD of virus were recorded in Ethiopia. The four identified serotype were O, A, C and SAT2. SAT2 was first identified in 1989 from bovine sample collected from Leben Ranch, Borena area, southern Ethiopia. Similarly, serotype C identified in 2005 from virus was identical to a virus identified in 1971. Serotype SAT1 and 3 have not been identified until 2005 (Esayas et al., 2005). Similarly, from the sample recover in 2005 by the WRL for FMD at institute of animal health, pirbright (UK), 22 types O,9 types A and 4 types C were recovered from Ethiopia.

Therefore, FMD is an highly contiguous disease, it is a very serious disease as it spreads rapidly, causes large scale economic losses and halt exports of all animals products as well as agricultural products used as animal feed in the country (Bouxton, 1977). Although, numerous researches were conducted on sero prevalence of FMD in the country, still there is lack of information in the study area. This is due to the controlling of FMD in endemics area that requires a good understanding of the status of the disease within the zones. Hence, this study was conducted to meet the following objectives:

1. To determine the Sero prevalence of foot and mouth disease in selected districts of West and South West Shoa zones.
2. To identify major risk factors of the disease.

MATERIALS AND METHODS

Study areas description

The study was conducted in South West and West Shoa zones of Oromia regional state, Ethiopia which located in West of Addis Ababa. The Zones have got a total land area of about 2.17 million hectare of land, and divide into three agro climatic zone. The low land located below 1500 m a.s.l which caver 17% of the total land area, the mid high land attitude from 1500 to 2500 m a.s.l covers 61% of the total land area and the high land cool temperature located above 2500 m a.s.l that covers 22% of the study area .

The study area has two rainy seasons, the long rainy season covering most of the place and occurs from June to September and the short rainy season occurs March to April with an average annual rain fall being 2900 mm. It is presumed generally that the climate of the study area is suitable for both agriculture and livestock production. The livestock population of the study area is estimated at 2.3 million of cattle, 619,000 Sheep, 172,000 Goat, 283,000 Equine and 1.4 million poultry. Agriculture, which is the main economy sector of activities of the zones, provides livelihood for more than 90% of the population. Almost 85% of the total land coverage used for crop production where 15% is used for animal grazing.

Animal health problems specially infections disease such as FMD, pasteurellosis, lumpy skin disease are important in the study area due to increase livestock population, transhumance way of movements from high land to low land area during long rainy season for season for grazing and low level of veterinary services. In addition external, internal parasites and tryp.\anomiasis are of considerable economic importance of veterinary concern in the area.

The study animals

The study conducted on cattle that were kept under majority of livestock production system in the Zones. Study animals were selected from West Shoa Zone of cattle population in ten (10) districts of West Shoa Zone namely: Welmera, Dendi, chelia, Ejere, Ambo, Nano, Metarobi, Jaldu Ada'aBarga, and Bake and from South West Shoa Zone cattle in seven (7) districts namely: Kersa Kondaltit, Alemgana, Dawo, Kokir, Wonchi,Weliso and Hamaya from which 180 and 241 animals were selected, respectively. Approximately 15 animals from each peasant associations (PAs) were selected randomly to be included in the study. Accordingly, 28 Pas and 421 animals were included in the study.

Sample size determination

The study was conducted on cattle that were kept under mixed farming system in which the sample size was determined by considering a prevalence of 50% to get the maximum number required to determine the prevalence in simple random sampling because there was no previous work of FMD in the study area. The precision was decided to be 5 to 95% confidence level. The sample size was estimated by the formula described by Thrusfield, (1995).

$$n = \frac{1.96^2 \times pexp\ (1-pexp)}{d^2}$$

Where:

n = required sample size

pexp = expected prevalence

d^2 =desired absolut precision

$$n = \frac{1.96^2 \times 0.5\ (1-0.5)}{(0.05)^2}$$

=384 cattle.

Even if 384 were the minimum sample size required, 421 cattle from West and south West Shoa zones area were considered in the study prevalence of FMD.

Study Animals and Characterization

A total of 421 samples were randomly collected from animals presented to grazing area. Animals were grouped into three categories based on agro climatic zone, age groups and sex. The animals were classified into three age groups (6 month to 2 years, 2 to 4years and >4years) according to Ken and Tony (1993).

Study design and methods

Study design

A cross sectional study was under taken from December, 2008 to April, 2009. During the laboratory work, a total of 421 sera samples collected from herds of West and South West Shoa zones of cattle, and were examined using 3 ABC ELISA for detection of FMD antibodies.

Sample collection and submission

Cattle blood samples were collected from mixed farming system of herds of cattle in South West and West Shoa zones for analysis of foot and mouth disease antibody. Blood samples were collected form jugular veins of individual animals using plain vacutainer tube of 10 ml capacity, 38 mm length and $1^{1/2}$ gauge sterile vacutainer needle. The owners handled the animals properly. After taking the sample code was given to test tube which contains the sample. Then blood/sample was allowed to clot by lacing it over night at room temperature. The serums were collected from clotted blood and transported using an icebox to national Animal health diagnostic and investigation center (NAHDIC) Sebeta, then transferred in a single sterile cryo vials and labeled with specific laboratory number. The sera sample was stored at -20°C until

Table 1. Sero prevalence of FMD in cattle of different origin/zones.

Zone	No. of samples	No. of sero positive	Sero prevalence
West Shoa	180	10	5.6
South West Shoa	241	53	22.0
Total	421	63	15.0

χ^2=21.875 ρ=0.000.

laboratory investigation

Laboratory analysis

During laboratory work, total of 421 sera were examined by the SVANOVIR foot and Mouth disease virus 3 ABC- EILSA kit to detect foot-and-mouth disease virus (FMDV) specific antibodies in bovine serum samples. The kit procedures were based on a solid phases indirect ELISA. In this procedure, samples were exposed to non structural FMDV antigen (NSP 3 ABC) coated wells on micro titer plates. FMDV antibodies (if present in their sample bind to the antigen in the well) horseradish peroxidase (HRP) conjugate added subsequently forms a complex with the FMDV antibodies. Unbound materials were removed by raising PBS-buffer before the addition of substrate solution, subsequently a blue-green color was developed which is due to the conversion of the substrate by conjugate.

The reaction was stopped by addition of stop solution. Within 15 min, the result was read by micro plate photometer, where the optical density (OD) was measured at 405 nm. The diagnostic relevance of the result was obtained by comparing the optical density (OD) which develops in wells containing the samples with the OD from the wells containing the positive control as it was read by the ELISA reader.

Data analysis

The data collected was entered into M-excel and coded for analysis, the laboratory investigation for prevalence result were analyzed using statistical package for the social sciences (SPSS) statistical package. Variation for the prevalence between the two different zones of Shoa (West and South West Shoa), districts, sex, age and altitude were analyzed by using chi-square (χ^2) test. In all the analysis, confidence level was at 95% and ρ<0.05 set for significance.

RESULTS

Sero prevalence result of total 421 cattle sera from West and South West Shoa zones of Oromia regional state were assessed for the presence of non structural FMDV protein (antibodies) (Table1). The overall sero prevalence of FMD in cattle was 15.0% (63/421). The prevalence rate was higher in the South West Shoa zone 22.0% (53/241) as compared to West Shoa 5.6% (10/180) was significantly different (ρ<0.05).

From seventeen district investigated, 10 were from West Shoa seven, 7 were from South West Shoa (Table 2). The highest sero prevalence were recorded at Dawo (26.7%), Alemgana (26.2%), kokir (24.4%) and Hamaya (21.4%) districst of South West Sho,a and no sero positivity was recorded in Enjere, Dendi, Bake and Ada Berga in West Shoa zone. The difference among district is statistically significant (ρ<0.05). The sero prevalence rate of FMD at West and South West Shoa zones are statistically significant difference (ρ<0.05) were recorded between the three age groups. Being highest in >4 years (Table 3).

The sero prevalence male and female were 16.0 (30/187) and 14.1% (33/234), respectively. However, statistically significant difference were not observed between the sexes (ρ>0.05) (Table 4). On the other hand, higher disease prevalence 16.8% (58/346) was observed in mid-high highland than cool highland 6.7% (5/75) with statistically significant variation (ρ < 0.05) (Table 5).

DISCUSSION

According to this study the sera prevalence of FMD in the study area was high, and statistically significance difference was observed between the two zones districts, age and altitude but not in sexes Although, knowledge on the serotyping of the FMD is very important, this study has limitation in identifying the types FMD Sero types circulating in the study area.

Currently Ethiopia exports beef and live animals to Egypt and Middle East from different parts of Ethiopian in which foot and mouth disease is one the most important diseases that cause restriction on trade of animals both locally and internationally thereby threatening the livelihood of mixed farming system pastoralists area and national agricultural economy in general (Rufael *et* al., 2007)

The overall sero prevalence rate of FMD in West and South West Shoa zones were recorded (15%) in individual animals. The study was less prevalence with previous findings from Ethiopia (Sahle et al., 2004) in which seropositivity of 26.5% (Rufael, 2006) reported 21.0% in Borana pastoral system. The increased in prevalence from the previous study may be associated to pastoral production system that with nature of increased live stock movement result in high rate of contact between animals at common grazing places as well as at watering point (Rufael et al., 2007)

The sero prevalence of South West Shoa Zone (22.0%)

Table 2. Sero prevalence of FMD in cattle at different districts of west and south wets zones.

Zone	District	No. of samples	No. of sero positive	Sero prevalence
West shoa	Welmera	15	1	6.7
	Ejere	15	0	0.0
	Meta Robe	30	3	10.0
	Dendi	15	0	0.0
	Bake	15	0	0.0
	Ambo	15	1	6.7
	Chelia	30	1	3.3
	Nono	15	2	13.3
	Jaldu	15	2	13.3
	Ada'a Berga	15	0	0.0
			16	26.2
South West Shoa	Alemgana	61	4	26.7
	Dawo	15	11	24.4
	Kokir	45	13	21.3
	Kersa	61	5	16.7
	Kondaltit	-	1	6.7
	Welliso	30	3	21.4
	Wanchi	15	-	-
	Hamaya	14	-	-
Total	-	421	63	15.0

χ^2=31.044, ρ= 0.013.

Table 3. Sero prevalence of foot and Mouth disease across age groups.

Age in years	No. of samples	No of sero positive	Sero prevalence (%)
0.6-2	54	5	9.3
2-4	97	6	6.2
Greater than 4	270	52	19.3
Total	63	15.0	15.0

2 =9.285,ρ= 0.010.

was higher as compared to west shoa zone (5.6%) (Table1). The different is statistically significant (ρ<0.05). This is probably due to the fact that South West Shoa zone has long border with the Southern Nations Nationalities and Peoples' Regional State (SNNPR) region and western part of Ethiopia which have two broad roads passing through it, and where free cattle movement across the boundaries for grazing and watering, and also by illegal trade thus promoting the concept that FMD peaked in cattle associated with cattle movement (Rufeal et al., 2007)

Among the sampled districtes, the highest sero prevalence was found in those districts of Alemgana, Kersa kondaltit, Dawo and kokir that are found in the south West Shoa Zone. These districts are located on the road of livestock trade root passed through, and found close to Addis Ababa. This is probably due to fact that South West Shoa Zone has long border with the SNNP and western part of Ethiopia. That has two cattle trek roots for trade from SNNP and western part of Ethiopia to Addis Ababa cattle Market. In this zone, it can cause high concept that FMD peaked in cattle associated with cattle movement (Rufael et al., 2007). But this is in agreement with the previous study indicating that all age groups are susceptible to the disease (Oluthemi and Mastiga, 1988).

A significant difference was observed in seroprevalence of FMD among age group of animal in the west Shoa Zones (Table 3). This may be due to the fact that those cattle with age group over four years had practiced more exposures to FMD at grazing, watering point and at market than in age group less than 2 years. Therefore, adult animals might have acquired infection from multiple sero type, and could produce anti bodies against all serotypes of FMD. The low prevalence in young and calves may be indicative of persistence passive immunity and less frequency of exposure of the animal to the disease as the farmers keep their calves around the home areas (Rufael et al., 2007).

Table 4. Sero prevalence of FMD in cattle of different sex groups.

Sex	No. of samples	Positive	Sero prevalence (%)
Male	187	30	16.0
Female	234	30	14.1
Total	421	63	15.0

$\chi 2$ =0.078, ρ=0.780.

Table 5. Distribution and sero prevalence of foot and mouth disease across altitudes.

Attitude (in meters)	No. of sample	No. of sero positive	Sero prevalence
<2500	346	58	16.8
>2500	75	5	6.7
Total	421	63	15.0

$\chi 2$=5.125, ρ=0.024.

Although, the variation in sero prevalence was seen in between sexes there was no significant different observed (Table 4), and the observation of statistical insignificant difference on prevalence rate across the sex was supported in the study of Rufael (2006). This observation could be due to both sex groups are equally exposed to the environment at same time and place in addition, significant difference found between areas of different altitude with the prevalence of 16.8 and 6.6% at mid high land and high lands altitude respectively on (Table 5). This variation may be due to the fact that in low land and mind high lands, cattle have to move long distance in search of good pasture and source of water (Rufael, 2006) tend to be contacted at different origin, which is the predominant factor for the transmission of the disease.

Therefore, from this study the level of sero prevalence indicated that FMD is one of the economically important diseases in the study areas which needs further attention to reduce the economic impact of the disease on the country's economy.

Conclusion

The presence of sero prevalence of 15.0% of FMD in the study area shows that FMD is one of the economically important diseases in the region. The study has proven that FMD is highly contagious, and a serious impediment for cattle production. Moreover, the study shows that age and altitude are major risk factors for the distribution of FMD in the study area. Movements of animal in the border regions and Zones freely due to illegal trade and seasonal movements of animal are also the major contributing factor for FMD virus transmission, and circulating in the Zones.

Based on this study high prevalence of FMD in adult indicates that it causes loss of production that has significant economic impact on the country.

Recommendations

1. Further study on FMD virus isolation should be conducted. Recommendation and sero typing should be conducted to fill the gap of informational on the incidence of FMD.

2. Presence of foot and mouth disease in livestock population affects the economy at large by limiting international trade of live animals and animal by products, and consideration of this situation is important in controlling the disease.

3. Policymakers and economy analysts have to be provoked to put their relentless effort in the control of such disease that has serious impact on international trade.

4. Active surveillance should be conducted in all regions of the country so as to control the disease on time before its outbreak.

5. Control measures through vaccination and restriction of animal movements remain the mast important to minimize the risk of FMD in the study area.

ACKNOWLEDGEMENTS

The authors are grateful to the management of the National Animal Health Diagnostic and Investigation Center (NAHDIC) for providing an enabling environment for conducting this study. The authors also acknowledge the NAHDIC laboratory personnel for their support at all levels.

REFERENCES

Asseged B (2005). Review of foot mouth disease: An in depth discourse of Global, Sub Saharan and Ethiopian status; Addis Ababa University. FVM. Research and graduate studies Debrezeit, Ethiopia. pp.3-49

Burrows R, Mann JM, Greig A , Goodridge D (1981). The pathogenesis of natural and simulated natural foot and mouth disease infection in Cattle. J. Comp. Pathol. 91:599-609.

Bouxton A , Faser G (1977). Animal microbiology. Black well scientific publication Ltd, Ed. In burgh. 2:611-619

Desta S (1999). Diversification of livestock assets for risk management in the Borana pastoral system of southern Ethiopia, PhD thesis Utah state University, Logan Utah. Pp10-31: Cited in ; Rufael T. (2006). Participatory appraisal and seroprevalence study of foot and mouth disease in borana pastoral system, southern Ethiopia, Msc theis FVM, AAu, debrezeit, Ethiopia pp.1-89

Esayas G, Berhanu B, Gelagay A (2005). Foot and mouth disease serotypes identified in Ethiopia. Ethiop. Vet. Assoc. J. 9(1):75-77.

FAO EMPRES and EUFMD commission (2007) Foot and mouth disease distribution Worldwide and major epidemiological events in 2005- 2006.Contributors; sumption K,Dinto J., Lubroth J., morzaria S., Murray T., Dela Racquet S., Nijeumi F., No 1:1-9.

Gibbs PJ (1981). Foot and Mouth Disease in: Viral diseases of food animals. Aworld geography of epidemiology and control. Vol II Academic press Inc.

Hirsh DC , Zee YC (1996). Foot and Mouth Disease in: Tropical animal health. Kluwer Academic Publisher, Netherlands. pp. 426-431

Hussen BM (2006). Seroprevalence study of Foot and disease in Export Bulls of Borana and Jimma origin, Ethiopia, DVM Thesis Faculty of Veterinary Medicine. AAU.Pp.1-21

Kahrs FF (2001).Foot and Mouth Disease in :Viral diseases of cattles. IOWA state Universitypress Pp.271-275

Kahan CM, Scottline (2005). Foot and Mouth disease in: The merck veterinary manual.9th Edition. Merck and Co. Inc. Whitehouse Stations. NJ USA Pp 509-511.

Ken, Tony P (1993). Feedlot ting: A guid for beef producer s. National Library of Australia Cataloguing –in- Publication dat. P17.

Kitching RP, Donaldson AI (1987). Collection and transportation of specimens for vesicular. Virus investigation. Rev. Sci. Tech. Off. Int. Epiz., 6,Pp.263-272.

Lennette EH, Nathalie MD, Schmidit J (1979). Foot and Mouth Disease in: Diagnostic procedures for viral, Rickettsial and Chlamydial infections. 5th Ediion. Washington Dc. Am. Public Health Assoc. Inc Pp.1013-1016

Murphy AF, Gibbs JE, Horzinec CM, Studdert JM (1999). Foot and Mouth Disease in: Veterinary virology 3rd Edition California, Academic press USA. pp. 521-537

OIE (2000). World organization for Animal health. Manual of standards for diagnostic test and vaccines. Office International des Epizooties (OIE), Paris, France, pp. 77-86.

OIE (1990). Recommended Diagnostic techniques and requirements for Biological products. Office international des Epizooties (OIE), Paris, France. pp. 1-7

Oluthem AW, Mastiga WN (1988).Viral Disease of Animals in Africa OAU/ST, RC, Scientific publication, Legos, Nigeria. pp. 178-199.

Radostits OM, Gay CC, Blood , Hinchliff KW (2000). Veterinary Medicine A textbook of the diseases of cattle, sheep, pigs, goats and houses. Foot and Mouth Disease, 9th Edition China Elsevier LTD Pp. 1059-106

Richard P (1998) Foot and Mouth Disease. The mark veterinary manual 8th Edition mark and Co Inc. White house station NJ, USA, 457-459

Reid SM, Ferris NP, Hutchings GH, Zhang Z, Belsham GJ, Alexanderson S (2002). Detection of all seven serotype of FMDV by real time fluorogenic reverse transcription polymerase chain reaction assay. J. Virol. Methods. 105:1-80.

Rufael T (2006).Participatory appraisal and seroprevalence study of Foot and Mouth Disease in Borana pastoral system, Southern Ethiopia, MSc thesis FVM AAU, Deberezeit, Ethiopia. pp.1-89.

Rufael T, Catley A, Bogale A, Sahle M, Shiferaw Y (2007). Foot and Mouth Disease in the borana pastoral system southern Ethiopia and implication for livelihoods and international trade. Trop. Anim. Health Prod. 40:29-38.

Sahle M, Venter EH , Warka RM, Voslo W (2004). Molecular epidemiology of serotype of foot and mouth disease viruses isolated from cattle in Ethiopa between 1979-2001. Onderstepoort. J. Vet. Res. 71(2):129-38.

Sainsbury D (2000). Foot and mouth Disease in: Animal Health. 2nd Edition Blackwell science Pp. 142-160.

Seifert HSH (1990). Tropical Animals Health. Kluwer Academic Publisher Netherlands. pp. 410-425.

Solomon H (1980). Animal health review Ethiopia 1979 Ministry of agricultural livestock research development department veterinary service division Pp. 275-276.

Thrusfield M (1995). Veterinary Epidemiology 2nd ed. Black well science Ltd. pp. 178-198.

Woodbury EL (1995). A review of the possible mechanisms for the persistence of Foot and Mouth Disease virus. Epidemiol. Infect. 114:1-13.

27

Detection of *Mycobacterium avium* subspecies *paratuberculosis* excretion in bovine feces, using quantitative real time polymerase chain reaction (Q-PCR)

Adriana Guadalupe Martínez-Covarrubias[1], Marco Antonio Santillán-Flores[1*], Dionicio Córdova-López[1] and Claudia Celic Guzmán-Ruíz[2]

[1]Instituto Nacional de Investigaciones Forestales, Agrícolas y Pecuarias-CENID Microbiología Carretera México -Toluca Km. 15.5, Colonia Palo Alto, CP. 04110, Delegación Cuajimalpa, México.
[2]Universidad de Guanajuato, División Ciencias de la Vida, Campus Irapuato –Salamanca, Exhacienda, El Copal Km. 9, Carretera Irapuato-Silao, CP 36820, Irapuato, Guanajuato, Mexico.

Mycobacterium avium subspecies _paratuberculosis_ (Map) causes paratuberculosis, an infectious enteritis that affects domestic ruminants. The main source of infection for herds comes from the elimination of the bacilli through feces. The objective of this study was to determine Map excretion in bovine feces. The study included forty, one-year-old bovine, Holstein breed females, from a herd that had >25% paratuberculosis prevalence. Samples of blood and feces were obtained four times with three-month intervals. Feces samples were subjected to bacteriological culture and DNA extraction for IS900 quantitative real time polymerase chain reaction (Q-PCR). Enzyme-linked immunosorbent assay (ELISA) was done from serum samples to detect the presence of anti-Map antibodies. Correlation between IS900 Q-PCR, culture and ELISA was established by the Kappa (K) test; statistical analysis was carried out by the Pearson Chi^2 test. On the first sampling, five animals were detected by IS900 Q-PCR, shed 1×10^2 to 2.6×10^3 Map copies per gram of feces; on the second sampling, 6 animals shed 3.25×10^4 to 8.5×10^8; on the third sampling two animals shed 2.03×10^5 to 1.10×10^6 and on the fourth, three animals shed 7.92×10^4 to 1.4×10^7 Map copies. Correlation between tests in samplings first, second and fourth, was 0.53 to 0.73, and for third was 0.22. With the use of IS900 Q-PCR, it was possible to detect animals that were eliminating Map in feces from 12 months of age without clinical manifestations. The IS900 Q-PCR is an alternative method to carry out programs of control of paratuberculosis that allow the detection of animals that shed Map in the early stages of the infection.

Key words: Paratuberculosis, *Mycobacterium avium* subspecies *paratuberculosis*, excretion, quantitative polymerase chain reaction (Q-PCR), bacteriological culture, enzyme-linked immunosorbent assay (ELISA).

INTRODUCTION

Paratuberculosisis is a chronic infectious disease, caused by *Mycobacterium avium* subspecies *paratuberculosis* (Map) that affects domestic and wild ruminants. Map is classified within the *Mycobacterium avium-intracelullare* complex (*M. avium* subspecies *avium, M. avium* subspecies *paratuberculosis, M. avium* subspecies *silvaticum* and *M. intracelullare*) and it differs from other subspecies of the complex by its dependence on mycobactin for *in vitro* growth (Stevenson et al., 2002). Map is an intracellular bacteria characterized by resistance to the environmental conditions; it can remain viable for 270 days in stagnant waters, 47 months in dry desiccated organic matter, 45 days in milk and 60 days in fresh cheese (Abalos, 2001; Cirone et al., 2007).

The disease has a chronic course and mainly affects adult animals of two to three years of age. It is characterized by progressive loss of body condition due to the lesions produced in the ileum, ileocecal, cecum and proximal colon mucosa and mesenteric lymph nodes; diffuse hypertrophy of the jejunum and ileum mucosa is developed, which acquire a rough appearance, causing low nutrient absorption (Valentin-Weigand, 2002).

Paratuberculosis has an important impact on animal production by generating a reduction in milk and meat production, early discarding of animals and low fertility with predisposition for mastitis (Eda et al., 2006). With this disease, carcasses have a lower commercial value and there is an increase in control program costs (Soto et al., 2002a). Map is excreted intermittently and animals are infected by consuming feed and water contaminated with paratuberculosis microorganisms shed by infected animals. Map concentration in feces may surpass 10^8 colony forming units (CFU)/g (Valentin-Weigand, 2002).Young animals less than six months of age are the most susceptible to infection; calves that are in subclinical stages of the disease shed the bacilli in feces without showing the characteristic signs of the disease (Park et al., 2006). The disease distribution is worldwide, especially in domestic ruminants confined rearing conditions; prevalence of the disease varies between 5 and 55% (Milian-Suazo et al., 2015; Avila et al., 2011).

To confirm diagnosis, bacteriological culture is carried out, although its disadvantage is that it is a slow process that needs more than six weeks to have a positive Map culture (Soto et al., 2002b). Currently, there are molecular tests developed to diagnose paratuberculosis and the most used is the polymerase chain reaction (PCR). It had been mainly applied as a qualitative method, but there is also the option to do the PCR test in real time or quantitative PCR (Q-PCR) that is a variation of the standard PCR used for quantification of DNA or messenger RNA (mRNA) of a sample. It is possible to determine the number of copies or the relative amount of a specific DNA or RNA sequence by using specific sequencing primers. The amount of amplicon produced in each PCR cycle is used for quantification. Product quantification occurs by the addition of fluorophores that join the amplicon in a directly proportional manner, and therefore, the higher amount of product there is, the higher fluorescence emission. Real time PCR programs detect the amount of fluorescence produced in each PCR cycle and the analysis programs represented the said fluorescence in graphs, in relation to the number of cycles (UCV, 2012; Vinueza-Burgos, 2009). Most of the PCR protocols, for DNA/RNA Map detection, use primers that amplify the 900-insertion sequence (IS900), and therefore it is been accepted as a standard Map marker. IS900 is a 1451 base-pair sequence that codifies for a hypothetical transposase of 399 amino acids, with 14 to 20 copies in the MAP genome inserted in a consensus region within highly conserved loci in the Map genome (Kralik et al., 2011; Bull et al., 2000). It is thought that, for every animal diagnosed with the clinical profile of paratuberculosis, there are approximately 25 other individuals that have a subclinical profile and that these will intermittently shed the bacillus through feces. It is therefore important that the diagnosis of this disease be done using diagnostic techniques, such as q-PCR, that can detect animals that are shedding the bacillus before clinical signs are present, in order to establish control measures within the herd. The purpose of this study was to determine the shedding of Map in bovine feces using Q-PCR.

MATERIALS AND METHODS

The work was carried out using 40 Holstein breed female cows at least 1-year-old that originated from a dairy herd with previous clinical history of paratuberculosis (>25% prevalence) in Hidalgo Mexico, confirmed with microbiological culture IS900 nested PCR and ELISA. Follow up was done by taking four samples of blood and feces, every three months. Blood was obtained from the caudal vein using vacutainer tubes and centrifuged at 180 × *g* for 10 min; the resulting serum was then divided into aliquots in microtubes. Feces were collected directly from the rectum using palpation gloves. All samples were stored at -20ºC until analyzed (Martínez et al., 2012).

DNA extraction

Two grams of feces were decontaminated using 50 ml of 7.6% 1-hexadecylpyridinium chloride (HCP) (Sigma Aldrich) for 18 h. DNA extraction was then carried out following the protocol described by Jaimes et al. (2008). DNA was stored at -20°C until used in q-PCR.

Real time Q-PCR

The Q-PCR reaction was done using the primers for ISIS IS900 PTB FP 5´AATGACGGTTACGGAGGTGGT3´ and PTB RP 5´GCAGTAATGGTCGGCCTTACC 3´ (Kim et al., 2002). Each 25-µl q-PCR reaction contained 3 µl DNA (45 ng/µl), 12.5 µl Maxima

*Corresponding author. E-mail: mayco1768@gmail.com, santillan.marco@inifap.gob.mx. .

Table 1. IS900 q-PCR, culture and ELISA of Map for each sampling (n=40).

Sampling	IS 900 Q-PCR (%)		Map culture (%)		ELISA (%)	
	Postive (+)	Negative (-)	Postive (+)	Negative (-)	Postive (+)	Negative (-)
1st	5 (12.5)	35 (87.5)	2 (5.0)	38 (95.0)	2 (5.0)	38 (95.0)
2nd	6 (15.0)	34 (85.0)	4 (10.0)	36 (90.0)	3 (7.5)	37 (92.5)
3rd	2 (5.0)	38 (95.0)	2 (5.0)	38 (95.0)	3 (7.5)	37 (92.5)
4th	3 (7.5)	37 (92.5)	2 (5.0)	38 (95.0)	2 (5.0)	38 (95.0)

SYBR green / ROX q-PCR Master mix (3 mM $MgCl_2$, 200 µM each dATP, dGTP, dCTP, 400 µM dUTP, 1.25 IU DNA polymerase and 0.5 IU Uracil-N-Glycosylase (UNG) (Thermo)), 1 µl each PTBFP and PTBRP primers (0.05 µM each/one), and 7.5 µl water. DNA from a standard Map strain (ATCC #43545) was used as positive control, while distilled water was used as the negative control.

The Q-PCR was carried out in a SmartCycler ® (Cepheid) with the following cycling conditions: 95°C/10 min, 40 cycles of 95°C/15 s, 60°C/30 s and 72°C/10 s, followed by a final cycle of 72°C/30 s. Samples were worked in duplicate and the results were analyzed following the guidelines in the SmartCycler operating manual. A linear regression was performed on *CT* versus log IS*900* copy number and *R2* was 0.99. The standard error of *y* was used to create two equations to estimate the upper and lower concentration, for calculation of *M. avium* subsp. *paratuberculosis* IS900 copy number; this was done following the protocol described previously by Moravkova et al. (2012), Slana et al. (2008) and Kim et al. (2002).

Bacteriological culture

Feces from all animals were cultured in duplicate following the technique described by Aly et al. (2010). All samples were decontaminated using 0.5% Zephiran and sowns in Herrold's egg yolk solid media with and without 2 mg/L mycobactin J (Allied Monitor INC) and incubated at 37°C for 6 months. Ziehl-Neelsen acid-fast stain was carried out on cultures that showed positive growth; DNA was also extracted and nested PCR carried out using primers that amplify a 210 bp region of IS900 (Jaimes et al., 2008).

Enzyme linked immunosorbent assay (ELISA)

Protoplasmic antigen of the 3065 Map strain was adhered to ELISA microplates following the protocol described by Martínez et al. (2012). Sera were diluted to a working concentration of 1:160 using a solution of 0.02% *Mycobacterium phlei* (Allied Monitor INC). A Map positive serum was used as positive control and a negative serum as negative control (Allied Monitor INC). The bovine anti-IgG conjugate tagged with horseradish peroxidase (Sigma-Aldrich) was used at a 1:2000 dilution, while 2, 2'-Azino-Bis-3-Ethylbenzothiazoline-6-Sulfonic acid (ABTS, AMPRESCO) was used as substrate, and 1.5 mM sodium nitrate (sigma-Aldrich) in 0.1 M citric acid was used as stop solution. Plate reading was done at 650 nm using a spectrophotometer (ELx800, BioTek). The cut-off was established at 0.22 optical deviations (OD).

Statistical analysis

Statistical analysis was carried out using the STATA® 7.0 software package (StataCorp LP, College Station, TX, USA). Cohen's Kappa test (k) or inter-rater agreement index was used to establish the association between the results obtained with the IS900 Q-PCR, culture and ELISA. Differences between diagnostic techniques were tested using Pearson's Chi^2 (χ^2). The scale proposed by Prieto et al. (2014), was used to determine the concordance among techniques. Range (%) to <0.000 is poor; to 0.00 and 0.20 is slight; to 0.21 and 0.40 is fair; to 0.41 and 0.60 is moderate; to 0.61 and 0.80 is substantial; to 0.81 and 1.0 is perfect.

RESULTS

Follow-up of the 40 female cows was done every three months starting at 12 months of age and continued until they reached 21 months, to determine the age at which the animals begin shedding the bacilli in feces. All cows came from a herd with a history of >25% prevalence of paratuberculosis. The results obtained in the work are shown in Table 1, with the use of IS900 Q-PCR, amplification curves of the Map positive control and samples that were found to be positive were present from cycle 20 up to cycle 30 of the Q-PCR run (Figure 1). Animals that were shedding the bacteria could be identified from the first sampling, which corresponded to 12 months of age. Map shedding in feces is intermittent, since only one animal was detected as positive in all samplings.

The presence of anti-Map antibodies was lower (2.5 to 7.5%); tests based on the detection of humoral immune response are not feasible during early stages of infection (subclinical stage), because the concentration of anti-Map antibodies in early stages of infection are low.

Bacterial growth could only be observed in tubes that had mycobactin added from five weeks on. Ziehl-Neelsen stain revealed the presence of acid-fast bacilli, and the nested PCR amplified the expected 210 bp amplicon which is specific to Map. The sensitvity of the bacteriological culture was less than 10%, the animals that were positive to the bacteriological culture in all the samplings were also positive to the IS900 Q-PCR.

Association between the three diagnostic tests used in this study was determined with Cohen's Kappa test (Tables 2 and 3). When comparing IS900 Q-PCR with bacteriological culture and ELISA, first, second and fourth samplings showed moderate to substantial concordance, while in third sampling the concordance was fair.

Results of the negative predictive values (VP-) indicate that IS900 Q-PCR is a highly specific test since the

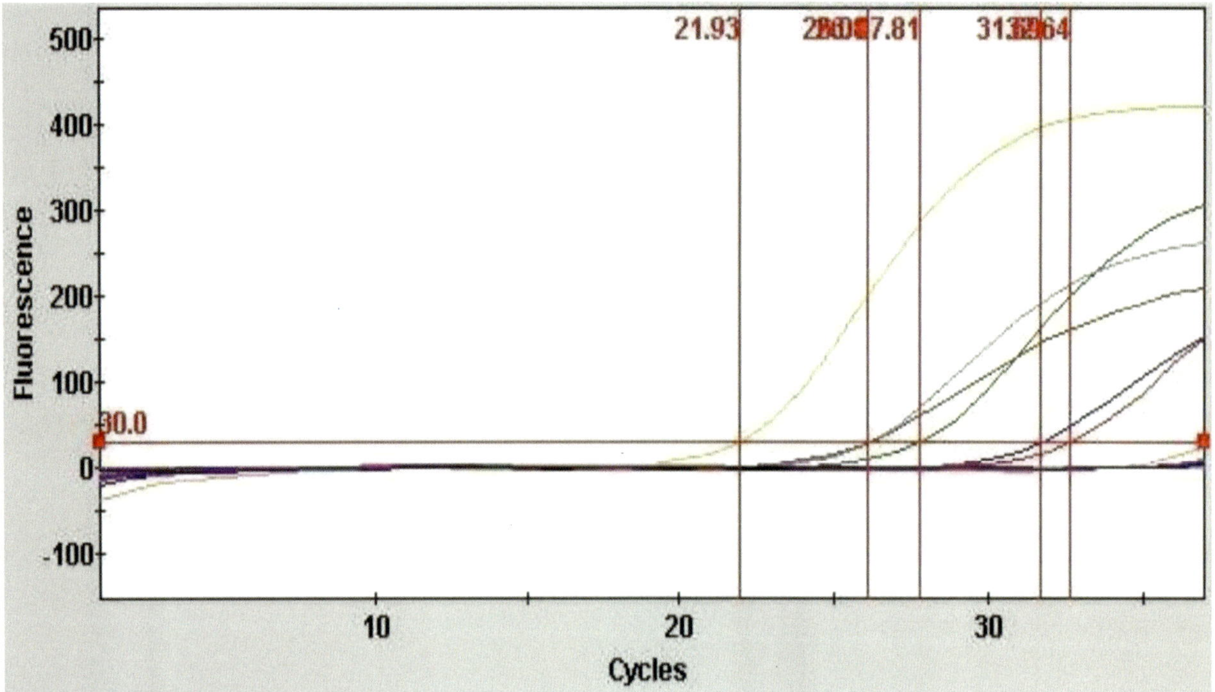

Figure 1. IS900 Q-PCR carried out from genomic DNA obtained from bovine feces of the first sampling.

Table 2. Cohen's Kappa (K), positive predictive value (VP+), negative predictive value (VP-) and χ^2 for each sampling, comparing IS900 q-PCR and Bacteriological culture (n=40).

Sampling number	IS900 Q-PCR *vs.* bacteriological culture			
	K	VP+ (%)	VP- (%)	χ^2
1st	0.538	40	100	0.0001
2nd	0.771	66	100	0.0000
3rd	0.294	33	92	0.0000
4th	0.411	33	100	0.0001

average VP-reached 98% when compared with the microbiological culture and 97.5% when compared with ELISA. As such, individuals that had a negative result in the IS900 Q-PCR test had been correctly diagnosed as they were true negatives. The positive predictive value (VP+) reached 43 and 47.5% when comparing IS900 Q-PCR with the microbiological culture and ELISA, respectively (Tables 2 and 3).

Quantification of Map shedding

Map shedding is intermittent and starts in the early stages of the infection. The IS900 Q-PCR detected bovine from 12 months of age, that were already excreting the bacillus in feces, and as the samplings advanced, the elimination increased logarithmically (bovine 1, 10 and 36). On the first sampling, it was detected that five animals shed between 1×10^2 and 2.6×10^3 copies of the IS900 from Map per gram of feces. In the second sampling, six animals shed between 3.25×10^4 and 8.5×10^8. On the third sampling, two animals were detected that shed between 2.03×10^5 and 1.10×10^6, while in the fourth sampling three animals shed between 7.92×10^4 and 1.4×10^7 (Table 4).

DISCUSSION

Forty dairy cows, which had a mean of 12 months of age at the first sampling, were followed for a year in order to determine the time of shedding of Map using IS900 Q-PCR and bacteriological culture. From the first sampling, animals that shed Map were detected, demonstrating that bovines infected with paratuberculosis can shed the bacillus even in early infection stages without any clinical

Table 3. Cohen's Kappa (K), positive predictive value (VP+), negative predictive value (VP-) and χ^2 for each sampling, comparing IS900 q-PCR and ELISA (n=40).

Sampling number	IS900 q-PCR *vs.* ELISA			
	K	VP+ (%)	VP- (%)	χ^2
1st	0.53	40	100	0.0001
2nd	0.62	50	100	0.0000
3rd	0.22	33	89	0.0001
4th	0.73	66	100	0.0000

Table 4. Quantification of amplicon copies by q-PCR in DNA samples taken from bovine feces positive to IS900.

Sampling	Mean age in months	Identification number	Number of IS900 map copies/g of feces
1st	12	1	5.30×10^2
		10	3.50×10^2
		25	2.60×10^3
		32	1.90×10^2
		41	1.50×10^3
2nd	15	1	5.11×10^4
		10	5.00×10^4
		25	3.25×10^4
		32	6.50×10^6
		41	8.50×10^8
		36	7.00×10^4
3rd	18	1	1.10×10^6
		36	2.03×10^5
4th	21	1	1.40×10^7
		10	7.92×10^5
		36	4.77×10^6

signs of the disease (Park et al., 2016; Fang et al., 2002).

Previously, Khol et al. (2010), had followed for 380 days a 2.5 year-old cow that had become naturally infected with Map, sampling feces on 9 occasions. Their results showed that the number of IS900 copies that were detected increased between 10^5 and 10^7 copies per gram of feces throughout the study, although in their third sample a slight decrease was observed, demonstrating that Map shedding is intermittent and can start from early infection stages (subclinical phase) before the infected animal becomes positive to the serological test. The results agree with those of Khol et al. (2010) in that Map shedding was detected from 12 months of age and that as time advances shedding increased logarithmically from 10^2 to 10^6 copies of IS900 of Map (bovines 1, 10 and 25; Table 4). Kralik et al. (2011) developed a predictive model to determine the shedding of Map using Q-PCR with DNA extracted from feces, establishing that the minimum detectable shedding is 10^2 copies of IS900 of Map per gram of feces. The results obtained agree with those of kralik et al. (2011), because in the first sampling three animals were detected as positive and the quantification was obtained as 1.9 to 5.30×10^2 copies of IS900 of Map per gram of feces.

Several authors have carried out studies on the correlation of q-PCR tests, bacteriological culture and ELISA with the diagnosis of paratuberculosis, with varying results. Pinedo et al. (2008) found that when comparing PCR tests with bacteriological culture and ELISA, Kappa values were 0.39 and 0.01, respectively. In contrast, Fang et al. (2002), when correlating IS900 Q-PCR with bacteriological culture, a Kappa value of 0.94 was found. In this study, Kappa values in the first, second and fourth samplings ranged from 0.53 to 0.73 indicating a moderate correlation, although the Kappa value in third sampling reached 0.22 indicating a fair correlation. It is possible that the latter is due to the fact that in this disease shedding of bacilli is intermittent and at the time of collecting the sample, it could have been absent from feces. Nevertheless, mistakes in DNA extraction or sample contamination could also explain the results and it cannot be excluded (Khol et al., 2010). Correlation between bacteriological culture and Q-PCR depends on the stage of the infection present in the individual at the time of sample collection which has an effect on the amount of bacilli shed (Kralik et al., 2011; Aly et al., 2010; Pinedo et al., 2008). The ELISA used in the study detected less number of animals as positive, this is because, in early infection stages the predominant immune response is cell type, and the elimination of bacillus in feces begins in an intermediate way. Other reason for which the antibody production may be affected, is the cause of loss of immune response after infection. This suppressor activity is known as anergia. Animals in early infection stages, even if they excrete the bacteria in their feces, may not necessarily be detected by the ELISA test, since it may take several months, or years, before the level of circulating antibodies is sufficient to trigger a positive reaction (Soto et al., 2002a).

Bacteriological culture from tissues, feces, milk, and semen, among others, is considered the gold standard for the diagnosis of paratuberculosis. Nevertheless, such testing has its limitations since, although it has a 100% specificity, it has very low sensitivity mainly due to the intermittent nature of the shedding of bacilli through feces, milk and semen (Khol et al., 2010). Furthermore, the culture media needs to be enriched by mycobactin to improve the development of the bacillus and the incubation times are more than six-weeks long for isolating Map. Another important disadvantage of bacteriological culture is the high risk of contamination with other microorganisms, especially fungi, and the decrease in viable bacilli after the sample decontamination process. By using Q-PCR, results are obtained within at least two days, depending on the amount of samples to be processed, representing a clear advantage in time-to-diagnosis when compared with bacteriological isolation allowing the quantification of bacilli shedding in feces (Kralik et al., 2011; Khol et al., 2010). With the simultaneous use of IS900 Q-PCR, fecal culture, and the ELISA test, it is possible to detect a greater number of infected animals.

In control and diagnostic testing, the probability that an individual that has a positive result is indeed positive is known as the positive predictive value, while the negative predictive value is the percentage of individuals with a negative test that do not have the disease. It is important to note that the predictive value is closely related with the sensitivity and specificity of a test, as well as with the prevalence of the disease in the population where the test is to be carried out (Martínez et al., 2012). The positive predictive values (VP+) obtained in this study, ranging between 43 and 47.5%, are considered low and are probably due to the long sampling interval (90 days) and the intermittent shedding of bacilli. Nevertheless, the negative predictive values (VP-) where high (97.5-98%) which demonstrates that the IS900 q-PCR is highly specific and that negative tests were appropriately classified.

The IS900 marker is considered the standard for endpoint PCR and Q-PCR since there are between 14 and 20 copies of the sequence within the mycobacterium genome improving the sensitivity for detecting Map. Other genetic markers have been evaluated for detecting Map, such as the SF57, IS*Mav2* and HspX sequences, but they have the limitation that they are only present in 1 to 6 copies within the Map genome, therefore sensitivity is reduced, although specificity is increased. To increase specificity when using primers for IS900, these should be designed so that they amplify regions that are close to the 5' end of this inserted sequence since it is highly conserved (Cook and Britt, 2007; Tasara and Stephan, 2005; Kim et al., 2002; Fang et al., 2002).

In this study, the IS900 Q-PCR detected that 12.5% of animals of the 12 months of age that were included in the first sampling where shedding bacilli through feces. This is important since the majority of the paratuberculosis clinical cases are observed in animals with two to six years of age and young animals, in general, do not show clinical signs but are already shedding the bacillus through their feces. As such, it is important that diagnostic tools are available that can detect the shedding of bacilli in the subclinical stage of the disease. In this sense, the IS900 Q-PCR is a good diagnostic alternative for detecting animals that are shedding the pathogen and prevent the spread of the disease by allowing the implementation of control and eradication measures for paratuberculosis.

Conclusion

The IS900 Q-PCR allows the diagnosis of early-stage paratuberculosis in animals from 12 months of age that do not have clinical signology of paratuberculosis. The technique is an alternative to carry out programs of control of paratuberculosis that allow the detection of animals that eliminate Map in early stages of infection.

ACKNOWLEDGEMENT

This study received financial support from CONACYT-SAGARPA research grantnumber48176.

REFERENCES

Abalos P (2001). News in Paratuberculosis Tecnovet. 7(3). Available at: http://www.tecnovet.uchile.cl

Aly SS, Mangold BL, Whitlock RH, Sweeney RW, Anderson RJ, Jiang J, Schukken YH, Hovingh E, Wolfgang D, Kessel JAS, Karns JS, Lombard E, Smith JM, Gardner IA (2010). Correlation between Herrold egg yolk medium culture and real-time quantitative polymerase chain reaction results for *Mycobacterium avium* subspecies *paratuberculosis* in pooled fecal and environmental samples. J. Vet. Diagnos. Invest. 22:677-683.

Avila GJ, Blando GE, Cruz HGE (2011). Paratuberculosis. Available at: http://fmvzenlinea2-7.fmvz.unam.mx/

Bull TJ, Harmon-Taylor J, Pavlik I, Zaatari E, Tizard M (2000). Characterization of IS900 loci in *Mycobacterium avium* subspecies *paratuberculosis* and development of multiplex PCR typing. Microbiology 146:2185-2197.

Cirone K, Morsella C, Romano M, Paolicchi F (2007). *Mycobacterium avium* subsp. *paratuberculosis* in food and its relationship with Crohn's disease. Rev. Argent. Microbiol. 39:57-68.

Cook KL, Britt JS (2007). Optimization of methods for detecting *Mycobacterium avium* subspecies *paratuberculosis* in environmental samples using quantitative, real-time PCR. J. Microbiol. Method 69:154-160.

Eda S, Bannantine JP, Waters WR, Mori Y, Whitlock RH, Scott MC, Speer CA (2006). A Highly sensitive and subspecies-specific surface antigen enzyme-linked immunosorbent assay for diagnosis of Johne´s Disease. Clin. Vaccine Immunol. 13(8):837-844.

Fang Y, Wu W-H, Pepper JL, Larsen JL, Marras SAE, Nelson EA, Epperson WB, Christopher-Hennings J (2002). Comparison of real-time, quantitative PCR with molecular beacons to nested PCR and culture methods for Detection of *Mycobacterium avium* subspecies *paratuberculosis*in bovine fecal samples. J. Clin. Microbiol. 40(1):287-291.

Jaimes NG, Santillán FMA, Hernández COA, Córdova LD, Guzmán RCC, Arellano RB, Díaz AE, Tenorio GVR, Cuellar OA (2008). Detection of *Mycobacterium avium* subspecies paratuberculosis by nested-PCR of ovine fecal samples. Rev. Vet. Méx. 39(4):377-386.

Khol JL, Kralik P, Slana I, Beran V, Aurich C, Baumgartner W, Pavlik I (2010). Consecutive excretion of *Mycobacterium avium* subspecies *paratuberculosis* in semen of a breeding bull compared to the distribution in feces, tissue and blood by IS900 and F57 quantitative real-time PCR and culture examinations. J. Vet. Med. Sci. 72(10):1283-1288.

Kim SG, Shin SJ, Jacobson RH, Miller LJ, Harpending PR, Stehman SM, Rossiter CA, Lein DA (2002). Development and application of quantitative polymerase chain reaction assay based on the ABI 7700 system (Taqman) for detection and quantification of *Mycobacterium avium* subspecies *paratuberculosis*. J. Vet. Diagnos. Invest. 14:126-131.

Kralik P, Slana I, Kralova A, Babak V, Whitlock RH, Pavlik I (2011). Devolopment of predictive model for detection of *Mycobacteiumavium* subspecies*paratuberculosis* in faeces by quantitative real time PCR. Vet. Microbiol. 149:133-138

Martínez CAG, Santillán FMA, Guzmán RCC, Favila HLC, Córdova LD, Díaz AE, Hernández AL, Blanco OM (2012). Development of an enzyme-linked immunosorbent assay (ELISA) for the diagnosis of bovine paratuberculosis. Rev. Mex. Cienc. Pecu. 3(1):1-18.

Milian-Suazo F, Santillán-Flores MA, Zendejas-Martínez H, García-Casanova L, Hernández-Andrade L, Canto-Alarcón GA (2015). Prevalence and associated risk factors for *Mycobacterium avium* subspecies *paratuberculosis* in cattle in México. J. Vet. Med. Anim. Health 7(10):302-307.

Moravkova MV, Babak V, Kralova A, Pavlik I, Slana I (2012). Culture-and quantitative IS900 real-time PCR-based analysis of the persistence of *Mycobacterium avium*subspecie*paratuberculosis* in a controlled dairy cow farm environment. Appl. Environ. Microbiol. 78(18):6608-6614.

Park HT, Shin MS, Park HE, Cho YI, Yoo HA (2016). PCR-based detection of *Mycobacterium avium* subspecies *paratuberculosis* infection in cattle in South Korea using fecal samples. J. Vet. Med. Sci. 78(9):1537-1540.

Park KT, Ahn J, Davis WC, Koo HC, Kwon NH, Jung WK, Kim JM, Hong SK, Park YH (2006). Analysis of the seroprevalence of bovine paratuberculosis and the application of modified absorbed ELISA to field sample testing in Korea. J. Vet. Sci.7(4):349-354.

Pinedo PJ, Rae DO, Willians JE, Donovan JE, Melendez P, Buergelt CO (2008). Association among results of serum ELISA, fecal culture and nested PCR on milk, blood and feces for detection of paratuberculosis in dairy cows. Transbound. Emerg. Dis. 55:125-133.

Prieto A, Lago N, Díaz JM, Pérez I, Guarddon M, Díaz P, López C, Fernández G (2014). Diagnosis of bovine paratuberculosis: Comparison between fecal culture and Q-PCR on field samples. XIX International Congress ANEMBE of bovine medicine. Ovideo, Spain, pp. 65-70

Slana I, Kralik P, Kralova A, Pavlik I (2008). On-farm spread of *Mycobacterium avium*subspecies*paratuberculosis* in raw milk studied by IS900 and F57 competitive real time quantitative PCR and culture examination. Int. J. Food Microbiol. 128:250-257.

Soto JP, Kruze J, Leiva S (2002a). Isolation of Mycobacteriumaviums subspecies paratuberculosis of faeces in dairy herds infected by the modified Cornell method. Arch. Med. Vet. 34(2):1-5

Soto JP, Kruze J, Leiva S (2002b). Comparison of three different methods for the diagnosis of bovine paratuberculosis in infected dairy herds. Arch. Med. Vet. 34(2):10-15

Stevenson K, Hughes VM, de Juan L, Inglis NF, Wright F (2002). Molecular characterization of pigmented and nonpigmented isolates of *Mycobacterium avium*subspecie paratuberculosis. J. Clin. Microbiol. 40:1798-1804.

Tasara T, Stephan R (2005). Development of an F57 sequence-based real-time PCR assay for detection of *Mycobacterium avium* subspecie *paratuberculosis* in milk. Appl. Environ. Microbiol. 71(10):5957-5968.

University of the Vasco Country (UVC) (2012). Análisis de expresión génica mediante PCR a tiempo real o Q-PCR. Available at: www.ehu.es/SGIker//expresion_genica//analisis_de_expresion.pdf

Valentin-Weigand P (2002). Johne's Disease: Pathogenesis and Problems Related to Diagnosis. In Recent Developments and Perspectives in Bovine Medicine. XXII World Buiatrics Congress, Hanover, pp. 18-23.

Vinueza-Burgos C (2009). Real Time PCR: The new era of celular genetic information. Rev. Elect. Vet. 10(2):1-13.

Microbiological quality of frozen raw and undercooked Nile tilapia (*Oreochromis niloticus*) fillets and food safety practices of fish handlers in Arba Minch town, SNNPR, Ethiopia

Wendwesen Teka[1*], Dagmar Nölkes[2], Yitbarek Getachew[2] and Matusala Mulachew[3]

[1]Zonal Veterinarian, Wolaita Sodo Zone Agricultural Office, Wolaita Sodo, SNNPR, Ethiopia.
[2]Haramaya University, College of Veterinary Medicine, Haramaya, Ethiopia.
[3]Wolaita Sodo Agricultural TVET College, Wolaita Sodo, SNNPR, Ethiopia.

The study was designed to assess the microbiological quality of Nile tilapia (Oreochromis niloticus) fillets and food safety practices of fish handlers in Arba Minch town, SNNPR, Ethiopia. A questionnaire survey was conducted to assess the food safety practices of fish handlers. The microbiological quality of frozen raw and undercooked (Asa leb-leb) tilapia fillets was assessed by determining the total plate count and isolating hygiene indicator bacteria that is, Escherichia coli and other major foodborne pathogens that is, Salmonella spp. and Staphylococcus aureus. Among interviewed fish handlers, 32.6% and 55.8% were not found to use overcoat and hair cover, respectively. Moreover, 30.2% of the fish handlers didn't take training regarding sanitary handling of fish food. The highest mean bacterial count was observed in frozen raw tilapia fillet sample (4.63x106 cfu/g), which was significantly (p=0.037) different from undercooked tilapia fillet (4.92x103 cfu/g). From 40 frozen raw samples of tilapia fillet examined, 42.5% had E. coli, 7.5% had Salmonella spp. and 65% had S. aureus. In contrast, from 40 undercooked samples of tilapia fillet examined, 7.5% had E. coli and 17.5% had S. aureus whilst Salmonella spp. was not detected. A significant (p=0.000) difference in frequency of bacterial isolates were also observed between frozen raw and undercooked tilapia fillet. Generally, the study revealed that there was a gap on food safety practices and high microbial profile were observed. Hence, it could be wise to advice the government to improve the food safety practices and quality standards of fish sold in the town.

Keywords: Fish, food safety, microbiological quality, Nile tilapia, pathogens, undercooked.

INTRODUCTION

Fish products are essential to food security, providing over 1 billion people with their main source of protein and more than 4.3 billion people with about 15% of their average per capita animal protein intake (FAO, 2012). In

*Corresponding author. E-mail: doyetekatero@gmail.com; doyeteka@yahoo.com;

2010, wild capture fisheries and aquaculture supplied the world with about 148 million tons of fish, worth US $ 217.5 billion. Approximately, 128 million tons or 86% were used for human consumption. Preliminary data for 2011 indicates that production has increased to 154 million tons, of which about 131 million tons, or 85%, were consumed as food (FAO, 2012; World Bank, 2010).

Ethiopia has only inland freshwater capture fisheries. Total annual fish production potential in the country is estimated to be 51,481 tons (FAO, 2012). In 2010/11 the total landing was about 18,058 tons, which is about 35% of the calculated potential (MoA, 2012). But the country overall per capita fish production is less than 240 g per person per year (FAO, 2006). However, in areas and communities where there is regular and sufficient supply, annual fish consumption can exceed 10 kg/person (FAO, 2012). This implies that fish consumption in the country is more highly influenced by supply factors (FAO, 2012). This supply factor is indirectly related to lack of preservation and processing techniques. In the country most (about 73%) of the total fish landed is marketed fresh in nearby markets. The rest reaches distant consumers chilled or frozen (26%), or as dried, smoked and canned (1%) forms (FAO, 2012).

Fish is one of the best protein sources available to the human body in quality and quantity. It is also a valuable source of vitamin A and B, iodine and oils containing polyunsaturated fatty acids (Adebayo et al., 2012). However, the increasing demand for fish and fish products all over the world is greatly challenged by microbial infection of fish and contamination of fish products (Pyatkin and Krivoshein, 1986).

Studies indicate that there are several bacteria that have been isolated from three main parts of fresh fish: slime layer, gills and the gastrointestinal tract. According to Cahill (1990) the microbiological diversity of the fresh fish muscle depends on the fishing grounds and environmental factors around it. Fish from warm waters mostly harbor mesophilic gram-negative bacteria while cold waters harbor mostly psychrophilic, gram-positive bacteria. These bacterial isolates are classified into two groups: indigenous and post-harvest bacteria. Previous studies have also demonstrated the presence of indicator microorganisms of fecal pollution, opportunistic and pathogenic bacteria to humans in fish (Tsai et al., 2002; Ferreira and Pinho, 2006; Tzikas et al., 2007).

The origin of most microbes in fish and fish products may not be precisely known, some workers have related microbial infections and/or contamination of fish and fish products to a number of factors including unfavorable conditions in the fish culture system (Okpokwasili and Ogbulie, 1993), pollution and seasonal changes (Obiajuru et al., 2010), fish handling and processing including personnel and processing equipment (Pelczer and Chan, 1986). Fish contains protein and nutrients favorable for microbial attack even after processing. This often leads to fish spoilage and nutritional deterioration. Recent studies in Owerri, Imo State of Nigeria, showed 20% prevalence of Salmonella in frozen fish (Ohalete et al., 2011). In developing countries like Ethiopia where there is a poor infrastructure for the sector, fish spoilage from microbial contamination is believed to be a critical problem of fisheries and public health (FAO, 1993). Hence, this study was designed to elucidate the microbiological quality of fish meat retailed at Arba Minch town in Southern Ethiopia.

Lake Abaya and Chamo, the two large rift valley lakes, are located about 10 km North and Southeast of Arba Minch town, respectively. The total annual average commercial catch from Abaya and Chamo Lake based on surface area was estimated at 10,100 and 5,500 tons, respectively (FAO, 1993). These two lakes supply fish for local and national markets, and Nile Tilapia (*Oreochromis niloticus*) is the common fish species harvested from them.

According to the data obtained from Arba Minch Zurya Woreda Marketing and Cooperative Office, authorized fishermen associations are the main supplier of fish to hotels and restaurants in Arba Minch town. Fish is transported to the town at the back of pick-up track. However, illegal fishermen have to walk daily to the town carrying fish in sacks on their heads in the sunny and hot weather conditions. Factors that could degrade the safety and quality of fish, such as lack of proper transportation facilities, poor handling and processing are common.

In Arba Minch, fish is processed and presented to the consumer in different types of dish. Among that, Asa leb-leb is the most famous and highly consumed fish dish in the town. The dish Asa leb-leb is lightly fried (undercooked) fish fillet, thus it may contain some pathogenic bacteria of great concern to public health (example, *Escherichia coli*) and their toxic metabolites (example, *Staphylococcus* toxins) which tolerate the temperature and time combination at which this dish is prepared. Moreover, several studies assured that cooking of sea food products would not destroy their toxic metabolites like thermostable enterotoxin of *Staphylococcus aureus* and thermostable enterotoxin of *E. coli* (Vieira et al., 2001; Ayulo et al., 1994). Even if this dish is prepared at the correct temperature and time combination which eliminate the above risks, there may be also a risk of recontamination from improper post-process handling. Therefore, consumers could be at risk of acquiring zoonotic pathogens and/or their toxic metabolites from consumption of Asa leb-leb dish.

Therefore, the general objective of this study was to assess the microbiological quality of Nile tilapia fillets and food safety practices of fish handlers in Arba Minch town, SNNPR, Ethiopia. The specific objectives of the study were:

1. To determine the microbial load of frozen raw and undercooked (Asa leb-leb) Nile tilapia fillets.
2. To isolate hygiene indicator bacteria that is, *E. coli* and

other pathogenic bacteria of great concern to public health that is, *Salmonella* spp. and *S. aureus* from frozen raw and undercooked (Asa leb-leb) Nile tilapia fillets.
3. To assess food safety practices of fish handlers working in the kitchens of different hotels.

MATERIALS AND METHODS

Description of the study area

The study was conducted from June to December, 2013 in Arba Minch town. Arba Minch is the capital town of Gamo Gofa Zone of Southern Nations, Nationalities and People's Regional State (SNNPR). It is located 505 km far from the capital city of Ethiopia, Addis Ababa, in the coordination of 5°57' N latitude and 37°32' E. The area has an average annual temperature of 29.7°C and rain fall of 700 mm (CSA, 2007). Arba Minch is presently experiencing rapid population growth. As a result, the number of commercial food establishments in the town has visibly increased. According to the data obtained from Trade and Industry Office of the town, about 20 registered hotels are currently present in the town. The sources of fish for all these commercial food establishments are fish harvested from Abaya and Chamo Lakes.

Study design

The study involved a questionnaire survey and a laboratory assessment of the microbiological status of frozen raw and undercooked (Asa leb-leb) Nile tilapia fillets collected from the different hotels in Arba Minch town. A questionnaire survey was used to assess the current status of food safety practiced by fish handlers working in the kitchens of different hotels in the town.

Sample and sampling method

In the present study, frozen raw and undercooked (Asa leb-leb) Nile tilapia fillets were collected from selected registered hotels in Arba Minch town. The subjects for this study were fish handlers in the kitchens of hotels, registered under the Trade and Industry Office of the town. Due to limited resources, only representative hotels were selected by purposive sampling strategy.

Sample collection, handling and transportation

A total of 80 (40 frozen raw and 40 undercooked (Asa leb-leb)) Nile tilapia fillets were collected in 10 trips from 10 (50% of total hotels) selected registered hotels of Arba Minch town. In each trip, two hotels were visited to take a total of eight samples of Nile tilapia fillets (two frozen raw and two undercooked from each hotels) to assess their microbiological quality. To make sure that samples were taken without being contaminated, inverted plastic bags were used for collection. The inner surface of the bag was used to touch nothing else but the sample. All samples were labeled with the type of the sample, the place, date of sampling and given an identification code and transported to Wolaita Sodo Regional Veterinary Laboratory in icebox containing ice packs for microbiological analysis. Upon arrival, the samples were immediately processed or stored at -20°C in a refrigerator until use and processed within 24 h of collection.

Microbiological analysis

Sample preparation

The frozen samples were thawed at room temperature for 5 to 6 h before processing (APHA, 2005). T10 g of each Nile tilapia fillet sample was weighed and placed into sterile stomacher bags, diluted with 90 ml of 0.1% sterile peptone water (HiMedia, India) and homogenized in a stomacher for 2 min per procedure describe by Fawole and Oso (2001).

Total plate count (TPC)

From the 10-fold dilutions of the homogenates, 0.1 ml of 10^{-2}, 10^{-3}, 10^{-4}, 10^{-5} and 10^{-6} dilutions of the homogenates were pour-plated in duplicates on fresh standard plate count agar (HiMedia, India). The plates were then incubated at 37°C for 24 to 48 h. At the end of the incubation period, plates exhibiting 30 to 300 colonies were counted using illuminated colony counter. The counts for each plate were expressed as colony forming unit of the suspension (cfu/g) (Fawole and Oso, 2001).

Isolation and identification of bacteria

Isolation and identification of Salmonella

Salmonella was isolated from 10 g fish samples homogenized in 90 ml of 0.1% sterile peptone water. Aliquots of 1 ml were added to 10 ml of selenite broth (Difco, France). These were incubated at 37°C for 24 h. After gentle mixing, a loopful of culture from the enrichment broth was streaked on to xylose lysine desocholate (XLD) agar (HiMedia, India) and incubated at 37°C for 24 to 48 h. Typical *Salmonella* colonies which were pink with or without black centers were isolated. The colonies were purified on fresh nutrient agar (HiMedia, India), then streaked and stabbed into the butt of triple sugar iron (TSI) (HiMedia, India) slants. These were incubated at 37°C for 24 h. The test tubes that had alkaline (red) slants and acidic (yellow) butts, with or without the production of H_2S (blackening) were presumed to be *Salmonella* isolates. Moreover, two or more colonies from pure isolate were inoculated on urea broth (SRL, India) and incubated at 37°C for 24 h. All test tubes that were urease negative were treated as suspects of *Salmonella* (FDA, 1992). In addition, isolates that were Gram-negative rod, oxidase negative, citrate positive, methyl red positive, indole negative, voges-proskauer negative and lactose and sucrose non-fermenter were accepted putatively as *Salmonella* (Fawole and Oso, 2001).

Isolation and identification of E. coli

For the isolation of *E. coli*, a loopful of homogenized sample was streaked on to eosin methylene blue (EMB) agar (HiMedia, India). The plates were incubated at 37°C for 24 to 48 h. Typical *E. coli* colonies which are blue-black with a green metallic sheen were isolated. The colonies were purified on fresh nutrient agar (HiMedia, India) and then streaked and stabbed into the butt of triple sugar iron (TSI) (HiMedia, India) slants. These were incubated at 37°C for 24 h. All test tubes that had acidic (yellow) slants and acidic (yellow) butts, without the production of H_2S (blackening) were treated as suspects of *E. coli* (FDA, 1992). In addition, isolates that were gram-negative rod, oxidase negative, citrate negative, indole positive, urease negative, methyl red positive, voges-proskauer negative and lactose and sucrose fermenter were accepted putatively as *E. coli* (Fawole and Oso, 2001).

Isolation and identification of S. aureus

For the isolation of *S. aureus*, a loopful of homogenized sample was streaked on to mannitol salt agar (HiMedia, India). The plates were incubated at 37°C for 24 to 48 h. Typical *S. aureus* colonies which are yellow with a yellow halo around the colony were isolated. The colonies were purified on fresh nutrient agar (HiMedia, India) and then transferred into small tubes with 0.5 mL of rabbit plasma (NVI, Ethiopia). The tubes were rotated gently to mix the content and incubated at 37°C for 2 to 24 h, after which tubes that had clotted plasma were treated as suspects of *S. aureus* (APHA, 2005). Moreover, the smear was prepared from the isolated culture on clean grease free microscopic glass slide and stained with Gram's Method of staining. The stained smears were observed under microscope. Smear that revealed gram positive, spherical cells arranged in irregular clusters resembling to bunch of grapes were considered for *Staphylococci* presumptive. The isolates were further characterized by catalase, voges-proskauer and sugar (mannitol and maltose) fermentation test (Fawole and Oso, 2001).

Questionnaire survey and observation

Hygiene and sanitation conditions were determined by the use of semi-structured questionnaire. Moreover, direct observation was employed to assess the hygienic status and practices by the fish handlers working in the kitchens of different hotels found in Arba Minch town. All fish handlers observed in all 10 purposively selected hotels for this study were interviewed by the use of detailed and semi-structured questionnaire in order to obtain relevant information on food safety practices and fish food handling. Personal information, like educational status and training of fish handlers on sanitary handling of fish food and practices were collected through questionnaire and observation. Informed consent was obtained from owners/managers of the hotels and fish handlers after a brief explanation about the benefits of the study. Confidentiality of the respondent was maintained by assuring that his/her answers would not be released to anyone and would remain anonymous and his/her name would not be written on the questionnaire or be kept in any other records.

Data quality control

The quality of the data was kept by preparing and using standard operational procedures for laboratory investigation and media preparation. Semi-structured questionnaire was tested using pretest before conducting the study. Sample collection and processing were carried out using aseptic techniques. The samples were labeled properly. Culture and bacterial colony count were carried out under supervision of experienced laboratory personnel. All media were prepared according to the manufacturer's specification and sterilized at 121°C 15 psi pressure unit for 15 min. The sterility test of prepared media was checked by incubating at 37°C (APHA, 2005).

Statistical analysis

Basic data entry and handling was done by Microsoft Excel database system. The data were then analyzed using statistical package for social sciences (SPSS) (2012). Descriptive statistics such as, means and frequencies were used to present the findings of both questionnaire survey and laboratory assessment. Also, a *t*-test was used to check whether the mean of two different groups under comparison were significantly different in the normally distributed population from which the samples were drawn.

RESULTS AND DISCUSSION

Practices of fish handlers

Since food handlers may be the source of food contamination either as carriers of pathogen or through poor hygienic practices. Thus all food handlers have basic responsibility to maintain a high degree of personal cleanliness and implement hygienic and safe food handling practices. Among the precautions that a food handler must maintain the major ones are; keeping hands clean and fingernails short, wearing clean working garment and hair cover (hair net and cap) (Kaferstein, 2003). However, the result of this study showed that 32.6% of the fish handlers did not wear appropriate overcoat (Table 1). This finding is higher than the result of similar study done on food handlers in Hawassa (14%) (Teklemariam et al., 2000) but lower than the finding of Fisseha et al. (1999) in Addis Ababa (45.8%). Moreover, 44.2% of fish handlers were also found with covered hair, which is consistent with that of Kumie et al. (2000) done in Zeway (40.1%) but better than the result of Teklemariam et al. (2000) assessed in Hawassa (11.8%).

In addition, nail of 46.5% of the fish handlers in this study were not shortly trimmed and clean (Table 1). This finding is higher than the result of Teklemariam et al. (2000) who found that 21.2% of food handlers in Hawassa city hotels did not trim their nail shortly. It was also observed that 72.1% of fish handlers in this study wore rings on their finger during food preparations, which was markedly higher than the report of Kumie et al. (2000) done in Zeway (28.7%). As food handlers can be the probable sources of contamination for micro-organisms, it is important to take all possible measures so that such contaminations would be reduced or eliminated (Muinde and Kuria, 2005).

Training of fish handlers on sanitary handling of food

According to Adams and Moss (1997), training of food handlers regarding the basic concepts and requirements of personal hygiene and sanitary handling of food play an integral part in ensuring a safe product to the consumer. But, the result of this study showed that 30.2% of the fish handlers have taken no training concerning sanitary handling of food. This result is lower than the previous result of Mekonnen et al. (2012) who obtained 61.5% of meat handlers not to take training on sanitary and food hygiene.

Total plate count (TPC)

Bacterial growth is the main cause of fish spoilage and public health concern therefore total bacterial count is used as a general index of fish quality. In this study the mean bacterial count (cfu/g) was found to be 4.63×10^6 in frozen raw Nile tilapia fillet samples (Table 2). This value was found to be higher than the result of Dhanapal et al. (2012) who found 4.9×10^4 in frozen raw Nile tilapia fillet samples. This high load is mainly the result of poor handling during the transportation, and/or poor personal

Table 1. Practices of fish handlers in relation to food safety, (n=43).

Practice at a time of visit		Frequency	Percentage (%)
Wear of appropriate overcoat	Yes	29	67.4
	No	14	32.6
Wear of appropriate hair cover	Yes	19	44.2
	No	24	55.8
Short trimmed and cleaned nail	Yes	23	53.5
	No	20	46.5
Cleanness of overcoat and visible body part	Kept	20	46.5
	Not Kept	23	53.5
Wear of jewelry or ring	Observed	31	72.1
	Not observed	12	27.9
Nail paint during visit	Observed	24	55.8
	Not observed	19	44.2
Washing of hand before starting work	Yes	43	100
	No	0	0
Discharge from nose, eye, ear and coughing	Observed	5	11.6
	Not observed	38	88.4
Any visible skin rash, boil, cut and wound	Observed	1	97.7
	Not observed	42	2.3

Table 2. Mean bacterial count of frozen raw and undercooked sampled Nile tilapia fillet.

Samples type	Mean bacterial count	Minimum bacterial count	Maximum bacterial count
Frozen raw fillet	4.63×10^6	1.5×10^3	6.5×10^7
Undercooked fillet	4.92×10^3	TFTC	8.5×10^4

TFTC = Too few to count.

hygiene during filleting.

In the current study, the mean bacterial count (cfu/g) was found to be 4.92×10^3 in undercooked Nile tilapia fillet samples. This result indicated that low mean value of bacterial load was found in the undercooked Nile tilapia fillet samples, which was significantly different from frozen raw Nile tilapia fillet samples (p=0.037). This is due to the exposure to heat during processing for the undercooked Nile tilapia fillet samples. Almost similar result has been` reported by Salaudeen et al. (2010) and Dhanapal et al. (2012). For ready to eat seafood, the microbiological limit for human consumption proposed by the International Commission on Microbiological Specifications for Foods (ICMSF) (1986) is 5×10^5 to 10^7 cfu/g in aerobic plate count analysis, which is also in line with this study result.

Bacterial isolation

Table 3 summarizes the frequency of bacterial isolate from frozen raw and undercooked Nile tilapia fillet samples. As it is shown, the lowest frequency of bacterial isolates were observed in undercooked Nile tilapia fillet samples which was significantly different from frozen raw Nile tilapia fillet samples (p=0.000). This could be due to the negative effect of heat on the growth of bacterial contaminants. Regarding the frequency of bacterial

Table 3. Frequency of bacterial isolate from frozen raw and undercooked sampled Nile tilapia fillet.

Samples type	Number of samples processed	Bacterial Isolates (%)		
		E. coli (%)	*Salmonella* spp. (%)	*S. aureus* (%)
Frozen raw fillet	40	17 (42.5)	3 (7.5)	26 (65)
Undercooked fillet	40	3 (7.5)	0 (0)	7 (17.5)
Total	80	20 (25)	3 (3.75)	33 (41.25)

isolate from heat treated fish and other ready-to-eat food stuffs similar observations were reported by other researchers (Mezgebu and Mogessie, 1998; Thailambal, 2006; Omenwa et al., 2012).

Finding of this study indicated that 42.5% of frozen raw Nile tilapia fillet samples carried *E. coli*. This result is higher than the result of Vieira et al. (2001) who reported that 12.5% of all samples from Brazilian markets had *E. coli*. The detectable presence of *E. coli* in the present study is a sign of faecal contamination of fish. This is in accordance with results obtained by Monzur-Hassan et al. (1994) and Yousuf et al. (2008) those associated with the detectable presence of *E. coli* in fish to the faecal contamination of fish sourced from the warm blooded animal.

Moreover, this study indicated that 7.5% of undercooked Nile tilapia fillet samples had *E. coli*. This result complies with previous report by El-Gohany (1994) that foods of animal origin either cooked or uncooked were predominantly contaminated with *E. coli*. Besides, Ohalete et al. (2013), reported 58.3% of *E. coli* contamination in fried fish samples from different bars and eating houses in Owerri, Nigeria. This is also in accordance to the assertion of Okonko et al. (2008, 2009a,b) that improper handling and improper hygiene might lead to the contamination of ready-to-eat foods and this might eventually affects the health of the consumers.

The result of this study further depicted that 65% of frozen raw and 17.5% of undercooked Nile tilapia fillet samples to harbor *S. aureus*. The occurrence of *S. aureus* in frozen raw Nile tilapia samples in this study was higher than the result of Mhango et al. (2010) who isolated *S. aureus* in 41% of the frozen gutted Nile tilapia samples studied and Ayulo et al. (1994) who isolated *S. aureus* in 20% of fresh fish and fish fillets (*Cynoscion leiarchus*). However, the presence of *S. aureus* in undercooked (Asa leb-leb) Nile tilapia samples in this study indicated that this type of heat treatment was not sufficient to eliminate the pathogen and/or the risk of recontamination from improper post-process handling. Generally, the high prevalence of *Staphylococcus* in the fish samples indicated the unhygienic handling of the fish since this species is found on human skin.

The frequency of isolation of *Salmonella* spp. from frozen raw Nile tilapia fillet samples in this study was 7.5%. This result is lower than the result of Ohalete et al. (2011) who isolated 20% of *Salmonella* spp. from frozen fish samples. Moreover, while in this study *Salmonella* spp. was detected, Rokibul and his team didn't isolate *Salmonella* spp. from frozen fish samples (Rokibul et al., 2012).

In contrast, no *Salmonella* spp. was isolated from undercooked Nile tilapia fillet samples in this study. The absence of *Salmonella* spp. in undercooked Nile tilapia samples in this study agrees with the result of Odu and Ameweiye (2013) that isolated no *Salmonella* spp. from ready-to-eat bole fishes.

But the presence of *E. coli* in undercooked Nile tilapia samples in this study indicated that *Salmonella* could also survive the heat treatment if it was there.

CONCLUSION AND RECOMMENDATIONS

The findings of this study revealed the presence of gap on food safety practices by fish handlers who work in different hotels of the Arba Minch town. The microbiological examination of frozen raw and undercooked (Asa leb-leb) Nile tilapia fillet samples revealed that the frozen raw Nile tilapia fillets are more contaminated than the undercooked Nile tilapia fillets. However, the detection of some zoonotic pathogens in undercooked (Asa leb-leb) Nile tilapia samples in this study indicated that this type of heat treatment was not sufficient to eliminate all zoonotic pathogens and/or the risk of recontamination from improper post-process handling.

In the light of these major findings, the following recommendations are made to safeguard the public against the risks of foodborne infections and intoxication:

1. Fish handlers should be trained on the adverse effect of lack of proper personal and environmental hygiene and sanitation.
2. Proper attention should be paid to the safety of both frozen raw and undercooked (Asa leb-leb) fish through proper handling and use of adequate processing procedures such as proper heating method.
3. Public health authorities in the state should ensure adequate supervision and monitoring of fish handling and sales especially ready-to-eat products like Asa leb-leb dish.
4. Further investigations should be conducted to assess the issues that are not addressed through this study.

ACKNOWLEDGEMENTS

The authors would like to thank their advisers, Dr. Yitbarek Getachew, Dr. Amare Berhanu, Dr. Dagmar Nölkes and Dr. Matusala Mulachew for their invaluable guidance, encouragement and support without limitation of time for successful completion of this study. They also would like to extend their appreciation to staff members of Wolaita Sodo Regional Veterinary Laboratory, especially to Endashaw Fikeru, Mulualem Almazu and Banciwosen Dejene

REFERENCES

Adams MR, Moss MO (1997). Food Microbiology. Royal Society of Chemistry. Science Park, Cambridge.

Adebayo BC, Odu NN, Igiwiloh NJ, Okonko IO (2012). Microbiological and Physicochemical Level of Fresh Catfish (Arius hendelotic) from Different Markets in Akwa Ibom State, Nigeria. New York Sci. J. 5(4):46-52.

Agric. Nutr. Dev.10:4202-4218.

American Public Health Association (APHA) (2005). Compendium of methods for microbiological examination of foods, 2nded. American Public Health Association, Washington, DC, USA.

Ayulo AM, Machado RA, Scussel VM (1994). Enterotoxigenic Escherichia coli and Staphylococcus aureus in fish and seafood from the southern region of Brazil. Int. J. Food Microbiol. 24:171-178.

Babalola ET, Ogun AA (2008). Microbial studies on frozen shrimps processed in Ibadan and Lagos, Nigeria. Sci. Res. Ess. 3(11):537-546.

Cahill MM (1990). Bacterial flora of fishes: a review. J. Microbial Ecol. 19(1):21-41.

Central Statistics Agency (CSA) (2007). Central Statistics Agency of Federal Democratic Republic of Ethiopia; Summary and statistical report of population and housing.

Dhanapal KG, Vidya SL, Binay BN, Venkateswarlu G, Devivaraprasad AR, Basu S (2012). Effect of cooking on physical, biochemical, bacteriological characteristics and fatty acid profile of Tilapia (Oreochromis mossambicus) fish steaks. Arch. Appl. Sci. Res. 4(2):1142-1149.

El-Gohany AH (1994). Sausage and minced meat as a source of food poisoning microorganisms to man. Assiut. Vet. Med. J. 30:146-215.

Fawole MO, Oso BA (2001). Laboratory manual of microbiology: Revised edition. Ibadan: Spectrum books Ltd, p. 127.

Ferreira IM, Pinho O (2006). Biogenic amines in Portuguese traditional foods and wines. J. Food Prot. 69(11):2293-2303.

Fisseha G, Berhane Y, Teka GE (1999). Food Handling Practice in Public Caterings in Addis Ababa, Ethiopia. Ethiop. Med. J. 37(1):1-10.

Food and Agricultural Organization (FAO) (1993). Contribution to the formulation of a short-medium term plan for the fisheries sector in Ethiopia. Technical report, part 1: Sector review, Rome.

Food and Agricultural Organization (FAO) (2006). Fishery Information, Data and Statistics Unit. Capture production: quantities 1950-2004. Rome. Retrieved from http://www.fao.org/fi/statist/FISOFT/FISHPLUS.asp.

Food and Agricultural Organization (FAO) (2012). The State of World Fisheries and Aquaculture 2012. Food and Agricultural Organization of the United Nations. Available at: http://www.fao.org/docrep/016/i2727e/i2727e.pdf

Food and Drug Administration (FDA) (1992). Bacteriological Analytical Manual. 7th Edition. AOAC international 2200 Wilson Blvd, Suite 400, Arlington, VA.

International Commission on Microbiological Specifications for Foods (ICMSF) (1986). Sampling plan and recommended microbiological limits for Seafood.

Kaferstein FK (2003). Food Safety: The fourth pillar in the Strategy to prevent infant Diarrhea. Bulletin of the WHO 81(11):842-843.

Kumie A, Genete K, Worku H, Kebede E, Ayele F, Mulugeta H (2000). The Sanitary Conditions of Public Food and Drink Establishments in the District town of Zeway, Southern Ethiopia. Ethiop. J. Health Dev.16(1):95-104.

Mekonnen H, Habtamu T, Kelali A, Shewit K (2012). Food safety knowledge and practices of abattoir and butchery shops and the microbial profile of meat in Mekelle City, Ethiopia. Asian Pac. J. Trop. Biomed. 3(5):952-957.

Mezgebu T, Mogessie A (1998). Microbial load and incidence of Salmonella spp. in 'kitfo', a traditional Ethiopian spiced, minced meat dish. Ethiop. J. Health Dev.12(2):135-140.

Mhango M, Mpuchane SF, Gashe BA (2010). Incidence of indicator organisms, opportunistic and pathogenic bacteria in fish. Afr. J. Food

Ministry of Agriculture (MoA) (2012). Ethiopian Ministry of Agriculture (MoA). National summary of agricultural production in Ethiopia. Annual report. pp. 56-72.

Monzur-Hassan MM, Rahman KM, Nahar A (1994). Studies on the bacterial flora of fish which are potential pathogens for human. Bangladesh Med. Res. Council Bull. 20(2):43-51.

Muinde OK, Kuria E (2005). Hygienic and sanitary practices of vendors of street foods in Nairobi, Kenya. Afr. J. Food Agric. Nutr. Dev. 5:1.

Obiajuru IOC, Ozumba UC (2009). Laboratory Methods for Medical Microbiology and Parasitology. Lifeway Amalgamations, Owerri. P 183.

Odu NN, Ameweiye NB (2013). Microbiological Quality of Street-Vended-Ready-to-Eat "Bole" Fish In Port Harcourt Metropoplis. New York Sci. J. 6(2):92-101.

Ohalete CN, Dozie INS, Obiajuru IOC, Ekeh IH (2011). Studies on the ecology of Salmonella bacilli in Owerri metropolis Imo State, Nigeria. GRJS 1:109-116.

Ohalete CN, Obiajuru IOC, Obiukwu CE, Uwaezuoke JC, Nwaehiri UL, Daniel UN (2013). Microbiological quality of fried and smoked fish in Owerri, Imo State Nigeria. WJPPS. 2:1-19.

Okonko IO, Donbraye E, Babatunde SOI (2009b). Microbiological Quality of Seafood processors and water used in two different sea processing plants in Nigeria. EJEAFche 8(8):621-629.

Okonko IO, Ogunnusi TA, Ogunjobi AA, Adedeji AO, Adejoye OD,

Okonko IO, Ogun AA, Adejoye OD, Ogunjobi AA, Nkang AO, Adebayo-Tayo BC (2009a). Hazards analysis critical control points (HACCP) and Microbiology qualities of Sea-foods as affected by Handler's Hygiene in Ibadan and Lagos, Nigeria. Afr. J. Food Sci. 3(1):035-050.

Okpokwasili GC, Ogbulie JN (1993). Bacterial and Metal quality of Tilapia (Oreochromis niloticus) aquaculture systems. Int. J. Environ. Health Res. 13:190-202.

Omenwa VC, Ansa EJ, Agokei OE, Uka A, George OS (2012). Microbiological quality of raw and processed farm-reared periwinkles from brackish water earthen pond Buguma, Nigeria. Afr. J. Food Agric. Nutr. Dev.11:4623-4631.

Pelczer MJ, Chan ECS (1986). Elements of Microbiology. McGraw – Hill Book co. New York.

Pyatkin KD, Krivoshein YuS (1986). Microbiology. MIR Publishers, Moscow. P 167.

Rokibul H, Mrityunjoy A, Eshita D, Kamal KD, Tasnia A, Muhammad AA, Kazi KF, Rashed N (2012). Microbiological study of sea fish samples collected from local markets in Dhaka city. Int. Food Res. J. 20(3):1491-1495.

Salaudeen M, Akande G, Oguntade O, Afolabi O, Olusola A, Ezekiel M (2010). Effect of preservatives on microbial safety and quality of smoked catfish (Clarias gariepinus) during ambient storage. Acta SATECH 3(2):81-86.

Statistical Package for Social Science (SPSS) (2012). SPSS for Window (Version 19) SPSS, Chicago, IL, USA.

Teklemariam S, Roma B, Sorsa S, Worku S, Erosie L (2000). Assessment of Sanitary and Hygiene Status of Catering Establishments of Awassa Town. Ethiop. J. Health Dev. 14(1):91-98.

Thailambal AS (2006). Effect of processing on bacterial population of cuttle fish and crab and determination of bacterial spoilage and rancidity developing on frozen storage. J. Food Process Preserv. 31(1):13-31.

Tsai YH, Chang SC, Kung HF, Wei C, Hwang DF (2002). Histamine Production by E. aeregenes in Salifish and Milkfish at Various Storage Temperatures. J. Food Prot. 68(8):1690-1695.

Tzikas Z, Amvrosiadis I, Soultos N, Georgakis SP (2007). Seasonal size distribution, condition status and muscle yield of of Mediterranean Horse Mackerel (Trachurus mediterraneus) from the North Aegean Sea Greece. J. Fish. Sci. 73(2):453-462.

Vieira RHSF, Rodrigues DP, Gocalves FA, Menezes FGR, Aragao JS, Sousa OV (2001). Microbicidal effect of medicinal plant extracts (Psidium guajava Linn. and Carica papaya Linn.) upon bacteria isolated from fish muscle and known to induce diarrhea in children. Rev. Inst. Med. Trop. S. Paulo 43:145-148.

World Bank (2010). The hidden harvests: the global contribution of capture fisheries. World Bank, Washington. Available at: http://siteresources.worldbank.org/EXTARD/Resources/3366811224775570533/TheHiddenHarvestsConferenceEdition.pdf

Yousuf AHM, Ahmed MK, Yeasmin S, Ahsa N, Rahman MM, Islam MM (2008). Prevalence of Microbial Load in Shrimp, Penaeus monodon and Prawn, Macrobrachium rosenbergii from Bangladesh. World J. Agric. Sci. 4(5):852-855

Permissions

All chapters in this book were first published in JVMAH, by Academic Journals; hereby published with permission under the Creative Commons Attribution License or equivalent. Every chapter published in this book has been scrutinized by our experts. Their significance has been extensively debated. The topics covered herein carry significant findings which will fuel the growth of the discipline. They may even be implemented as practical applications or may be referred to as a beginning point for another development.

The contributors of this book come from diverse backgrounds, making this book a truly international effort. This book will bring forth new frontiers with its revolutionizing research information and detailed analysis of the nascent developments around the world.

We would like to thank all the contributing authors for lending their expertise to make the book truly unique. They have played a crucial role in the development of this book. Without their invaluable contributions this book wouldn't have been possible. They have made vital efforts to compile up to date information on the varied aspects of this subject to make this book a valuable addition to the collection of many professionals and students.

This book was conceptualized with the vision of imparting up-to-date information and advanced data in this field. To ensure the same, a matchless editorial board was set up. Every individual on the board went through rigorous rounds of assessment to prove their worth. After which they invested a large part of their time researching and compiling the most relevant data for our readers.

The editorial board has been involved in producing this book since its inception. They have spent rigorous hours researching and exploring the diverse topics which have resulted in the successful publishing of this book. They have passed on their knowledge of decades through this book. To expedite this challenging task, the publisher supported the team at every step. A small team of assistant editors was also appointed to further simplify the editing procedure and attain best results for the readers.

Apart from the editorial board, the designing team has also invested a significant amount of their time in understanding the subject and creating the most relevant covers. They scrutinized every image to scout for the most suitable representation of the subject and create an appropriate cover for the book.

The publishing team has been an ardent support to the editorial, designing and production team. Their endless efforts to recruit the best for this project, has resulted in the accomplishment of this book. They are a veteran in the field of academics and their pool of knowledge is as vast as their experience in printing. Their expertise and guidance has proved useful at every step. Their uncompromising quality standards have made this book an exceptional effort. Their encouragement from time to time has been an inspiration for everyone.

The publisher and the editorial board hope that this book will prove to be a valuable piece of knowledge for researchers, students, practitioners and scholars across the globe.

List of Contributors

Lizzet Corona-Gómez, Laura Jaramillo-Meza and Fernando Díaz-Otero
Departamento de Inmunología, Centro Nacional de Investigación Disciplinaria en Microbiología Animal, INIFAP, Toluca, Mexico

Rafael Pérez-González and Fernando Diosdado-Vargas
Facultad de Estudios Superiores Cuautitlán, Universidad Nacional Autonoma de México, México City, Mexico

Julio Santiago-Cruz
Departamento de Microbiología y Parasitología, Facultad de Medicina, Universidad Nacional Autonoma de México, México City, Mexico
Instituto Nacional de Enfermedades Respiratorias Ismael Cosío Villegas, Secretaria de Salud, Mexico

Clara I Espitia-Pinzón
Instituto de Investigaciones Biomédicas, Universidad Nacional Autonoma de México, México City, Mexico

Ricardo Lascurain
Departamento de Bioquímica, Facultad de Medicina, Universidad Nacional Autonoma de México, México City, Mexico

Seblewongel Ayichew Megerrsa and Taddesa Bezu Ashine
School of Veterinary Medicine, Wolaita Sodo University, Ethiopia

Alsácia Atanásio-Nhacumbe, Maria Consuêlo Carybé Ayres, Sabrina Mota Lambert and Bárbara Paraná Souza
School of Veterinary Medicine-Federal University of Bahia (UFBA), Av. Adhemar de Barros, 500, Ondina, Salvador-Bahia, CEP: 40.170-110, Brazil

Alsácia Atanásio-Nhacumbe
National Centre for Biotechnology and Biosciences (CNBB), Ministry of Science and Technology, High Education and Vocational Training (MCTESTP), Av. Patrice Lumumba, 770, Maputo, Mozambique

Getnet Fekadu
College of Veterinary Medicine, Haramaya University, Dire Dawa, Ethiopia

Gelagay Ayelet
National Veterinary Institute, Bishoftu, Oromia, Ethiopia

Fufa Abunna
College of Veterinary Medicine and Agriculture, Department of Clinical Studies, Addis Ababa University, Bishoftu, Oromia, Ethiopia

Golo Dabasa, Wubishet Zewdei, Tadelle Shanko, Gete Gurmesa and Garu Lolo
Yabello Regional Veterinary Laboratory, Yabello, Ethiopia

Kula Jilo
School of Veterinary Medicine, College of Agriculture and Veterinary Medicine, Jimma University, Jimma, Ethiopia

Abriham Kebede, Jiregna Dugassa and Geremew Haile
School of Veterinary Medicine, College of Medical and Health Science, Wollega University, Nekemte, Ethiopia

Berhanu Wakjira
School of Veterinary Medicine, College of Agriculture and Veterinary Medicine, Jimma University, Ethiopia

Migbaru Keffale Bezabih
Department of Biomedical Science, College of Veterinary Medicine, Haramaya University, Haramaya, Ethiopia

Mabure Shille Bisho
Debre-Tsehay District Agricultural Office, Southern Nations Nationalities and Peoples Region, Ethiopia

Getaw Yeshitila and Dejene Bekele
Ministry of Livestock and Fisheries, Ethiopia

Anteneh Wondimu and Getachew Sharew
College of Veterinary Medicine, Haramaya University Dire Dawa, Ethiopia

Rukayya Hussain Abubakar, Darshana Morar-Leather and Folorunso O. Fasina
Department of Veterinary Tropical Diseases, Faculty of Veterinary Sciences, University of Pretoria, South Africa

Evelyn Madoroba
Bacteriology Section, Agricultural Research Council–Onderstepoort Veterinary Research, South Africa
College of Agriculture and Environmental Sciences, University of South Africa, Florida Campus, South Africa

Olubukola Adenubi
Department of Paraclinical Sciences, Faculty of Veterinary Sciences, University of Pretoria, South Africa

Folorunso O. Fasina
Emergency Centre for Transboundary Animal Diseases (ECTAD), Food and Agriculture Organization of the United Nations (FAO), UNON, Gigiri, Kenya

Guash Abay, Hailai Hagos, Minister Berhanie and Tsegay Teame
Abergelle Agricultural Research Center, Abyi-Adi, Ethiopia

Mulalem Zenebe and Daniel Desta
Shire-Mytsebri Agricultural Research Center, Shire, Ethiopia

Andualem Yimer and Sisay Fanta
School of Veterinary Medicine, Wollo University, Dessie, Ethiopia

Zekarias Fantaye
Field staff, Ministry of Livestock Development and Fisheries, Ethiopia

Berhanu Mekibib Melake
School of Veterinary Medicine, Hawassa University, Hawassa, Ethiopia

Jesca Nakayima, Daniel Aleper and Duke Okidi
National Livestock Resources Research Institute (NaLIRRI), Tororo, Uganda

Mary L. Nanfuka
National Animal Disease Diagnostics and Epidemiology Centre (NADDEC). Entebbe, Uganda

A. A. Raji
Department of Veterinary Pathology, Faculty of Veterinary Medicine, Usmanu Danfodiyo University, Sokoto, Nigeria

S. B. Oladele
Department of Veterinary Pathology, Faculty of Veterinary Medicine, Ahmadu Bello University, Zaria, Nigeria

L. Saidu
Veterinary Teaching Hospital, Ahmadu Bello University, Zaria, Nigeria

A. H. Jibril
Department of Veterinary Physiology, Faculty of Veterinary Medicine, Usmanu Danfodiyo University, Sokoto, Nigeria

C. Cazaban
Innovation Strategy Department, Ceva Santé Animale, France

Desie Sheferaw
Faculty of Veterinary Medicine, Hawassa University, Hawassa, Ethiopia

Anteneh Wondimu, Endeshaw Reta and Asnake Fekadu
Haramaya University College of Veterinary Medicine, Dire Dawa, Ethiopia

Agegnehu Ashinde, Abebaw Gashaw and Nejash Abdela
School of Veterinary Medicine, College of Agriculture and Veterinary Medicine, Jimma University, Jimma, Jimma, Ethiopia

Temesgen Kassa Getahun and Tihune Zeleke Kassa
Ethiopian Institute of Agricultural Research, Holeta Agricultural Research Center, Holeta, Ethiopia

M. Sylvestre, Ramneek Verma, Ravi Kant Agrawal and Dipak Deka
School of Animal Biotechnology, Guru Angad Dev Veterinary and Animal Sciences University Ludhiana-141004, Punjab, India

Mohamed, M. Ibrahem
Department of Zoology, Faculty of Sciences, University of Zawia, Zawia, Libya

Wafa, M. Ibrahem
Department of Parasitology, Faculty of Medicine, University of Zawia, Zawia, Libya

Kawther, M. Ibrahem
Department of Medicinal Chemistry, Faculty of Pharmacy, University of Zawia, Zawia, Libya

Badereddin, B. Annajar
National Centre for Disease Control, Ain Zara, Tripoli, Libya

Egbe-Nwiyi T. N. and Sherrif G. A.
Department of Veterinary Pathology, University of Maiduguri, Maiduguri, Nigeria

Paul B. T.
Veterinary Teaching Hospital, University of Maiduguri, Maiduguri, Nigeria

Mohammed Hussen
School of Veterinary Medicine, Wollo University, Dessie, Ethiopia

Alebachew Tilahun and Alemu Aylate
School of Veterinary Medicine, Wolaita Sodo University, Sodo, Ethiopia

Ashenafi Kiros
Ministry of Livestock and Fisheries, National Animal Health Diagnostic and Investigation Center

Addisu Awukew Yegoraw
School of Veterinary Medicine, Wolaita Sodo University, Wolaita, Ethiopia

Addis Kassahun Gebremeskel
School of Veterinary Medicine, Hawassa University, Hawassa, Ethiopia

Tesfaye Sisay Tesema
Unit of Health Biotechnology, Institute of Biotechnology, College of Natural and Computational Sciences, Addis Ababa University, Ethiopia

Biruk Tesfaye Birhanu
College of Veterinary Medicine and Agriculture, Addis Ababa University, Debrezeit, Ethiopia

Jesca Nakayima, Daniel Aleper and Duke Okidi
National Livestock Resources Research Institute (NaLIRRI), Uganda

William Kabasa
College of Veterinary Medicine, Animal Resources and Bio-security (CoVAB), Kampala, Uganda

Kebede Shanko Hordofa, Tesfaye Rufael Chibsa and Enquibaher Kasaye
Mekelle University, Ethiopia

Adriana Guadalupe Martínez-Covarrubias, Marco Antonio Santillán-Flores and Dionicio Córdova-López
Instituto Nacional de Investigaciones Forestales, Agrícolas y Pecuarias-CENID Microbiología Carretera México -Toluca Km. 15.5, Colonia Palo Alto, CP. 04110, Delegación Cuajimalpa, México

Claudia Celic Guzmán-Ruíz
Universidad de Guanajuato, División Ciencias de la Vida, Campus Irapuato -Salamanca, Exhacienda, El Copal Km. 9,Carretera Irapuato-Silao, CP 36820, Irapuato, Guanajuato, Mexico

Wendwesen Teka
Zonal Veterinarian, Wolaita Sodo Zone Agricultural Office, Wolaita Sodo, SNNPR, Ethiopia

Dagmar Nölkes and Yitbarek Getachew
Haramaya University, College of Veterinary Medicine, Haramaya, Ethiopia

Matusala Mulachew
Wolaita Sodo Agricultural TVET College, Wolaita Sodo, SNNPR, Ethiopia

Index

A
Actinobacillosis, 79, 85-86, 89
Actinomycosis, 85-87, 89
Acute Respiratory Distress Syndrome (ARDS), 93
African Horse Sickness, 48-49, 52
Albendazole, 15-20, 165, 167-168
Anthelmintic Resistance, 15-16, 19-21
Anthrax, 63, 84-87, 89
Aparasitaemic, 43, 46, 128-129

B
Body Condition Score (BCS), 44
Bovine Herpesvirus Type-1, 153
Bovine Schistosomosis, 38-42, 177, 180
Bovine Tuberculosis (BTB), 1-2
Brucellosis, 37, 59, 76, 78, 90
Bursa of Fabricius, 112, 115-118
Bursal-body Index, 112

C
Chi-square, 5, 17, 22, 25-27, 45, 134, 146, 178, 195
Colibacillosis, 57-58, 64, 66, 68, 72, 76-77, 85-87, 89
Conjunctivitis, 60, 63, 87, 154
Coproculture, 144
Coproscopy, 176, 178
Cross Border Diseases, 30-31, 36
Culture Filtrate Protein Extract, 2-3

D
Debilitating Disease, 43
Degree of Lameness, 134, 136-137
Delayed Type Hypersensitivity, 1, 7
Dermatophilosis, 99-105

E
Ear Necrosis, 58
Echinococcosis, 160-168
Ectoparasites, 88-89, 99-100, 105, 136, 175
Enteroaggregative, 57, 65, 75, 78
Enterohaemorrhagic, 57, 64-65
Enteropathogenic, 57, 64, 66, 68, 75, 77
Enterotoxigenic, 57, 64-66, 70, 76-79, 212
Enzyme Linked Immuno Sorbent Assay, 48
Epidemiological Investigation, 22
Equine Piroplasmosis (EP), 106

F
Faecal Egg Count Reduction Test, 15-16
Faeco-oral Route, 61, 66
Flea Infestation, 84-87, 89
Foot and Mouth Disease (FMD), 192

G
Gastrointestinal Nematode Infection, 55
Gastrointestinal Tract Parasitism, 84-85, 88-89
Glycoprotein D, 153, 158-159

H
Hepatomegaly, 59, 106

I
Infectious Bovine Rhinotracheitis (IBR), 159
Infectious Bursal Disease (IBD), 112-113, 115
Infectious Pustular Vulvovaginitis, 153

L
Lice Infestation, 84-87, 89, 99, 101-103
Lumpy Skin Disease, 99, 102-104, 194

M
Madin-darby Bovine Kidney (MDBK), 153
Middle East Respiratory Syndrome Corona Virus, 22, 91

O
Orchitis, 59, 63

P
Parasitaemic, 43, 45-46, 128-129
Parasitic Bronchitis, 85-88
Paratuberculosis, 199-205
Pastuerellosis, 84, 86, 88-89
Pathotype, 64-67, 78
PCV, 43-46, 127-129, 170-174
Petechial Haemorrhages, 59, 114
Pleurisy, 59-60, 63
Polyarthritis, 59-60, 63
Polymerase Chain Reaction, 22, 25, 75, 78-79, 93, 95-96, 107, 164, 168, 198-200, 205
Post-weaning Diarrhea, 66, 78
Praziquantel, 39, 165-166, 180
Prophylaxis, 57, 72, 78, 158, 166, 190
Pseudoparticle Neutralization Assay, 24, 28
Purified Protein Derivative, 2

S

Septicaemia, 59-61, 64-65
Sero Prevalence, 26-27, 92, 95-96, 192, 194-197
Seroepidemiology, 48
Serogroup, 60, 66, 68
Serotype, 52, 67-68, 193, 198
Severe Acute Respiratory Syndrome (SARS), 23, 92, 98
Single Intradermal Comparative Tuberculin Test, 1
Small Ruminant Production, 15, 21, 88, 171
Stomoxy, 127
Swine Erysipelas, 59, 78

T

Tick-borne Haemoparasitic Diseases, 37, 105, 170, 172, 174-175
Trypanosomosis, 9, 43-47, 126-130, 151, 175, 185
Tuberculin Skin Test, 1-2, 5

V

Vegetative Endocarditis, 59, 61